Essentials of Paediatric Gastroenterology

Essentials of Paediatric Gastroenterology

Edited by

J. T. Harries, M.B.B.S., D.C.H., M.R.C.P., M.D., M.Sc.

Senior Lecturer in Paediatric Gastroenterology, Institute of Child Health, University of London; Honorary Consultant Physician, The Hospital for Sick Children, Great Ormond Street, London

CHURCHILL LIVINGSTONE
EDINBURGH LONDON AND NEW YORK 1977

CHURCHILL LIVINGSTONE
Medical Division of Longman Group Limited

Distributed in the United States of America by Longman Inc., 19 West 44th Street, New York, N.Y. 10036 and by associated companies, branches and representatives throughout the world.

First published 1977

ISBN 0 443 01645 3

Library of Congress Cataloging in Publication Data
Main entry under title:

Essentials of paediatric gastroenterology.

Bibliography: p.
Includes index.
1. Pediatric gastroenterology. I. Harries, John Thomas.
RJ446.E87 618.9′23 77-4440

Printed in Great Britain by T. & A. Constable Ltd., Edinburgh

To
My Colleagues, and
Waveney, David and Thomasy

Preface

The purpose of this book is to present a volume of moderate size which attempts to cover the important areas of a rapidly growing specialty, paediatric gastroenterology. It is written primarily for the practising general paediatrician, but hopefully it will also be a useful source of information to the paediatric surgeon, the undergraduate and postgraduate student, as well as to those with a special interest in paediatric gastroenterology. To this end moderately extensive bibliographies have been included in selected parts of the book, providing an opportunity for readers to pursue certain subjects in greater depth.

The book is arranged in three parts. The first deals with the prenatal development of structure and function, the interrelationships between structure and function with particular emphasis on the small gut, and an account of the currently available investigatory techniques. The pre- and postnatal development of hepatic, pancreatic and alimentary tract structure and function represents a relatively neglected, albeit extremely important, area of paediatric gastroenterology which has major implications with regard to nutritional practices in the newborn as well as in the older infant. In recent years major advances have been made in our understanding of the intricate and subtle relationships which exist between the structure and function of biological tissues involved in the digestion, transport and metabolism of nutrients, and an understanding of these interrelationships can only lead to the enhanced clinical care of patients. A wide range of techniques are now available for investigating children with gastroenterological problems, and these are described in Chapter 3.

The second part of the book considers a variety of conditions but, in the main, is orientated towards the alimentary tract. It begins with an account of the surgical conditions which can affect the newborn and older child, and of chronic inflammatory bowel disease. It continues with chapters on the long-term effects and management of children following intestinal resections, and on the effects of malnutrition on the structure and function of the alimentary tract, liver and pancreas. The important area of small intestinal enteropathies is covered in detail, as is infective diarrhoea and vomiting; both represent major world problems. The selective inborn errors of absorption are 'accidents of nature' and represent a unique group of disorders which are only rarely encountered in paediatric practice. Nevertheless they are important, since early diagnosis and treatment may be life-saving as, for example, in congenital glucose-galactose malabsorption; diagnosis is also important in terms of genetic counselling. Moreover, there is much to be learnt about 'alternative' transport systems from these genetically determined disorders of absorption, since the clinical manifestations invariably improve with age. For these reasons, a brief account is included. Parasitic infestations, protein-losing enteropathies and gastrointestinal disturbances related to psychological disturbances conclude this section of the book.

The third and final part of the book is devoted to disorders of the liver and pancreas in childhood. The inborn errors of hepatic metabolism, persistent neonatal jaundice, infections of the liver and chronic liver disease are considered in some detail; tumours of the liver and disorders of the pancreas are discussed in the two concluding chapters.

The role of gastrointestinal hormones and disturbed immune function in the pathogenesis of gastrointestinal disturbances have been integrated into the appropriate sections of the book, rather than given individual attention.

The clinical conditions encountered in paediatric gastroenterology pose fundamentally different problems to those encountered in adult patients, and this is particularly the case during the first few years of life. For example, during the first year of life a variety of biological processes are immature, and disease may have irreversible and permanent effects. Malnutrition secondary to malabsorption can interfere with brain cell replication and result in permanent intellectual defects. Acute infectious diarrhoea and/or vomiting, and its complications, may be a devastating event in the life of a young child and his family. Similarly, surgical procedures in the newborn and older infant present problems which are different to those encountered in the adult patient. The relationship between gastrointestinal symptoms and psychological disturbances in the child and its family, and the diseases which affect the liver in childhood, are other examples which emphasise some of the differences between paediatric and adult gastroenterology. These are some of the reasons why I accepted an invitation to edit a book which I thought should be concerned with the 'essentials' of paediatric gastroenterology, and why the above areas of paediatrics were selected as prominent items in the genesis of this volume. They delineate but do not separate the concept of adult from paediatric gastroenterology. Collaboration between paediatric and adult physicians and surgeons concerned with gastroenterological problems is critical to our understanding and to the clinical care of gastrointestinal disease at any age.

This book would not have been possible without the generous advice and support of my colleagues and family, to whom I am deeply grateful and to whom the book is dedicated. My interest in paediatric gastroenterology was born within myself, but was catalysed by Sir Wilfrid Sheldon and Dr Tony Dawson. The opportunity to establish a clinical and research team in paediatric gastroenterology resulted from the efforts, encouragement and support of Professor Otto Wolff and Professor June Lloyd. David Muller has been a constant source of intellectual and friendly inspiration. I am indebted to John Tripp, John McCollum and Peter Milla for many helpful discussions. I have been fortunate to be associated with the above mentioned people and have learnt much from them.

I wish to record my thanks to all the contributors for their tolerance and co-operation in my editorial duties, and I am indebted to my publishers for their patience and guidance. Last, but not least, I extend my gratitude to Miss Anna Curtis for an enormous amount of secretarial help.

1977 J. T. Harries

Contributors

J. A. S. Dickson, MB ChB, FRCSE, FRCS
Senior Lecturer in Paediatric Surgery, Institute of Child Health, and Honorary Consultant Surgeon, The Hospital for Sick Children, London.

G. J. Ebrahim, FRCPE, FRCP(Glas), DCH
Senior Lecturer/Tutor WHO-UNICEF Course for Senior Teachers of Child Health, Institute of Child Health, London.

Roy V. Howarth, MB ChB, MRCPsych, DCH
Consultant in Psychological Medicine, The Hospital for Sick Children, London.

J. T. Harries, MRCP, MD, MSc, DCH
Senior Lecturer in Paediatric Gastroenterology, Institute of Child Health, and Honorary Consultant Physician, The Hospital for Sick Children, London.

Jean W. Keeling, MB BS, MRCPath
Consultant Paediatric Pathologist, John Radcliffe Hospital, Oxford.

Anne Kilby, MA, MB BChir(Cantab), MRCP
Heinz Research Fellow in Paediatric Gastroenterology, Medical College of St Bartholomew's Hospital and The London Hospital Medical College at Queen Elizabeth Hospital for Children, and Honorary Senior Registrar, Royal Hospital of Saint Bartholomew, London.

June K. Lloyd, MD, FRCP
Professor of Child Health, St George's Hospital Medical School, and Honorary Consultant Physician, St George's Hospital, London.

W. C. Marshall, MD(Syd), PhD, MRACP, DCH
Senior Lecturer under Wellcome Trustees University Award Scheme, Department of Microbiology, Institute of Child Health, and Honorary Consultant Physician, The Hospital for Sick Children, London.

J. P. K. McCollum, MB BS, MRCP, MSc
Lecturer in Child Health, Institute of Child Health, and Honorary Senior Registrar, The Hospital for Sick Children, London.

Alex P. Mowat, MB ChB, FRCP, DObst RCOG, DCH
Consultant Paediatrician, Department of Child Health, King's College Hospital Medical School, and Bethlem Royal & Maudsley Hospitals, London.

P. J. Milla, MB BS, MRCP
Research Fellow, Department of Child Health, Institute of Child Health, London.

David P. R. Muller, BSc, PhD
Lecturer in Biochemistry, Department of Child Health, Institute of Child Health, London.

S. M. Packer, MB BS, FRACP
Research Fellow, University of Nottingham, and Honorary Senior Registrar, Nottingham Children's Hospital.

William L. Tift, MD
Chief, Pediatric Service, United States Naval Hospital, Cherry Point, North Carolina, U.S.A.

J. H. Tripp, MB BS, MRCP
Research Fellow, Department of Child Health, Institute of Child Health, London.

H. B. Valman, MD, MRCP
Consultant Paediatrician, Northwick Park Hospital, London.

John Walker-Smith, MD, MRCPE, MRCP, FRACP
Consultant Paediatrician, Royal Hospital of Saint Bartholomew, London, Senior Lecturer in Child Health, Medical College of St Bartholomew's Hospital and The London Hospital Medical College at Queen Elizabeth Hospital for Children, and Honorary Consultant Physician, The Hospital for Sick Children, London.

R. J. West, MD, MRCP
Senior Lecturer in Child Health, St George's Hospital Medical School, and Honorary Consultant Physician, St George's Hospital, London.

Brian A. Wharton, MD, FRCPE, MRCP, DCH
Consultant Paediatrician, Birmingham South and Central Health Districts, and Honorary Research Fellow in Child Nutrition, Institute of Child Health, Birmingham.

Contents

PART 1

Chapter 1.
Prenatal development of structure and function — 1
J. P. K. McCollum and P. J. Milla

Chapter 2.
Structure and function — 16
D. P. R. Muller

Chapter 3.
Investigatory techniques — 38
S. M. Packer, P. J. Milla and J. H. Tripp

PART 2

Chapter 4.
Surgical emergencies in the first few weeks of life — 63
J. A. S. Dickson

Chapter 5.
Surgical conditions in the infant and older child — 89
J. A. S. Dickson

Chapter 6.
Chronic inflammatory bowel disease — 105
J. A. S. Dickson

Chapter 7.
Long-term effects and management of intestinal resection — 119
H. B. Valman

Chapter 8.
The effects of malnutrition on structure and function — 130
B. A. Wharton

Chapter 9.
Small intestinal enteropathies — 141
J. A. Walker-Smith and Anne Kilby

Chapter 10.
Infective diarrhoea and vomiting — 164
J. H. Tripp and J. T. Harries

Chapter 11.
Selective inborn errors of absorption 199
J. T. Harries

Chapter 12.
Parasitic infections 210
G. J. Ebrahim

Chapter 13.
Protein-losing enteropathies 227
W. L. Tift

Chapter 14.
Gastrointestinal symptoms related to psychological disturbances 235
R. V. Howarth

PART 3

Chapter 15.
Inborn errors of hepatic metabolism 251
R. J. West and June K. Lloyd

Chapter 16.
Persistent neonatal jaundice 266
A. P. Mowat

Chapter 17.
Infections of the liver 286
W. C. Marshall and A. P. Mowat

Chapter 18.
Chronic liver disease 310
A. P. Mowat

Chapter 19.
Tumours of the liver 326
Jean W. Keeling

Chapter 20.
Disorders of the pancreas 335
J. P. K. McCollum and J. T. Harries

Index 355

PART 1

1. Prenatal development of structure and function

J. P. K. McCollum and P. J. Milla

Early development of the fertilised ovum
Morphological development
Functional development

Embryology is the study of the progressive development of an organism from its earliest stage and involves three fundamental processes, namely growth, differentiation and metabolism. Growth involves an increase in cell size and number, differentiation describes the ultrastructural organisation of the cell and metabolism relates to the development of cell biochemistry. These three processes are closely linked during development to produce an integrated functioning organism. In this chapter early embryological development will be discussed, together with subsequent development up to the time of birth. The morphological and functional development of the alimentary tract, liver and pancreas will be described, and embryological defects which result in postnatal disease will be discussed where appropriate. Although a considerable amount of information is available on developmental patterns in the experimental animal, information is limited with regard to the human fetus, which this chapter is concerned with.

EARLY DEVELOPMENT OF THE FERTILISED OVUM

The spherical fertilised ovum, within its trophoblastic covering embedded in the uterine wall, divides into numerous cells from which the different systems and organs of the body will develop. The germ layers are the inner endoderm, the outer ectoderm and between them the mesoderm. These layers are laid down in the first three weeks of prenatal life, and between three and eight weeks rapid growth and differentiation takes place during which time all the major systems and organs of the body are established. During the first seven days the fertilised ovum or blastocyst is embedding itself in the uterine wall. The primitive ectoderm separates from the trophoblast by the formation of a cavity, the amniotic cavity. On the opposite surface a single layer of primitive endoderm forms between the ectoderm and the blastocyst cavity. In the succeeding stages the blastocyst cavity becomes lined with mesodermal cells which are in continuity with the endoderm around its margins. These stages are shown in Figure 1.1. The cells of the primitive germ layers now become arranged in a more regular manner and the primary yolk sac undergoes a marked reduction in size, during which a cavity appears within the endoderm, the secondary

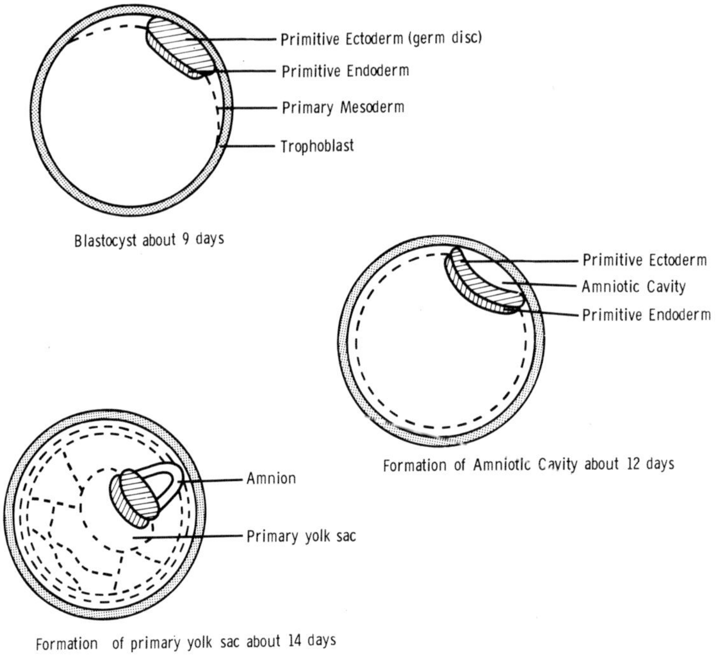

Fig. 1.1 Formation of amniotic cavity and primary yolk sac from the fertilised ovum.

yolk sac. In the roof of the sac the endoderm is in contact with the ectoderm and forms a bilaminar embryonic disc, which is roughly circular in shape. This stage occurs towards the end of the second week and is shown in Figure 1.2. Only the tissue of the embryonic disc contributes to the formation of the embryo.

The alimentary tract and its derivatives originate from the splanchnopleure of the embryonic disc. As shown in Figure 1.2, the splanchnopleure is composed of two layers, a mesodermal layer which gives rise to muscle and connective

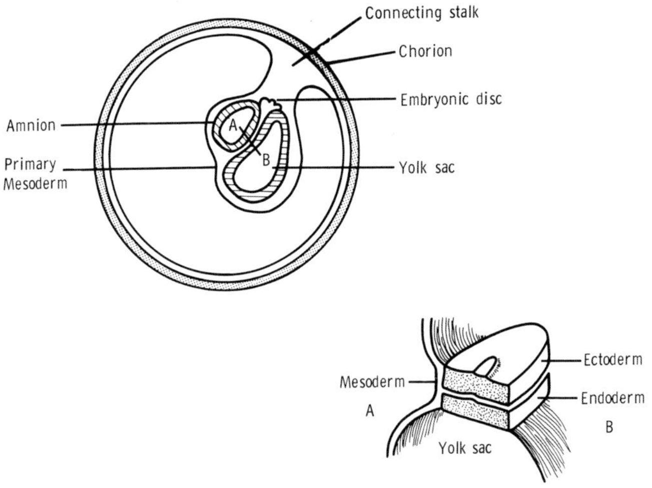

Fig. 1.2 Development of the splanchnopleure of the embryonic disc.

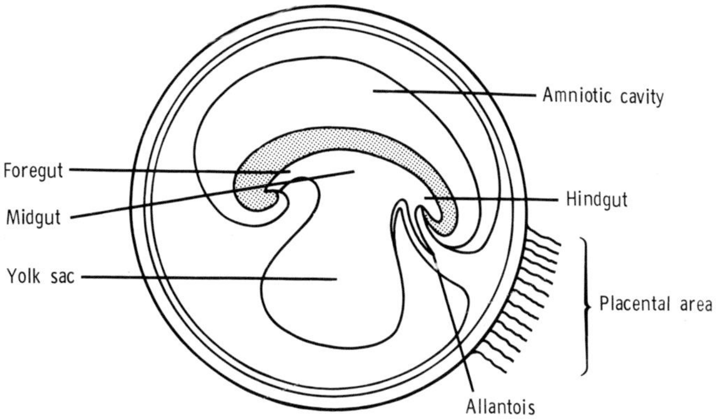

Fig. 1.3 Differentiation of yolk sac into fore-, mid- and hindgut.

tissue elements, and an endodermal layer which forms the epithelium of the intestinal tract and the parenchyma of the liver and pancreas.

From Figure 1.2 it will be seen that the yolk sac is an ovoid cavity with a roof of endoderm. With development of the cranial and caudal extensions of the embryonic disc the yolk sac becomes differentiated into fore-, mid-, and hindgut, as shown in Figure 1.3. The foregut gives rise to the pharynx, thyroid, thymus, parathyroid glands, respiratory tract, oesophagus, stomach, upper duodenum, liver and pancreas. The lower duodenum, small and large intestine as far as the distal third of the transverse colon are formed from the midgut. The remainder of the large bowel arises from the hindgut.

MORPHOLOGICAL DEVELOPMENT

Gross structural development

By four weeks the primitive gut is identifiable as a tubular structure extending from mouth to cloaca. It is suspended dorsally by the dorsal mesentery which extends along the whole length of the intra-abdominal gut, and ventrally by a thick mesentery which extends from the septum transversum to the intra-abdominal portion of the foregut. Between four and six weeks the cranial part of the foregut changes from a flattened tube into a complicated series of structures, the branchial arch system; in man this system is transitory and is almost entirely obliterated by seven weeks. Occasionally, however, epithelial-lined cysts, sinuses or fistulae may result from incomplete obliteration of the branchial arch system.

The pharynx and oesophagus

Concurrent with the development of the pharynx the cranial ends of the oesophagus and trachea become demarcated, growth of the former occurring at a later stage when the embryo grows cranially. Two events may result in congenital malformations. Partitioning of the foregut into oesophagus and trachea can result in one of the various types of tracheo-oesophageal fistulae, with or without oesophageal atresia. The formation of the cardia results from the co-ordinated development of the oesophagus, stomach, diaphragm and their autonomic innervation; failure of co-ordination may result in either a structural abnormality, such as an oesophageal web, or in a functional defect, such as achalasia.

The stomach

The rudimentary stomach appears at the caudal end of the foregut as a fusiform dilatation, and beyond this the gut opens into the yolk sac (see Fig. 1.3). At first the opening is wide but by the fifth week it has become narrowed into a tubular stalk, the vitellointestinal duct, following which the stomach soon loses its connection with the duct. Growth alterations lead to the final shape and position of the stomach. The dorsal mesentery increases in depth and folds upon itself to form the greater omentum, and the ventral mesentery forms the lesser omentum. During its development there is little alteration in the form of the stomach, and consequently malformations are very rare.

The small and large intestine

The terminal portion of the foregut and the cranial end of the midgut grow rapidly to form a loop which becomes the duodenum, the apex of the loop representing the junction between the fore- and midgut. During gastric growth the duodenum is carried dorsally and to the right, and the mesentery is ultimately approximated to and absorbed by the dorsal peritoneum rendering the duodenum retroperitoneal. While the stomach is growing, the midgut is increasing its length more rapidly than the embryo and forms a U-shaped loop which acquires a dorsal mesentery. At the apex of the loop is the vitellointestinal duct demarcating a cranial and caudal limb. As a result of this growth discrepancy, a series of manoeuvres occur which culminate in the final position of the gut within the abdomen, and these are depicted in Figure 1.4. From a simple straight tube the gut has undergone a counter-clockwise rotation of 270 degrees.

The dorsal mesentery from the duodenojejunal flexure to the ileocaecal junction remains as the mesentery of the small intestine, and the mesenteries of the ascending and descending colon become fused with the parietal peritoneum. The transverse colon retains its mesentery which later fuses with the greater omentum.

The majority of small intestinal and proximal large intestinal malformations are related to three events: (1) failure of the endoderm of the yolk sac to separate from the notochord during the third week, which results in a variety of reduplications of the intestine, (2) failure of the vitellointestinal duct to regress during the fifth week, which results in a Meckel's diverticulum and other vestigial abnormalities, and (3) failures in herniation, return and fixation of the intestine between the fifth and twelfth weeks; failure at any stage may result in anomalies such as malrotation, exomphalos or an undescended caecum.

The hindgut becomes established early and a ventral diverticulum, the allantois, arises from it (see Fig. 1.3). Just caudal to the junction of the allantois and hindgut the cloaca develops, and the junction between the allantois and hindgut becomes the cloacal membrane. During the sixth week the cloaca

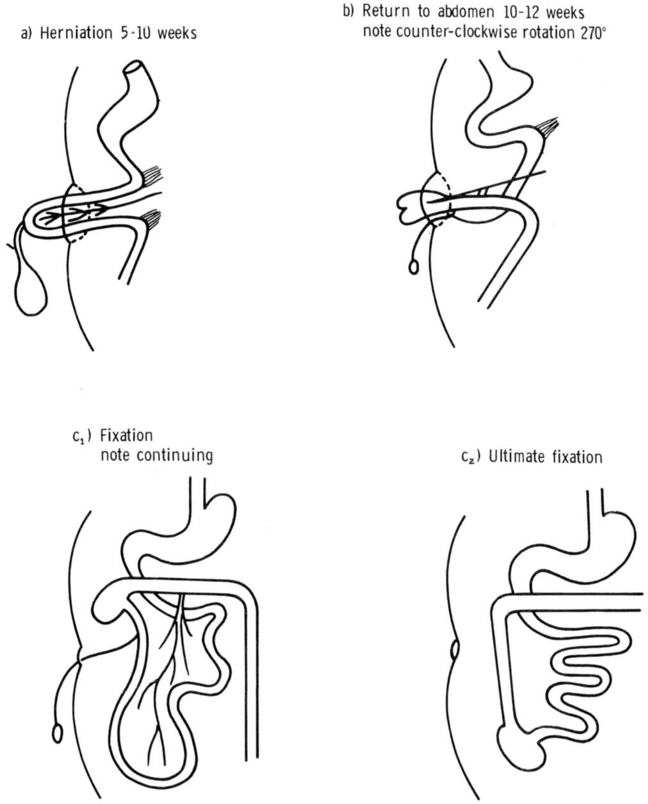

Fig. 1.4 Sequential events leading to the ultimate fixation and position of the gut within the abdomen.

becomes flattened from side to side and elongates in the sagittal plane. A septum forms to divide the cloaca dorsally into rectum and ventrally into the urogenital sinus. The part of the cloacal membrane sealing the rectum usually ruptures between the eighth and ninth weeks. Congenital defects of the anus and rectum resemble those of the oesophagus and are associated one with another more frequently than by chance; anal and rectal anomalies may arise from abnormalities occurring at several different stages of development. Duhamel (1961) has proposed a syndrome of caudal regression, with anorectal malformations as the milder expression, and sirenoid monsters as the most extreme form.

The liver and biliary system

The liver and biliary system arise from that region of the gut endoderm which also gives rise to the duodenum. At four weeks an hepatic diverticulum can be seen at the ventral aspect of the duodenum which has two portions, a cranial bud which differentiates into hepatic cells and bile ducts, and a caudal bud which becomes the gall bladder and cystic duct. These developmental events are depicted in Figure 1.5. The cranial bud divides into two main branches which form the right and left lobes of the liver. Initially these are of equal size,

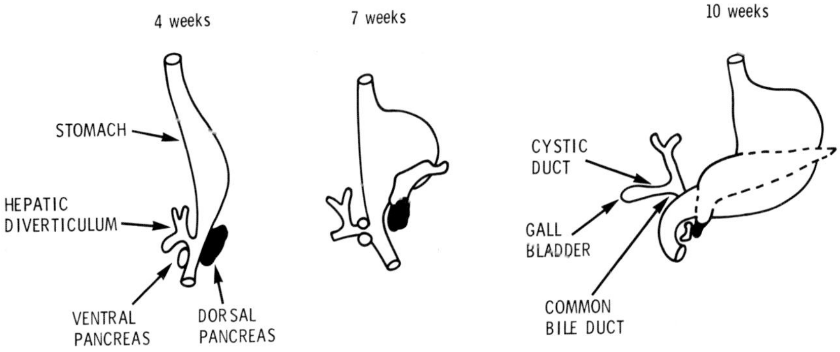

Fig. 1.5 Origin and development of the hepatic diverticulum and pancreas.

but after the third month the right lobe becomes larger and parts of this lobe then form the subordinate lobes. The hepatic cells divide rapidly so that the liver increases rapidly in size, and at 10 weeks it occupies most of the abdominal cavity. At the same time the original diverticulum elongates and differentiates into the hepatic duct and common bile duct. At birth the liver is relatively large in size but it is unusual for any anomalies to occur in its development. Occasionally an accessory lobe (Riedel's lobe) grows from the right lobe and can be easily palpated below the right costal margin.

Whilst the cranial bud of the hepatic diverticulum is developing into the liver and common bile duct, the caudal region of the diverticulum elongates to form the cystic duct during the fifth week of embryonic life. This expands at its distal end to form the gall bladder. Initially the gall bladder and hepatic ducts are hollow; proliferation of the epithelial lining temporarily converts them into solid cords and recanalisation takes place by seven weeks. The gall bladder usually lies in a shallow bed on the undersurface of the liver, but congenital anomalies involving the biliary tract are relatively common with a frequency of 10 per cent. The gall bladder may be absent, as in certain animals (e.g. the rat and the horse), a double gall bladder may be present and occasionally it may develop a mesentery of its own and hence be liable to torsion. Rarely a cystic dilation of the common bile duct (choledochal cyst) may develop. The commonest congenital anomaly is atresia of the bile ducts, which was considered to be due to failure of recanalisation of the ducts, but this is almost certainly not the sole explanation; for example, atresia may represent the end result of an inflammatory process during fetal development.

As soon as the cranial portion of the hepatic diverticulum is formed it rapidly proliferates to form cords of epithelial cells. These grow rapidly to develop into a network of branching epithelial strands. The intrahepatic bile ducts arise as tributaries of the hepatic duct at eight weeks, differentiating into interlobular ducts at points of contact with connective tissue. The bile canaliculi extend between the hepatic cells and are continuous with the interlobular bile ducts. The canaliculi and intrahepatic ducts are probably formed from the liver cells. The rich vascular network of the liver grows with the hepatic cells.

The pancreas

Like the hepatobiliary system the pancreas also develops from the gut endoderm. Between three and four weeks two outpocketings arise from opposite sides of the duodenum, representing the earliest signs of pancreatic development. The dorsal pancreas extends out from the duodenum just cranial to the level of the hepatic diverticulum, and the ventral pancreas appears in the caudal angle between the gut and hepatic diverticulum (Fig. 1.5). The dorsal pancreas grows rapidly into the dorsal mesentery, and by six weeks it is an elongated nodular structure. The ventral pancreas grows more slowly and remains closely associated with the developing hepatic diverticulum. The hepatic diverticulum forms the common bile duct and, as a result of this close relationship, a common exit into the duodenum develops for the biliary system and the pancreas.

As the duodenum grows the ventral pancreas and bile ducts are swept behind the duodenum to meet the dorsal pancreas, and at eight weeks the dorsal and ventral primordia fuse. The dorsal pancreas forms the tail, body and part of the head, whilst the majority of the head and the uncinate process arise from the ventral pancreas (Fig. 1.6). Failure of migration of the ventral pancreas may result in the formation of an annular pancreas, which in one study was found in 13·7 per cent of 410 autopsies (Feldman and Weinberg, 1952).

Both the dorsal and ventral pancreas have an axial duct. The dorsal duct arises directly from the duodenal wall, and the ventral duct unites with the common bile duct as it arises from the duodenum. At eight weeks when the pancreas is relatively mature, the dorsal duct drains the body and tail and unites with the ventral duct to form the main pancreatic duct of Wirsung. Thus, bile and pancreatic juice have a common outlet into the duodenum at the ampulla of Vater. A circular layer of muscle develops around this outlet to form the sphincter of Oddi. The proximal end of the dorsal duct may either become a tributary of the main pancreatic duct or retain its opening into the duodenum, when it is known as the accessory duct of Santorini. This accessory duct is patent in up to 70 per cent of adult subjects (Kleitsch, 1955), but in only 10

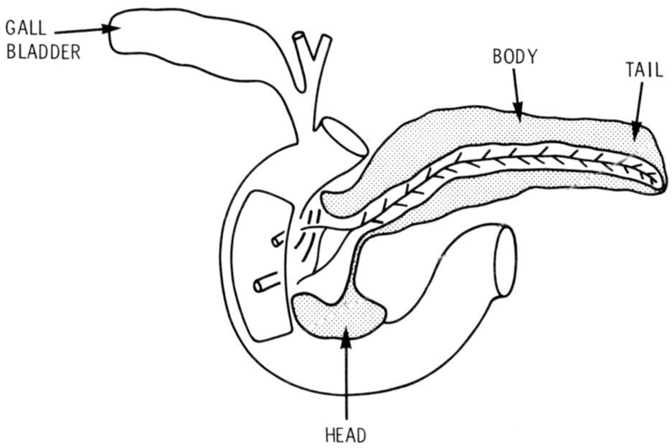

Fig. 1.6 Fusion of dorsal and ventral pancreas to form the head, body and tail of the pancreas.

per cent is it the only exit into the duodenum; in the remainder pancreatic juice reaches the duodenum through both openings.

The mature pancreas is an elongated lobular gland, the head lying in close proximity to the duodenal loop. It is covered by a thin layer of connective tissue derived from the dorsal mesenchyme; the dorsal mesenchyme also grows into the developing gland, giving the mature pancreas its characteristic lobular appearance.

Histological development

The oesophagus, stomach and intestine

Although the epithelium of most of the alimentary tract is of endodermal origin, differentiation varies according to the region of the tract. Thus in the oesophagus it differentiates to stratified squamous epithelium, in the stomach it forms gastric glands which contain a variety of secretory cells and in the small and large intestine both absorptive and secretory cells develop. Epithelial differentiation is initiated by exuberant proliferation of cells which may completely occlude the lumen, particularly in the oesophagus and small intestine; failure of recanalisation of the lumen may account for some congenital small gut atresias.

In the oesophagus a single lumen is restored by the ninth to tenth weeks and is lined by ciliated cells, which are replaced by stratified squamous cells during the fifth month.

The first glandular pits of the stomach appear at six weeks, and by 12 weeks parietal, chief and mucous cells have differentiated.

The histological development of the small intestine has been more extensively studied than any other region of the alimentary tract (Várkonyi, Gergely and Varró, 1974). Initially a single layer of cells is arranged radially towards the lumen; they contain large nuclei occupying most of the cytoplasm, the mitochondria are elongated and rough endoplasmic reticulum is present. Between eight and 10 weeks a transition takes place in a craniocaudal direction. The flat mucosal cells with short irregular microvilli develop into a columnar epithelium which lines the villi of the mucosa. Their cytoplasm contains apical vesicles, mitochondria, scattered glycogen-containing lysosomes and many ribosomes. By 10 to 12 weeks, the epithelial cells have become longer and narrower, and resemble mature enterocytes. The Golgi apparatus has expanded, the apical cytoplasm is dominated by a rapidly developing tubular system, particularly at the villous tips, and goblet, endocrine and Paneth cells are present.

In the large intestine villi and glandular cells appear in the colon during the third month, the villi reach their maximum development during the fourth month and thereafter gradually shorten and disappear; goblet and simple columnar cells appear by the eleventh week.

The musculature of the bowel arises from mesoderm and develops in a craniocaudal direction, differentiation of the inner circular layer preceding that of the outer longitudinal layer.

Innervation of the bowel also proceeds in a craniocaudal direction. The neuroblasts of the myenteric plexus migrate down the alimentary tract with the vagus nerve preceding formation of the longitudinal muscle layer. The neuroblasts reach the oesophagus at six weeks, the cranial loop of the midgut by seven to eight weeks and innervation is complete by 12 weeks. Arrest in the migration of ganglion cells down the developing gut results in aganglionosis distal to the level of arrest, and leads classically to Hirschsprung's disease.

The liver

The anatomy of the hepatic architecture is complex and includes the portal venous system, which accounts for 60 to 80 per cent of the total influx, the remainder being supplied by the hepatic artery. The vascular sinusoid spaces develop in the early weeks of embryonic life and serve to link the portal and hepatic venous systems. This venous network branches in a regular and uniform way to result in the formation of the hepatic lobules.

Layers of mesenchyme intervene between the endothelium of the sinusoids and the epithelial cells, and these layers give rise to blood-forming cells, haemocytoblasts. The haemocytoblasts rapidly proliferate to outnumber the hepatocytes and produce erythrocytes, which pass through the sinusoid walls to enter the general circulation. This source of haemopoietic activity subsides towards the end of gestation, and only small foci are present in the liver of the newborn.

The pancreas

The cells of the exocrine and endocrine pancreas develop from the cells which line the primitive pancreatic ducts, and at eight weeks the developing pancreas consists largely of a network of anastomosing ducts and ductules which are lined by a single layer of cells. Endocrine cells precede the development of exocrine cells, and there appear to be two generations of islet cells during embryonic life (Liv and Potter, 1962). The first generation arises during the eighth week from cells lining the primitive pancreatic ducts, and the second arises from the cells of the terminal ductules after the third month when the exocrine acinar cells have been formed. The islet cells disengage themselves from the ductular system and appear as irregular structures scattered throughout the gland being separated from the acinar cells by a thin reticular membrane; they are particularly prominent in the tail of the pancreas.

Acinar cells also develop from cells lining the embryonic pancreatic ducts and first appear in both the dorsal and ventral pancreas during the third month of intrauterine life. The acinar cells are pyramidal in shape and rest on a reticular membrane, to become arranged in a circular or tubular fashion around a central lumen, forming the intralobular ducts. These ducts drain into the interlobular ducts, which in turn drain into the main pancreatic duct.

FUNCTIONAL DEVELOPMENT

The alimentary tract

In utero the demands made by the fetus on the alimentary tract are relatively small compared to those at birth when the tract is required to initiate and sustain the rapid body growth of the newborn.

Swallowing
The fetus begins to swallow amniotic fluid during the second trimester of pregnancy at a rate of 2 to 7 ml per 24 hours, and at 20 to 21 weeks of gestation at a rate of 13 to 16 ml per 24 hours (Pritchard, 1966; Abramovich, 1970). Hydramnios often accompanies pregnancies in which fetal swallowing is impaired, such as in proximal small intestinal atresias (Lloyd and Clatworthy, 1958), and fetal swallowing is undoubtedly an important mechanism in the regulation of amniotic fluid volume.

The stomach
With the exception of hydrochloric acid gastric secretions may be found early in the second trimester. Hydrochloric acid is rarely present in the fetal stomach before the thirty-second week, and even at term the pH of gastric contents is only about 6 but decreases precipitously during the first 24 hours of life (Ebers, Smith and Gibbs, 1956; Ahn and Kim, 1963). Pepsin activity increases markedly during the third trimester but small preterm babies may have an impaired ability to digest dietary protein (Werner, 1948). However, impaired proteolysis may favour the absorption of macromolecules, such as antibodies present in colostrum, and in this way enhance passively acquired immunity. Although the hormone gastrin has been detected in the fetal stomach, it has not been quantitatively determined.

The small intestine
Transport. The fetal intestine can absorb intact macromolecules and this process may be important in the development of immune function (Walker and Isselbacher, 1974).

Everted sac studies have shown that both the human jejunum and ileum are capable of actively transporting glucose and L-alanine as early as the twelfth week, and separate studies measuring transmural potential difference changes have confirmed these findings (Koldovský *et al.*, 1965; Levin *et al.*, 1968).

Enzymes. The development of enzymes in the small intestinal mucosa has been extensively studied (see Grand, Watkins and Torti, 1976). Figure 1.7 shows the relative activities of the brush border disaccharidases at different stages of

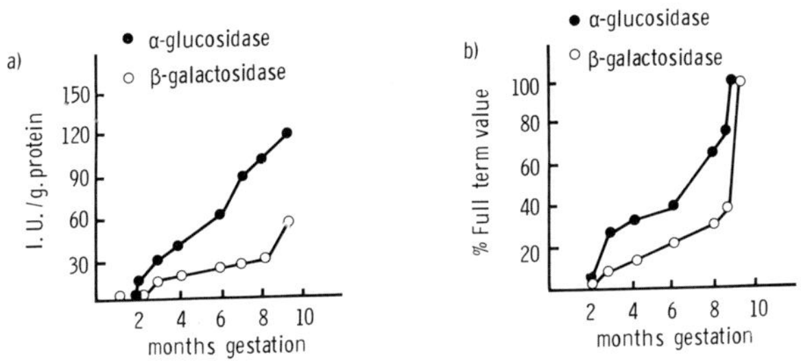

Fig. 1.7 Development of the brush border disaccharidases of the small intestine.

gestation. At 12 weeks the α-glucosidases (maltase, sucrase-isomaltase) possess considerable activity, whereas β-galactosidase (lactase) activity is very low and remains so until about the thirty-second week, when it rapidly increases to reach a maximum just before birth. This probably explains why some premature babies are intolerant to lactose. Topographically there exists an activity gradient for the disaccharidases, maximal activities occurring in the proximal small bowel.

Adult activities of a variety of mucosal dipeptidases are attained by 12 weeks and are maximal in the proximal small intestine (Lindberg, 1966). In contrast, leucine aminopeptidase activity increases with gestational age after 12 weeks (Jirosvá *et al.*, 1966).

Several lysosomal enzyme systems are fully developed as early as the twelfth week and may be detectable biochemically prior to the ultrastructural appearance of organised lysosomes.

Adenyl cyclase is an enzyme which is located in the basolateral membranes of the enterocyte, and the secretory effects of certain bacterial toxins (e.g. cholera toxin, heat-labile *E. coli* toxin and possibly others) result from activation of adenyl cyclase (see Ch. 10). Adenyl cyclase activity is present as early as 10 weeks and increases by more than two-fold by the seventeenth week of gestation (Grand, Torti and Jaksina, 1973). The same study also demonstrated that the fetal enzyme is activated by cholera toxin.

Immune systems. During recent years a great deal of attention has been focused on the role of the gut in the body's overall immune competence in man, and it has become clear that it is of great importance. Perhaps this is not surprising since it is continually exposed to foreign antigenic material to which it must react to ensure the balanced survival of the host. The prenatal development of the immune systems of the gut is therefore a critical preparatory event to the newborn baby being suddenly exposed to its postnatal hostile environment. Knowledge on this aspect of paediatric gastroenterology is fragmentary and represents an important area for future investigation.

The density of the lymphoid Peyer's patches in the small intestine increases distally, and they are concentrated in the ileum; they are well developed by about the twentieth week of gestation. IgA containing plasma cells are absent from the lamina propria of the fetal gut, and they first appear in the neonatal period preceding serum IgA. IgM-containing cells appear before birth during the third trimester. Of the specific immunoglobulin classes, only IgG can be transported across the placenta; this immunoglobulin represents an important source of passive immunity to the newborn against Gram-positive organisms but is relatively ineffective against Gram-negative species. There is no information on IgE or IgD immunoglobulins in the developing human fetus.

Bockman and Cooper (1975) have studied the fine structure of the human fetal appendix and found a relationship between the development of lymphoid follicles and the specialisation of the covering epithelium. They speculated that the follicle-associated epithelium provides a channel through which antigens can stimulate clonal proliferation and seeding of B lymphocytes in the lamina propria.

The colon

During the middle trimester the mucosal cells of the colon contain villi, disaccharidase, dipeptidase and alkaline phosphatase activity (Dahlqvist and Lindberg, 1966; Lev and Orlic, 1974). The significance of these findings is not clear but may indicate an absorptive function for the fetal colon. No information is available on colonic absorption of fluid and electrolytes in the fetus.

The liver

The metabolic development of the fetus is intimately associated with that of the liver and most of the available information has been derived from studies in the experimental animal. As with all other aspects of functional prenatal development, information on the human fetus is very limited.

Carbohydrate metabolism

Glucose is the major source of energy during fetal life and anaerobic metabolism the most important component of glucose metabolism (Stembera and Hodr, 1966; Villee *et al.*, 1958). Glycogen is stored solely in the liver, and rapid accumulation is initiated between 13 and 14 weeks' gestation (Capkova and Jirasek, 1968) continuing until term. Small for dates neonates have a disproportionately reduced liver mass and glycogen reserve, and this is a major factor in the aetiology of the hypoglycaemia which they may experience (Shelley and Neligan, 1966). Gluconeogenic and lipogenic pathways function from as early as the eleventh week of gestation (Villee *et al.*, 1958).

Protein metabolism

The fetal liver is a very active site with regard to protein synthesis, though some of this undoubtedly represents haematopoietic activity. Albumin synthesis commences at about 12 weeks and gradually increases throughout gestation. In contrast coagulation proteins and caeruloplasmin concentrations are frequently low at term.

Cystine is not formed by the fetal liver because the transsulphuration pathway is incomplete due to the absence of cystathionase which does not appear until after birth (Sturman, Gaull and Raiha, 1970). Cystine should therefore be regarded as an essential amino acid in the newborn, in contrast to older children and adults. The pathways involved in phenylalanine and tyrosine metabolism may also be immature at birth despite the fact that phenylalanine hydroxylase activity can be detected as early as eight weeks (Raiha, 1973) and the tyrosine oxidation system as early as the fourteenth week of gestation (Raiha, Schwartz and Lindroos, 1971). Premature infants may have an impaired dietary tolerance to these amino acids due to defective cofactor metabolism (Light, Berry and Sutherland, 1966).

Detoxication and excretion

The nitrogen-excreting mechanism, the urea cycle, is closely coupled to kidney development. Thus the human fetal liver is capable of synthesising urea at the same time as the mesonephric glomeruli are formed (Raiha and Suihkonen, 1968). Generally speaking, however, the fetus relies on maternal tissues for the detoxication of noxious substances, and the term infant has a limited capacity for detoxication.

The pancreas

The development of exocrine pancreatic function is not fully understood, but it is, nevertheless, clear that development is still incomplete at birth. Zymogen granules first appear in the acinar cells at three months' gestation (Keene and Hewer, 1929), but it is not clear which enzymes are contained in the granules at this stage nor how their subsequent development is controlled.

Proteolytic enzymes

The proteolytic enzyme which has been most studied is trypsin, and it has been detected in the fetal pancreas as early as 16 weeks (Keene and Hewer, 1929; Lieberman, 1966). This, however, is unusual and activity can only rarely be found in fetuses weighing less than 500 g. In fetuses weighing 1000 g, corresponding to about 28 weeks' gestation, tryptic activity can be detected in the pancreas of about 30 per cent; between 28 and 36 weeks a ten-fold increase in activity occurs, and activity is present in the vast majority by 36 weeks' gestation (Lieberman, 1966). There is little change in activity between 36 weeks and term. Following pancreatic stimulation with intravenous secretin and cholecystokinin-pancreozymin, tryptic activity in the duodenal juice of premature babies (32 to 34 weeks) is similar to that in full-term neonates; there is then a further ten-fold rise in activity between birth and nine months (see Grand *et al.*, 1976). Also, trypsin activity at one week after birth is significantly higher in preterm than in full-term infants, and activity can be stimulated in preterm infants by increasing the protein content of the diet.

The factors which regulate the increase in tryptic activity after 28 weeks are not clearly understood, but maturation of trypsinogen or enterokinase are likely possibilities. Little is known about the development of enterokinase, but recent studies suggest that it appears late in gestation (see Grand *et al.*, 1976).

Lipase

This enzyme has not been extensively studied in the fetal pancreas. In some studies it has been reported to be present as early as 16 weeks (Tachibana, 1928), whereas other studies have failed to detect the enzyme until 32 weeks' gestation (Keene and Hewer, 1929).

Lipase is undoubtedly present at 34 to 36 weeks of gestation, but its activity is only about half that seen in full-term infants (Zoppi *et al.*, 1972). Between birth and nine months a ten-fold increase in activity takes place. Lipase activity can be stimulated by a high protein diet both in preterm and full-term infants, but activity is independent of the quantity of fat in the diet (Zoppi *et al.*, 1972).

Amylase

Amylase has been detected in amniotic fluid as early as 16 weeks (Wolf and Taussig, 1973) and in fetal pancreas as early as 22 weeks' gestation (Keene and Hewer, 1929). However, amylase activity remains very low or even absent in the vast majority of infants until after birth (Auricchio, Rubino and Murset, 1965;

Zoppi *et al.*, 1972). Keene and Hewer (1929) could detect amylase in the pancreas of only about half of full-term infants. Between birth and the age of nine months a dramatic and 200-fold rise of pancreatic amylase activity occurs.

Knowledge of the functional development of the fetal pancreas is still very limited and represents an important area of future research. It is clear, however, that even in the full-term neonate the pancreas is still functionally immature and that this may have important clinical implications to feeding practices in the newborn, particularly in the premature baby.

References

Abramovich, D. R. (1970) Fetal factors influencing amniotic fluid volume and composition of liquor amnii. *Journal of Obstetrics and Gynaecology of the British Commonwealth*, **77**, 865.

Ahn, C. I. & Kim, Y. J. (1963) Acidity and volume of gastric contents in the first week of life. *Journal of the Korean Medical Association*, **6**, 948.

Auricchio, S., Rubino, A. & Murset, G. (1965) Intestinal glycosidase activities in the human embryo, fetus and newborn. *Pediatrics*, **35**, 944.

Bockman, D. E. & Cooper, M. D. (1975) Early lymphoepithelial relationships in human appendix. A combined light- and electron-microscopic study. *Gastroenterology*, **68**, 1160.

Capkova, A. & Jirásek, J. E. (1968) Glycogen reserves in organs of human fetuses in the first half of pregnancy. *Biologia Neonatorum*, **13**, 129.

Dahlqvist, A. & Lindberg, T. (1966) Fetal development of the small intestinal disaccharidase and alkaline phosphatase activities in the human. *Biologia Neonatorum*, **9**, 24.

Duhamel, B. (1961) From the mermaid to anal imperforation: the syndrome of caudal regression. *Archives of Disease in Childhood*, **36**, 152.

Ebers, D. W., Smith, D. I. & Gibbs, G. E. (1956) Gastric acidity on the first day of life. *Pediatrics*, **18**, 800.

Feldman, M. & Weinberg, T. (1952) Aberrant pancreas: a cause of duodenal syndrome. *Journal of the American Medical Association*, **148**, 893.

Grand, R. J., Torti, F. M. & Jaksina, S. (1973) Development of intestinal adenyl cyclase and its response to cholera enterotoxin. *Journal of Clinical Investigation*, **52**, 2053.

Grand, R. J., Watkins, J. B. & Torti, F. M. (1976) Development of the human gastrointestinal tract: A review. *Gastroenterology*, **70**, 790.

Jirsvá, V., Koldovský, O., Heringová, A., Hošková, J., Jirásek, J. & Uher, J. (1966) The development of the functions of the small intestine of the human fetus. *Biologia Neonatorum*, **9**, 44.

Keene, M. F. L. & Hewer, E. E. (1929) Digestive enzymes of the human foetus. *Lancet*, **1**, 767.

Kleitsch, W. P. (1955) Anatomy of the pancreas. A study with special reference to the duct system. *Archives of Surgery*, **71**, 795.

Koldovský, O., Heringová, A., Jirsová, V., Jirásek, J. E. & Uher, J. (1965) Transport of glucose against a concentration gradient in everted sacs of jejunum and ileum of human fetuses. *Gastroenterology*, **48**, 185.

Lev, R. & Orlic, D. (1974) Histochemical and radioautographic studies of normal human fetal colon. *Histochemistry*, **39**, 301.

Levin, R. J., Koldovský, O., Hošková, J., Jirsová, V. & Uher, J. (1968) Electrical activity across human foetal small intestine associated with absorption processes. *Gut*, **9**, 206.

Lieberman, J. (1966) Proteolytic enzyme activity in fetal pancreas and meconium. Demonstration of plasminogen and trypsinogen activities in pancreatic tissue. *Gastroenterology*, **50**, 183.

Light, I. J., Berry, H. K. & Sutherland, J. M. (1966) Aminoacidaemia of prematurity. *American Journal of Diseases of Children*, **117**, 96.

Lindberg, T. (1966) Intestinal dipeptidases: characterization, development and distribution of intestinal dipeptidases of the human foetus. *Clinical Science*, **30**, 505.

Liv, H. M. & Potter, E. L. (1962) Development of the human pancreas. *Archives of Pathology*, **74**, 439.

Lloyd, J. R. & Clatworthy, H. W. (1958) Hydramnios as an aid to the early diagnosis of congenital obstruction of the alimentary tract: a study of the maternal and fetal factors. *Pediatrics*, **21**, 903.

Pritchard, J. A. (1966) Fetal swallowing and amniotic fluid volume. *Obstetrics and Gynaecology*, **28,** 606.

Raiha, N. C. R. (1973) Phenylalanine hydroxylase in human liver during development. *Pediatric Research*, **7,** 1.

Raiha, N. C. R., Schwartz, A. L. & Lindroos, M. C. (1971) Induction of tyrosine and ketoglutarate transaminase in fetal rat and fetal human liver in organ culture. *Pediatric Research*, **5,** 70.

Raiha, N. C. R. & Suihkonen, J. (1968) Development of urea synthesizing enzymes in human liver. *Acta Pediatrica Scandinavica*, **57,** 121.

Shelley, H. J. & Neligan, G. A. (1966) Neonatal hypoglycaemia. *British Medical Bulletin*, **22,** 34.

Stembera, Z. K. & Hodr, J. (1966) Mutual relationships between the levels of glucose, pyruvic acid and lactic acid in the blood of the mother and of both umbilical vessels in hypoxic fetuses. *Biologia Neonatorum*, **10,** 303.

Sturman, J., Gaull, G. & Raiha, N. C. R. (1970) Absence of cystathionase in human fetal liver: is cystine essential? *Science*, **169,** 74.

Tachibana, T. (1928) Physiological investigation of fetus. 4. Lipase in pancreas. *Japanese Journal of Obstetrics and Gynecology*, **11,** *92.*

Várkonyi, T., Gergely, G. & Varró, V. (1974) The ultrastructure of the small intestinal mucosa in the developing human fetus. *Scandinavian Journal of Gastroenterology*, **9,** 495.

Villee, C. A., Hagerman, D. D., Holmberg, N., Lind, J. & Villee, D. B. (1958) The effects of anoxia on the metabolism of human fetal tissues. *Pediatrics*, **22,** 953.

Walker, W. A. & Isselbacher, K. J. (1974) Uptake and transport of macromolecules by the intestine: possible role in clinical disorders. *Gastroenterology*, **67,** 531.

Werner, B. (1948) Peptic and tryptic capacity of the digestive glands in newborns. *Acta Paediatrica Scandinavica*, **35,** (suppl. 70), 1.

Wolf, R. O. & Taussig, L. M. (1973) Human amniotic fluid isoamylases. *Obstetrics and Gynecology*, **41,** 337.

Zoppi, G., Andreotti, G., Pajno-Ferrara, F., Njai, D. M. & Gaburro, D. (1972) Exocrine pancreas function in premature and full term neonates. *Pediatric Research*, **6,** 880.

2. Structure and function

D. P. R. Muller

The oesophagus
The stomach
The small intestine
The large intestine
Digestive organs and glands associated with the alimentary tract
Aspects of the postnatal development of structure and function

For practical purposes the digestive system may be thought of as a long muscular tube beginning at the lips and ending at the anus with certain large glands and organs such as the salivary glands, gall bladder, pancreas and liver situated outside this tube but emptying secretions into it. This chapter considers the relationships between the structure and the function of the mature alimentary canal, placing particular emphasis on the small intestine, and briefly reviews the associated digestive glands and organs; where appropriate disturbances in the relationships between structure and function will be described in the context of disease states. In addition, some aspects of postnatal development of structure and function will be considered.

The major function of the alimentary canal is the absorption of food-stuffs; it is, however, also a secretory and defensive organ and its structure will be considered in relation to these different aspects. The gross anatomical arrangement of the alimentary tract is similar throughout its length and consists of four layers, the serosa, the submucosa, the muscularis mucosa and the mucosa. These will be discussed in detail when describing the small intestine, the most important absorptive region of the tract. The alimentary tract is taken as extending from the oesophagus to the rectum and other parts, such as the lips, tongue, teeth and pharynx, are not considered.

THE OESOPHAGUS

As with all parts of the alimentary tract the oesophagus consists of four layers, but because of its specialised function structural differences exist compared with the small intestine. For example, because of the rapid luminal transit of food there is no requirement for an absorptive surface epithelial layer or for the secretion of digestive enzymes. Similarly there is not the same requirement for lymphoid tissue as a protection against invading micro-organisms and, as it is well lubricated by saliva, mucous secreting cells are not plentiful. However, because of the relatively undigested nature of the food which passes along its length, a stratified squamous epithelium is provided.

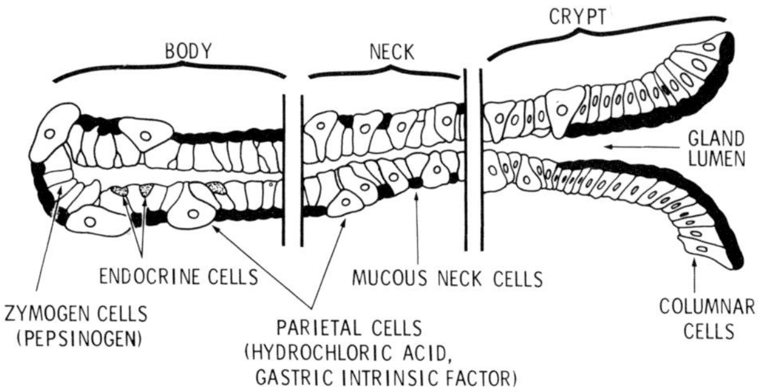

Fig. 2.1 The foveolae gastricae of the gastric mucosa showing the different regions and cell types.

THE STOMACH

Structure

The mucosa is relatively thick and contains many mucous-producing cells and, when the stomach is partially empty, the mucosa is principally arranged in longitudinal folds or rugae. The only glands present in the submucosa are found in the pyloric region, adjacent to the duodenum. The muscularis mucosa consists of three rather than the usual two layers: an outer longitudinal, a middle circular and an inner oblique layer. The pyloric sphincter is a thickening predominantly of the middle circular layer.

On close examination of the gastric mucosa many small pits (foveolae gastricae) can be identified which secrete the gastric juice; these pits can be delineated into a crypt, neck and body as shown in Figure 2.1. The crypts contain four important cell populations: zymogen or chief cells, parietal or oxyntic cells, mucous neck cells and endocrine cells; the parietal cells are concentrated in the fundi and body regions of the stomach. The zymogen cells are found in the deepest part of the pits and secrete digestive enzymes, principally pepsinogen. The parietal cells are interspersed among the zymogen cells and secrete hydrochloric acid and the gastric intrinsic factor which is necessary for the absorption of vitamin B_{12}. The mucous cells are located between the parietal cells in the neck region of the pits. The endocrine cells are scattered between the basement layer and the zymogen cells; they appear to be heterogeneous in nature and synthesise and secrete the gastric hormones.

The surface epithelium of the stomach is made up of tall columnar cells which start abruptly at the cardiac region. They form a membrane which is one cell thick and secrete the mucus which coats and protects the lining of the stomach. The cells appear to originate at the pit openings and migrate upwards to replace those lost by desquamation, complete renewal of the surface cells taking place approximately every one to three days.

Function

The stomach has several important functions, which are listed in Table 2.1.

It receives and stores food, mixes it to form chyme and delivers the chyme in a controlled fashion to the small intestine. The function of the proximal stomach

Table 2.1 Functions of the stomach

Storage, mixing and controlled emptying of food
Antibacterial properties of hydrochloric acid
Release of vitamin B_{12} from dietary protein
Synthesis of intrinsic factor
Initiation of protein digestion by pepsin
Initiation of fat digestion by lipase
Synthesis of hormones
Facilitation of iron absorption

(fundus and body) as a reservoir is facilitated by the elasticity of its walls. The process of gastric filling is poorly understood, but it is probably not a completely passive process since gastric muscle appears to contract or relax to maintain the intragastric pressure constant over a wide range of volumes, implying that the process is regulated by a control mechanism. Immediately following the entry of food the gastric contents are composed of a liquid and solid phase which undergoes mixing and digestion to form a semisolid fluid or chyme which has an even consistency. This is achieved by the muscular movements of the stomach and by the digestive properties of gastric juice.

Gastric emptying is regulated by many factors all of which, with the exception of distension, are inhibitory (Hunt and Knox, 1968; Cooke, 1975). Liquid meals are emptied faster than solid ones, the antrum appearing to prevent the exit of solid foods from the stomach. The osmolality of the gastric contents is a sensitive and important mechanism regulating gastric emptying, isotonic contents leaving the stomach faster than hypo- or hypertonic ones. The effects of osmolality on gastric emptying are mediated via sensitive osmoreceptors located in the proximal small intestinal mucosa. Acids, particularly hydrochloric acid, and fats (the longer the chain length of the fatty acids the greater the effect) both delay emptying. The mechanisms responsible for these inhibitory effects are likely to be both neural and humoral. Thus, pain or distension of the intestine inhibits gastric emptying by way of the sympathetic motor innervation to the stomach. Vagotomy has also been shown to abolish the inhibitory effect of hyperosmolar and fatty meals. In addition several gastrointestinal hormones liberated by the gastric and duodenal mucosa, such as gastrin, secretin, cholecystokinin as well as the 'candidate hormones' enterogastrone and motilin, affect gastric emptying. Despite the number and variety of the regulatory mechanisms the net result is that emptying occurs as a single exponential function, which implies a high degree of control between the various systems.

The acidity of gastric contents provides an important defence mechanism against ingested enteropathogenic bacteria, and patients with impaired gastric acid secretion are more susceptible to infective enteritis (Drasar *et al.*, 1969).

Vitamin B_{12} does not exist in the free form but is attached to dietary protein, and the first step in the digestion and absorption of the vitamin is its removal from dietary protein. Both the proteolytic enzymes and the acidic medium present in the stomach may contribute to the release of vitamin B_{12} from its protein bonds. The free vitamin then binds to intrinsic factor, which is secreted from the parietal cells, and is a glycoprotein with a molecular weight of about

50 000 to 60 000. The molecules of intrinsic factor aggregate to form a dimer and two molecules of vitamin B_{12} bind to the dimer. The complex stabilises and protects the vitamin during intestinal transit and binds to specific receptors in the distal ileum prior to the release and absorption of the free vitamin. In general, intrinsic factor and acid are secreted in parallel and patients with achlorhydria usually have a reduced secretion of intrinsic factor. However, a continued secretion of small amounts of intrinsic factor may be sufficient to prevent the development of pernicious anaemia.

An ordinary meal remains in the stomach for about four hours and during this time it undergoes some digestion. The principal enzyme found in gastric juice is pepsin (Samloff, 1971). This is formed from the inactive precursor pepsinogen, firstly by the action of hydrochloric acid and then by the autocatalytic action of free pepsin in the presence of hydrochloric acid. Pepsin is stable under acid conditions with a pH optimum at about 1·0 to 1·5. It initiates proteolysis in the stomach by hydrolysing peptide bonds at the amino groups of aromatic or acidic amino acids.

Gastric lipase may be of importance in initiating fat digestion in the normal individual (Cohen *et al.*, 1971). In patients with isolated lipase deficiency, gastric lipase probably accounts for the fat which can be absorbed (Muller *et al.*, 1975).

Gastrin is synthesised and secreted by the 'G' cells of the antrum of the stomach, and the reader is referred to an excellent review of this hormone (Walsh and Grossman, 1975). There are at least three human gastrins, 'big-', 'little-' and 'mini-' gastrin, with molecular weights of 3839, 2098 and 1647, respectively. The regulation of gastrin release from the 'G' cells is complex and is influenced by many factors. Stimulating factors include certain peptides and amino acids, gastric distention (acting via reflexes), vagal cholinergic stimulation (initiated from head or stomach), and blood-borne calcium or epinephrine. Inhibitory factors include acid and a variety of blood-borne peptide hormones such as secretin, gastric inhibitory peptide, vasoactive intestinal peptide and calcitonin. In addition to its stimulatory effect on gastric acidity, gastrin has a variety of other effects on gastric function and also on the function of other organs such as the small intestine, pancreas, colon and liver. These effects include secretion and inhibition of water and electrolyte transport, stimulation and inhibition of smooth muscle, enzyme secretion, release of hormones and trophic effects (see Walsh and Grossman, 1975).

The acidity of the stomach facilitates the absorption of inorganic iron. At an acid pH precipitation of iron is prevented and chelation by ascorbate, dietary carbohydrates and amino acids is enhanced (Conrad and Schade, 1968); both these effects result in increased solubilisation and absorption of iron.

THE SMALL INTESTINE

Basic structure and cell types (see Trier, 1973)

Before discussing the function of the small intestine in some detail it is important to consider its basic structure and the cell types present.

The wall of the small intestine consists of the four layers which are common to the whole alimentary tract (see Fig. 2.2). The outermost layer or serosa is an

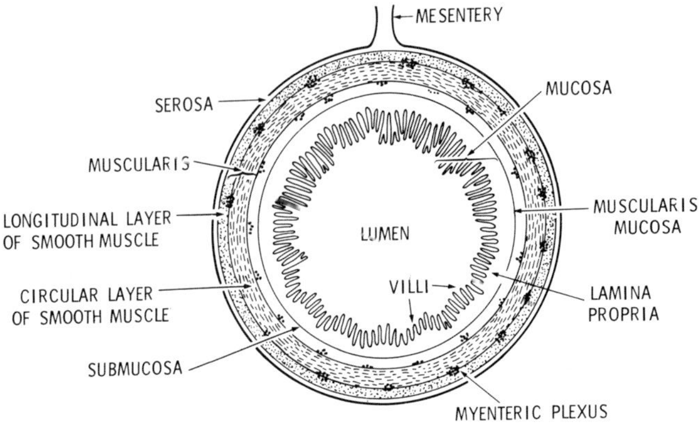

Fig. 2.2 Schematic cross-section of the small intestine showing its gross anatomical arrangement.

extension of the peritoneum and is made up of a single layer of flattened mesothelial cells which lie over some loose connective tissue. The muscularis comprises an outer longitudinal and an inner circular layer of smooth muscle, which together provide the primary mechanism for propelling the contents of the alimentary canal along its length. This is achieved by waves of constriction (peristalsis) which sweep downward, pushing the contents of the bowel ahead of them. Situated between the two muscle layers is a plexus of nerve fibres with numerous ganglia (myenteric plexus), which provides a conducting system for

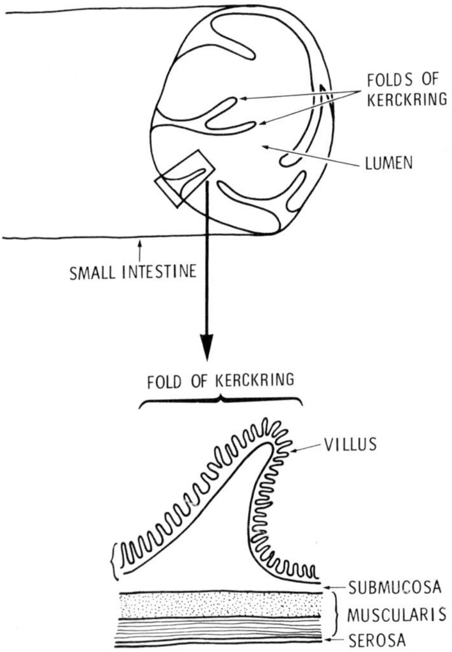

Fig. 2.3 Cross-section of the folds of Kerckring and the villi of the small intestine.

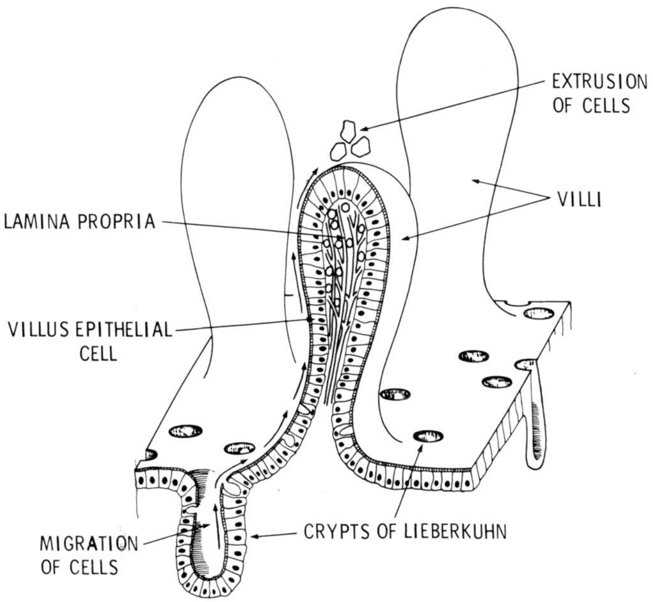

Fig. 2.4 The villi and crypts of the small intestinal mucosa.

peristalsis. The control of intestinal motility is a complicated and poorly understood field, but it is clear that the autonomic nervous system and certain gastrointestinal hormones play an important role (Harvey, 1975).

The submucosa consists largely of dense connective tissue sparsely infiltrated by lymphocytes, macrophages, eosinophils, mast cells and plasma cells. It contains elaborate venous and lymphatic plexuses which drain the respective capillaries of the lamina propria of the mucosa. In addition it contains an extensive network of arterioles, ganglion cells and nerve fibres which form the autonomic submucosal plexus. Branched acinar glands (Brunner's glands) are found in the submucosa of the duodenum; their secretions are rich in mucus and bicarbonate and may provide protection against acid-peptic digestion of the proximal duodenum.

The innermost layer or mucosa can be subdivided into three further layers, the muscularis mucosa, the lamina propria and the epithelium. With the exception of the ileum the mucosa is thrown into a series of folds (folds of Kerckring) from which slender villi (0·2 to 1·0 mm in height) project into the lumen of the gut (Fig. 2.3). As will be discussed later these folds and villi provide a mechanism to increase the absorptive surface area of the intestine. Between the villi are the crypts of Lieberkühn which dip down from the surface of the mucosa almost as far as the muscularis mucosa (Fig. 2.4). The villus:crypt length ratio is approximately 2:1, and there are about three times as many crypts as villi. The muscularis mucosa separates the mucosa from the submucosa and consists of a thin sheet of smooth muscle; one of the functions of the muscularis is to counteract stretching forces and so maintain the tall slender architecture of the villi.

The lamina propria

The lamina propria forms the connective tissue core of the villus, surrounds the crypts (Fig. 2.4) and has numerous functions. It provides structural support for the epithelium as well as for the many vascular and lymphatic channels that nourish the mucosa and transports absorbed material away to the systemic circulation. It contains numerous cell types, such as plasma cells, lymphocytes, mast cells, eosinophils and macrophages, and presents a defensive barrier to micro-organisms and other foreign substances which may penetrate the surface epithelium. The lamina propria of the small intestine, particularly the distal part, contains isolated collections of lymphoid nodules. The larger ones may occupy the whole thickness of the mucosa, bulge onto its surface and even extend through the muscularis mucosa into the submucosal layer. When groups of nodules are massed together they form Peyer's patches which occur predominantly in the ileum. Immunoglobulins (IgA, IgM and IgG) are synthesised by the plasma cells and act as a first line of defence against invasion by micro-organisms and other substances which may be involved in the production of local intestinal or systemic disease states (see Walker and Hong, 1973). About 80 to 90 per cent of the IgA in intestinal secretions is structurally and antigenically different to that found in serum, and the so called secretory IgA. Secretory IgA consists of two molecules of IgA stabilised by a glycoprotein, secretory piece. It is likely that IgA molecules synthesised in the lamina propria pass into the epithelial cells where they complex with secretory piece and pass into the lumen as secretory IgA. The presence of secretory piece protects the IgA molecule from enzymatic digestion by the proteolytic enzymes normally present in the intestinal lumen. Immunoglobulins produced in the lamina propria probably also make an important contribution to the serum immunoglobulins. Indeed, the gut can be considered as an organ which makes an important contribution to the immune competence of the host as a whole.

Small unmyelinated nerve fibres are present in the lamina propria, and these may play a role in regulating mucosal blood flow and possibly also mucosal secretory activity. Smooth muscle fibres are present which may control villus motility. The activity (contraction and relaxation) of the villi is low during periods of fasting and increases during the absorption of a meal. By contracting and relaxing, the villi act as a 'micromixer' assuring optimal conditions for absorption, and may also be of importance in forcing lymph along the lymphatics. A hormone, villikin, may be responsible for this activity (Grossman and others, 1974).

The surface epithelium

The crypt epithelium is composed of at least four distinct cell types: Paneth, undifferentiated, goblet and endocrine cells, none of which have a brush border. The Paneth cells are located at the base of the crypts, are similar to salivary acinar glands and secrete large amounts of protein-rich materials, including lysozyme (Peeters and Vantrappen, 1975). By virtue of the bactericidal activity of lysozyme, Paneth cells probably play a role in the overall defence system of the small gut. The most abundant cells in the crypts are the undifferentiated or principal cells which form the lateral walls of the crypts and are also dispersed between the Paneth cells. Their cytoplasm contains many secretory granules. Goblet cells are found on the lateral wall of the crypts and are so named because of their shape. The thin basal half of the cell contains the nucleus and the apical half is distended by secretory material having the staining characteristics of sulphated mucoprotein. The function of intestinal mucus has not been completely defined, but it is believed to be important in protecting and lubricating the intestinal mucosa. The endocrine cells, also termed enterochromaffin, argentaffin, basal granular or more recently APUD cells, are characterised by their inverted appearance compared to the other crypt cells. Their small secretory granules are distributed in the basal cytoplasm between the cell apex and the nucleus and are liberated into the lamina propria as opposed to the lumen of the gut. These cells synthesise and secrete the gastrointestinal hormones.

A major role of the crypt epithelium is that of cell proliferation and renewal of the intestinal epithelium (Creamer, 1967). Within the crypts the undifferentiated cells divide and, as replication proceeds, new cells migrate up the wall of the crypt and on to the base of the villus, where they begin to differentiate into mature cells. Differentiation continues as the cells migrate until the upper third of the villus is reached, where absorptive capacity is at a peak. At the extreme villus tip the cells degenerate, lose their absorptive capacity and are extruded into the intestinal lumen. The entire process of cell migration and maturation takes from four to five days in the ileum and five to seven days in the duodenum and jejunum. The epithelium covering the villus is composed of absorptive cells or enterocytes, goblet cells and a few endocrine cells. The latter types of cells closely resemble those found in the crypt epithelium. The enterocytes are the principal cells of the villus with the major role of digestion and absorption of the luminal contents.

Relationship between structure and function

Following the controlled emptying of chyme from the stomach, the duodenum is the area where neutralisation, mixing, equilibration and the continuation of digestion takes place. By the time the intestinal contents reach the jejunum conditions are optimal for absorption. The ileum provides reserve capacity for absorption, as well as possessing specialised functions such as the absorption of vitamin B_{12}, and the sodium-dependent active absorption of bile salts.

Surface area and absorptive efficiency

The structure of the small intestine is so arranged as to provide the maximum available functional surface area, and this is achieved in three ways (Laster and Ingelfinger, 1961; Trier, 1968):

1. The luminal surface is thrown into a series of spiral or circular horizontal folds (i.e. folds of Kerckring) which increase the surface area by a factor of about three (Fig. 2.3). They begin at the duodenum and end at the middle or distal third of the ileum, and are most abundant and highly developed in the distal duodenum and proximal jejunum where they may reach a length of 1 cm.

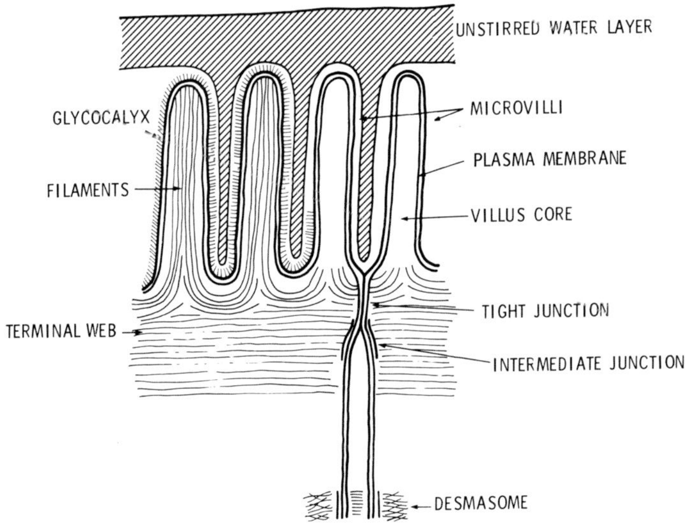

Fig. 2.5 The brush border of the absorptive cells of the small intestinal mucosa.

2. The numerous villi (Fig. 2.3) which extend from the mucosa amplify the surface area by a factor of eight to 10 and they are approximately 0·5 to 1 mm in length. In the proximal duodenum they are normally broad and ridge-shaped, in the distal duodenum and proximal jejunum they are commonly leaf-shaped, whereas in the distal jejunum and ileum they are normally finger-like in shape. The villi are tallest in the distal duodenum and proximal jejunum and become progressively shorter as the ileocaecal valve is approached.
3. Finally, the brush border of the individual absorptive cells lining the villus is made up of slender microvilli which project into the lumen (Fig. 2.5). In man the microvilli average 1 μ in length with a width of approximately 0·1 μ, and it has been estimated that they increase the absorptive surface of the cell by a further 15 to 40 times. Thus, the total surface area of the small intestine compared to a simple cylinder may be increased by a factor of up to 1200. Any reduction in villus size and/or number will result in a reduced surface area and impaired absorption. This mechanism partially explains the malabsorption in coeliac disease and intestinal resection.

The absorptive cell

The transport of dietary substances from the lumen to the bloodstream is regulated by the absorptive cell, which is represented schematically in Figure 2.6. Although the individual features of the enterocyte are not unique its general appearance is distinctive and readily permits identification; the cells are tall columnar cells with a basally located oval-shaped nucleus and a brush border.

The brush border. The brush border can be regarded as a subcellular organelle consisting of an apical plasma membrane surrounded by a surface coat or glycocalyx, a microvillous core and a terminal web (Fig. 2.5). The plasma membrane of the microvillus is both morphologically and biochemically different from the basal and lateral membranes of the absorptive cell; it is significantly wider (Palay and Karlin, 1959) and has a different phospholipid composition (Lewis *et al.*, 1975). The glycocalyx is composed of a sulphated, weakly acidic mucopolysaccharide which differs structurally and histochemically from the mucus secreted by the goblet cell. It is an integral part of the cell, synthesized by the particular epithelial cell on which it is found and cannot be removed either by proteolytic or mucolytic agents (Holmes, 1971). The microvillous core contains bundles of filaments which run parallel to the long axis of the microvillus and extend down into the cytoplasm of the cell where they interdigitate with the fibrils of the terminal web. The microvillous core and terminal web appear to provide important structural support for the brush border, thus ensuring that the maximum surface area is presented for absorption.

The microvilli together with the glycocalyx do much more than increase the available surface area. They actively participate in digestion and absorption in a number of ways. Firstly, intraluminal enzymes may be adsorbed on to the surface coat and thus some hydrolysis of substrates may take place at or in the glycocalyx with the theoretical advantage of releasing products near the microvillous plasma membrane (Ugolev, 1972). The physiological importance of this digestive process compared to intraluminal digestion is probably minor. Secondly, a number of enzymes, particularly disaccharidases and peptidases, are

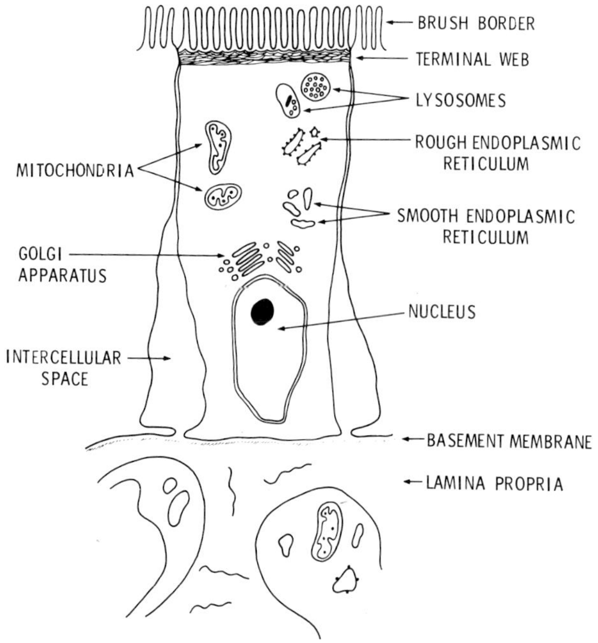

Fig. 2.6 The absorptive cell of the small intestinal mucosa.

located at or in the brush border membrane. The terminal digestion of carbohydrates.and proteins occurs at the microvillus membrane prior to monosaccharide, amino acid or peptide transport into the cells. Thirdly, there appear to be specific receptors on the microvillus membrane-glycocalyx complex. For example, ileal absorptive cells have been shown to have specific receptors for the vitamin B_{12}-gastric intrinsic factor complex (Donaldson *et al.*, 1967). Fourthly, there is evidence that certain transport carriers are also located in the microvillus membrane. These are essential components of the overall transport process if the hydrophilic (water-loving) products of digestion, such as monosaccharides, amino acids and dipeptides, are to be transported across the lipid bilayer of the membrane. The close proximity of the hydrolytic enzymes and specific carriers of the brush border confers a 'kinetic advantage' for the transport of the terminal products of digestion across the plasma membrane into the cell (Crane, 1968). For example, glucose is absorbed faster from sucrose than when presented to the mucosa as the free monosaccharide. Certain inborn errors of absorption are thought to result from a genetically determined defect or absence of protein carriers (see Ch. 11).

When considering the transport of substances from the lumen of the small intestine across the brush border there is a further barrier to take into account; for the brush border is exposed to a predominantly aqueous environment, and a series of water lamellae extend outwards from the brush border becoming progressively more stirred until they blend imperceptibly with the bulk phase of the luminal contents. These relatively unstirred water layers immediately adjacent to the brush border present a barrier to uptake of substances by the mucosal cell and may be a rate-limiting factor in fat absorption (Wilson and Dietschy, 1972).

The basolateral membranes. The basal and lateral membranes of the cell contain two enzymes which play a fundamental role in transport: sodium-potassium activated adenosine triphosphatase (Na^+–K^+)-ATPase and adenyl cyclase (Quigley and Gotterer, 1969; Parkinson *et al.*, 1972). The former enzyme catalyses the hydrolysis of adenosine triphosphate (ATP) to adenosine diphosphate (ADP) and inorganic phosphate, which results in the liberation of energy; this energy is utilised by the 'sodium pump' to actively extrude sodium out of the cell across the basolateral membranes. This process generates and maintains a sodium concentration gradient between the intestinal lumen and the interior of the cell and allows for the active sodium-coupled transport of glucose and galactose and certain amino acids (Crane, 1968); the resulting osmotic gradients result in water absorption. Thus the hydrolysis of ATP provides the cellular energy for the transport of electrolytes, certain sugars and amino acids against electrochemical gradients.

Adenyl cyclase catalyses the conversion of ATP to cyclic adenosine monophosphate (cAMP), and the role of this cyclic nucleotide in the regulation of water and electrolyte secretion has been increasingly recognised in recent years (Field, 1974). Any factor which increases the intracellular concentration of cAMP also induces secretion of fluid and electrolytes, particularly monovalent anions, into the intestinal lumen. For example, the enterotoxins elaborated by

Vibrio cholerae and certain strains of *E. coli* (Field, 1974), prostaglandins (Kimberg *et al.*, 1971) and vasoactive inhibitory peptide (Schwartz *et al.*, 1974) all appear to exert their secretory effects via this system.

An important morphological specialisation can be seen in the upper part of the lateral membrane where adjacent plasma membranes fuse for a short distance to form the so-called 'tight junction' (Fig. 2.5). It appears very likely that many small solutes, ions and water are able to traverse this junction (extracellular shunt pathway) during passive intestinal absorption or secretion. Other larger solutes, however, are unable to traverse this junction and must therefore cross the microvillus membrane, the cell cytoplasm and the lateral membrane before entering the intercellular spaces (Fordtran, 1973). Immediately below the tight junction the lateral membranes diverge to form the intermediate junction which is approximately 200 Å wide. Below this is the third type of junctional complex, the desmasome, which serves to bind adjacent cells firmly together (Weinstein and McNutt, 1972).

The basal membrane of the enterocyte is very close to the thin basement membrane on which the columnar cells lie and to the capillaries and lymphatics of the lamina propria. Absorbed material must always cross the basement membrane in order to reach these vascular and lymphatic channels. It has become increasingly clear that solute and water transport across the surface epithelium of the small intestine can occur via two routes, a transcellular route (i.e. the enterocyte) and an extracellular route (i.e. the extracellular shunt pathway), and the reader is referred to an excellent review by Schultz, Frizzell and Nellans (1974) for more detailed information.

Subcellular organelles. A variety of organelles, each with a specialised function, are distributed below the terminal web of the brush border; for example, mitochondria, lysosomes, the rough and smooth endoplasmic reticulum, and the Golgi apparatus (Fig. 2.6). As in other cells the mitochondria provide metabolic energy and the lysosomes degrade waste and toxic substances. The endoplasmic reticulum has important roles in synthetic and transport processes. For example, it synthesises the digestive enzymes of the enterocyte, it is responsible for the re-esterification of absorbed fatty acids and monoglycerides to triglyceride and the organelle also synthesises the protein moiety surrounding the discreet packets of lipid (chylomicra) which eventually pass into the lymphatic system. In Addison's disease mild fat malabsorption may occur due to a reduced activity of the enzymes necessary for triglyceride synthesis, and in abetalipoproteinaemia chylomicra cannot be formed owing to a defect in the synthesis of an essential apoprotein designated apo-B (Gotto *et al.*, 1971). The Golgi apparatus, located just above the nucleus, is thought to store and chemically modify material absorbed and synthesised by the cell (Ockner and Isselbacher, 1974).

THE LARGE INTESTINE

The wall of that part of the large intestine which lies within the peritoneal cavity consists of the four layers already discussed. The rectum, however, which lies outside the peritoneal cavity, has no serosa. The muscularis is composed of an inner circular and outer longitudinal muscle layer. The latter is distinctive because it is made up of three separate longitudinal strips (taeniae coli). The mucosa differs from that of the small intestine in that it has a flat absorptive surface with no villi; crypts are, however, present. The flat absorptive surface is lined by absorptive cells which have considerably less microvilli than the small intestine and which contain a moderate number of mucus-secreting goblet cells.

The main functions of the large intestine are the storage of intestinal contents prior to excretion, the absorption of water and electrolytes entering from the ileum and, in particular, the conservation of sodium ions and water (Cummings, 1975). The colonic mucosa is able to absorb sodium from luminal concentrations as low as 15 mmol/l and against a potential difference of as much as 40 mV (lumen negative compared to the serosa), whereas the maximum potential difference generated by the ileum and jejunum is about 5 mV. Unlike the jejunum the absorption of sodium by the colon is not stimulated by glucose or amino acids. Patients with established ileostomies provide indirect evidence of the importance of the colon in sodium and water conservation, since they are susceptible to water and salt depletion especially in hot climates. The mineralocorticoid aldosterone influences colonic conservation of fluid, sodium and chloride. It promotes net absorption and increases the transmural potential difference, and in addition reduces the sodium:potassium ratio in the effluent of patients with an ileostomy (Sladen, 1972). In patients with chronic inflammatory disease of the large bowel transport of water and electrolytes may be impaired, which also emphasises the importance of the large bowel in fluid conservation. The capacity of the large intestine to absorb declines progressively down the intestinal tract, with the rectum absorbing very little.

The factors which control the electrophysiology, the pharmacology and the motility of the large intestine and the act of defaecation are complex, and the reader is referred to the following reviews for detailed accounts of these processes: Duthie, 1971; Bennett, 1975; Edmonds, 1975; Misiewicz, 1975.

DIGESTIVE ORGANS AND GLANDS ASSOCIATED WITH THE ALIMENTARY TRACT

The salivary glands

There are three pairs of salivary glands, the parotid, mandibular and sublingual, all of which are of the compound tubuloalveolar type.

The parotid glands are the largest and are serous glands producing zymogen granules, which are precursors of salivary amylase. The submandibular glands are predominantly serous but also contain mucous cells; the sublingual glands are also mixed but mainly secrete mucus. These three types of glands secrete saliva, which has several functions. It lubricates the buccal mucosa and lips, washes the mouth clear of cellular and food debris, moistens food and converts it to a semisolid or liquid mass prior to swallowing and is involved in the initial stages of digestion; salivary amylase initiates starch digestion, and recent studies suggest that glands in or near the pharynx secrete a lipase which is able to hydrolyse triglyceride (Hamosh *et al.*, 1975).

Secretion of saliva is regulated by the autonomic nervous system and may be influenced by cephalic, mechanical or chemical factors.

The pancreas

The pancreas produces both exocrine and endocrine secretions, but in the context of intestinal function the exocrine secretion is of primary importance and its endocrine function will only be briefly mentioned.

Structure

The pancreas is a compound acinous gland containing lobules which are bound together by loose connective tissue that is traversed by blood vessels, lymphatics, nerves and secretory ducts. The predominant acinar cells produce the exocrine secretion of the gland. Dispersed within these cells are isolated clumps of other species of cells (i.e. islets of Langerhans) which synthesise and secrete certain peptide hormones. The acinar cells consist of a single row of pyramidal epithelial cells which rest on a delicate reticular membrane and converge towards a central lumen, the size of which varies with the functional condition of the organ; it is small when at rest but becomes distended with secretory material during active secretion. The lumen of the acinus connects with small intercalated ducts; these are surrounded by centroacinar cells that drain into intralobular ducts which are covered by low columnar cells similar to centroacinar cells. These anastomose to form the interlobular ducts, which in turn communicate to become the main pancreatic duct of Wirsung. The interlobular ducts are lined with a columnar epithelium containing goblet cells, and the occasional argentaffin cell and mucous gland. The duct of Wirsung runs the whole length of the pancreas gradually increasing in size before opening into the duodenum at the ampulla of Vater. The islets of Langerhans, which produce the endocrine secretions, are separated from the surrounding acinar tissue by fine reticular fibres and do not connect with the pancreatic ducts. They contain three types of cells, designated alpha, beta and delta cells, which liberate glucagon, insulin and an unknown secretion, respectively.

Function (see Beck, 1973; Brandborg, 1973)

The exocrine pancreas performs two important functions. Firstly the acinar cells synthesise and secrete a number of enzymes which take part in the luminal digestion of ingested protein, carbohydrate and fat.

The proteolytic enzymes are secreted as inactive precursors (zymogens) which, on entering the intestinal lumen, are activated by the action of a key enzyme, enterokinase. Enterokinase is a brush border enzyme which is released into the lumen and converts trypsinogen to trypsin, which in turn activates the other proteolytic zymogens. These enzymes convert proteins to amino acids and short-chain peptides, and these products are transported and further hydrolysed to enter the portal vein as amino acids. Salivary and pancreatic α-amylase hydrolyses starch to maltose, maltotriose and α-limit dextrins. Maltose and maltotriose are then split by brush border maltases to glucose, and α-limit dextrins are split by brush border sucrase-isomaltase to glucose; glucose then enters the cell by an active sodium-coupled transport system. The pancreas secretes three classes of enzymes which participate in the luminal digestion of lipids, phospholipases, lipase and esterase. The main function of the phospholipases is to convert lecithin (phosphatidyl choline) to lysolecithin. Lipase converts triglyceride to monoglyceride and free fatty acids, and esterase hydrolyses molecules such as cholesterol esters to free cholesterol. The products of pancreatic lipolysis are solubilised by bile salt micelles and transported to the brush border for absoprtion.

The second important function of the pancreas is to secrete an alkaline aqueous fluid which is isosmotic with plasma; this neutralises the acid chyme leaving the stomach and provides an optimal environment for luminal digestion. Sodium and potassium concentrations in pancreatic secretions are similar to those in plasma, and the chloride concentration is reciprocally related to that of bicarbonate and may reach 150 mmol/l. The intercalated ducts and centro-acinar cells are the sites of water and electrolyte secretion. Carbonic anhydrase, an enzyme involved in bicarbonate secretion, is found only in the ductular epithelium.

Exocrine pancreatic secretion is regulated by a complex series of neuro-humoral mechanisms (see Youngs, 1972; Brooks, 1973). The most important hormones involved in this regulatory process are gastrin, secretin and cholecystokinin-pancreozymin (CCK-PZ). Gastrin stimulates enzyme secretion, is under cholinergic control and a low intragastric pH is the principal inhibitory factor to gastrin release. Secretin-producing cells are located in the mucosa of the proximal small gut and its secretion results from the passage of acid from the stomach. Secretin stimulates pancreatic secretion of water and electrolytes, principally bicarbonate, and has relatively little effect on the secretion of enzymes. CCK-PZ is also synthesised and secreted by the proximal small intestinal mucosa in response to the arrival of chyme from the stomach. It stimulates the secretion of pancreatic enzymes and is approximately three times as potent as gastrin. The vagus appears to be involved in the release of secretin and CCK-PZ, but the presence of a local cholinergic mechanism is controversial. A cephalic phase of pancreatic secretion has also been demonstrated in man and results in stimulation of both bicarbonate and enzyme secretion.

Some implications of these control mechanisms are that hormonal stimulation of pancreatic secretion may be impaired because of (1) a reduction in the number of hormone-producing cells (i.e. APUD cells), as in coeliac disease or following gastric antrectomy; (2) a failure of hydrochloric acid and/or chyme to reach APUD cells, as is the case following gastrojejunostomy, or (3) a reduction in the number of pancreatic secretory cells, as may occur in cystic fibrosis, congenital pancreatic hypoplasia or pancreatitis.

The liver

The liver is the largest organ in the body and performs numerous functions, some of which are of fundamental importance in a consideration of intestinal function.

Structure

The liver is composed of lobules, the outlines of which are indistinct as a result of poorly developed connective tissue partitions between them. The central

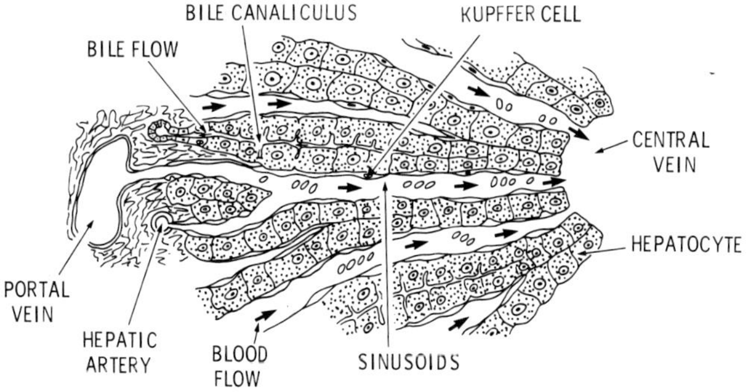

Fig. 2.7 The microstructure of the liver showing the arrangement of the hepatocytes, blood vessels and bile canaliculi.

hepatic vein runs through the centre of the lobules, whereas the branches of the portal vein, hepatic artery, interlobular bile ducts and lymphatics run together in the connective tissue of the portal tracts at the periphery of the lobules. The lobules are made up of hepatocytes which extend radially from the central vein to the periphery. In order for the hepatocytes to perform both an exocrine and endocrine function they are arranged in such a way as to form anastomosing thin plates (Fig. 2.7). Each cell therefore abuts on to a blood vessel into which it delivers its endocrine secretions, and on to a canalicular lumen into which its exocrine secretion (i.e. bile) passes. Between the plates of cells are vascular sinusoids which receive blood from the portal vein and hepatic artery and carry it to the centre of the lobule where it drains into the central vein. Lining the walls of the sinusoids are the Kupffer cells which have important phagocytic properties. The sinusoids and portal tracts also contain free round cells which are precursors of both red and white blood cells. Within the plates but between adjacent rows of hepatocytes are the bile canaliculi into which the bile is secreted. The canaliculi anastomose with each other and drain the bile to the periphery of the lobule and into the canals of Herring, which are bordered in part by hepatocytes and also by duct-type cells. These canals are short and connect with small bile ducts in the portal tract.

Function

With respect to intestinal function the prime function of the liver is the secretion of bile. Bile is an isosmotic alkaline solution (pH 7·5 to 9·5) which contains an abundance of organic solutes such as conjugated bile salts, bilirubin, cholesterol and lecithin. Its main function is the solubilisation of dietary lipids in the small intestine by bile salts prior to their absorption (see Ch. 7). Adequate intraluminal concentrations of bile salts are also important for other digestive events. For example, colipase and bile salts at concentrations above the critical micellar concentration are necessary for optimum activity of pancreatic lipase (Borgstrom and Donner, 1975). Similarly bile salts activate pancreatic esterase (Muller *et al.*, 1976) and amylase (O'Donnell *et al.*, 1975), and may promote the activation of trypsinogen by trypsin (Hadorn *et al.*, 1974). In addition, bile salts protect some of these enzymes against tryptic digestion and regulate the biosynthesis of cholesterol by the small gut mucosa.

There is a ductular and canalicular phase to the secretion of bile (Erlinger, 1972). The ductular epithelium actively secretes sodium and bicarbonate into the lumen of the ducts by a coupled pump, which is under the influence of gastrointestinal hormones such as secretin, CCK-PZ and gastrin, all of which increase bile flow and bicarbonate secretion. Vagal stimulation appears to enhance these humoral effects. The canalicular phase of secretion has two components, a bile acid-dependent and a bile acid-independent component. The active secretion of bile acids from the hepatocyte into the canaliculi establishes an osmotic gradient which results in the passive movement of water and cations to give an electrically neutral and isosmotic secretion. There is a linear relationship between bile flow and bile acid secretion rate, but if this is extrapolated to zero bile acid secretion, there is still significant bile flow. This and other evidence suggests that there is another mechanism for bile flow which is bile acid-independent. It is thought that the active transport of sodium ions may be responsible for this component, and this is supported by the fact that the bile acid-independent flow is suppressed or greatly decreased by inhibitors of the sodium pump. This component of bile flow can be stimulated by phenobarbitone, which produces no significant change either in the total bile acid secretion rate or in the relative output of individual bile acids.

In addition to synthesising and transporting bile, the hepatocytes are ideally situated to perform their numerous metabolic functions as they come into intimate contact with the absorbed dietary constituents present in portal blood.

The gallbladder

The gallbladder is a distendable sac with a mucosa which is thrown into numerous folds, thereby increasing its surface area for absorption. The epithelium of the mucosa is columnar with microvilli and thus resembles the absorptive cells of the small intestine. Its wall also has submucosal, muscularis and serosal layers. In addition it has a well-developed layer of smooth muscle which is arranged in an interlocking pattern of longitudinal and spirally arranged fibres. The gallbladder is drained by the cystic duct, which enters the common hepatic duct to form the common bile duct. This terminates in the duodenum close to the point of entry of the pancreatic duct at the ampulla of Vater. The complex of smooth muscle fibres associated with the ampula and the distal ends of the bile and pancreatic ducts form the sphincter of Oddi. The sphincter regulates the flow of bile into the intestine, inhibits the entry of bile into the pancreatic duct and prevents reflux of intestinal contents into the duct.

The function of the gallbladder is to concentrate and store bile and to deliver it to the duodenum during meals (Banfield, 1975). Hepatic bile is rapidly concentrated to the extent that about 90 per cent of the fluid is removed as an isotonic solution composed principally of sodium, chloride and bicarbonate; sodium and chloride are absorbed by an electrogenically neutral coupled transport process. The flow of concentrated bile from the gallbladder is initiated by predominantly hormonal stimuli. Cholecystokinin-pancreozymin is released from the mucosa of the proximal small intestine following a meal, and the hormone simultaneously stimulates gallbladder contraction and relaxation of the sphincter of Oddi. Vagal stimulation may enhance the action of CCK-PZ on gallbladder contraction. As the products of digestion are absorbed so the hormonal stimuli diminish, sphincter tone returns, the gall bladder relaxes and thus bile is again retained and concentrated. The effects of CCK-PZ appear to be mediated by the cyclic nucleotide, guanosine cyclic monophosphate.

ASPECTS OF THE POSTNATAL DEVELOPMENT OF STRUCTURE AND FUNCTION

As an organism adapts to extrauterine life its digestive and absorptive system undergoes many structural and functional changes. The vast majority of observations have been made in the experimental animal, and information on postnatal development in the human is limited. In the main, this section confines itself to certain aspects of postnatal development of structure and function in the human.

Structural changes

The relationship between the length of the intestine and body length changes with age. The relative length of the small intestine increases in the fetus, whereas it decreases postnatally. Autoradiographic studies have shown that turnover rates of small intestinal epithelial cells are reduced in the suckling rat compared with the adult (Koldovsky *et al.*, 1966), and a study in a newborn infant suggests that a similar situation exists in the human (Hebs *et al.*, 1969).

Functional changes

Enzymes

Brush border enzymes. The relative activities of the brush border disaccharidases at birth in the human are in general similar to those found in the adult (Dahlquist and Lindquist, 1971), which is in contrast to most animal species where adult activities are achieved after weaning. With regard to human brush border lactase, however, there are two distinct populations. Caucasians retain lactase activity at a relatively constant level throughout life. In non-Caucasian ethnic groups lactase levels decline after the first year or so of life at about the time of weaning; depending on the ethnic group, 50 to 100 per cent have clinical intolerance to lactose as judged by oral lactose load tests (Dahlquist and Lindquist, 1971). In a detailed study of 72 Bantu infants Cook (1967) showed that the blood glucose response to a lactose load gradually decreased during the first decade of life and that the majority were probably lactase-deficient by 4 years of age. In some exceptional cases lactose intolerance had already developed by six months.

In the developing fetus lactase activity does not reach adult levels until just before birth, which probably explains why premature babies may be more susceptible to lactose intolerance compared with the full-term infant.

Pancreatic enzymes. The activities of trypsin, lipase and amylase are all low at birth and increase with age (Zoppi *et al.*, 1972); pancreatic amylase takes the longest to reach adult levels (Hadorn *et al.*, 1968). The low levels of pancreatic lipase in the newborn may contribute to their reduced coefficient of fat absorption.

Gastric acidity

Gastric contents aspirated immediately after birth consist of material accumulated before birth or swallowed at birth, and are alkaline. Within about an hour of birth the contents have a mean pH of 3, which falls to between 2 and 3 by six hours (Ebers *et al.*, 1956). Gastric acidity then tends to fall further until the eighth to tenth day, after which it gradually rises (Miller, 1941).

Bile salts (see Murphy and Signer, 1974)

Qualitative changes. In the neonate, taurine-conjugated bile salts predominate over glycine conjugates (Poley *et al.*, 1964), but after only a few days of life the ratio approximates to that found in adults (i.e. about 3:1 in favour of the glycine conjugates). There is also an altered ratio of the primary bile acids in the neonate. During the first week of life the ratio of cholic to chenodeoxycholic acid is about 2·5:1·0 (Encrantz and Sjovall, 1959), but after a further few weeks this falls to the normal adult value of 1·2:1·0. These latter workers also reported the virtual absence of the secondary bile acid deoxycholic acid from the duodenal contents of infants up to the age of 12 months, whereas children between 4 and 10 years had near adult concentrations of this bile acid. Deoxycholic acid has been shown to appear at around the age of 13 months (Poley *et al.*, 1964), and this is presumably related to colonisation of the gastrointestinal tract by bacteria capable of 7 α-dehydroxylating the primary bile acid cholic acid.

Quantitative changes. The bile salt pool and the synthesis of the primary bile acids are reduced in the newborn compared with the older child or adult, and this is particularly the case in the premature neonate (Watkins *et al.*, 1973). It appears, however, that synthesis of bile salts exceeds their faecal loss in the newborn and that the bile salt pool therefore gradually increases (Weber *et al.*, 1972). As a result of the reduced bile salt pool in the neonate, duodenal bile salt concentrations frequently fall below the critical micellar concentration during digestion (Norman *et al.*, 1972). Solubilisation of dietary fat is therefore likely to be impaired and contribute to the reduced fat absorption observed in the newborn.

Absorption of macromolecules (see Walker and Isselbacher, 1974)

The gastrointestinal tract presents a barrier against the absorption of macromolecules such as proteins. There is, however, increasing evidence that the normal intestine, and in particular that of the neonate, is capable of absorbing macromolecules in quantities that may be antigenically or biologically important. It has been shown, for example, that the newborn can absorb measurable quantities of gamma globulin from maternal colostrum (Iyengar and

Selvaraj, 1972), and that bovine serum albumin present in infant milk formulas can be detected in serum (Rothberg and Farr, 1965). Other workers have shown that the serum of neonates contains a higher percentage of antibodies to food antigens than that of adults. The increased absorption of macromolecules in the neonatal period has important clinical implications, both favourable and unfavourable to the host. It provides a mechanism for the transfer of passive immunity from mother to offspring, as a result of the absorption of immunoglobulins from colostrum and breast milk. On the other hand, foreign antigens may be absorbed and elicit allergic responses. It is also possible that certain macromolecules may fix to target organs and result in autoimmune disease states.

Intestinal transit (see Koldovsky, 1969)

The transit of small intestinal contents is longer (three to six hours) in the newborn compared to the adult (about two and a half hours); transit through the large intestine is, however, much more rapid, ingested material appearing in the stools of the newborn after only 24 hours.

Bacterial flora

Meconium is usually sterile, but bacteria can be detected after about four hours. The faecal flora which subsequently develops differs according to whether the infant is breast- or bottle-fed. In both groups there is initially a high incidence of Gram-positive cocci, especially the coagulase-negative staphylococci. This flora is transient and by eight days a Gram-negative flora becomes established; this transition occurs earlier in breast-fed babies, but by eight days bottle-fed infants have a higher incidence of both numbers and frequency of Gram-negative bacilli. There is a more striking difference in the anaerobic flora present in the stools of breast-fed infants compared with bottle-fed infants (see Ch. 10).

References

Banfield, W. J. (1975) Physiology of the gallbladder. *Gastroenterology,* **69,** 770.

Beck, I. T. (1973) The role of pancreatic enzymes in digestion. *American Journal of Clinical Nutrition,* **26,** 311.

Bennett, A. (1975) Pharmacology of colonic muscle. *Gut,* **16,** 307.

Borgstrom, B. & Donner, J. (1975) Binding of bile salts to pancreatic colipase and lipase. *Journal of Lipid Research,* **16,** 287.

Brandborg, L. L. (1973) Pancreatic physiology. In *Gastrointestinal Disease: Pathophysiology, Diagnosis, Management,* p. 359, Sleisenger, M. H. & Fordtran, J. S. Philadelphia: Saunders.

Brooks, F. P. (1973) The neurohumoral control of pancreatic exocrine secretion. *American Journal of Clinical Nutrition,* **26,** 291.

Cohen, M., Morgan, R. G. H. & Hofmann, A. F. (1971) Lipolytic activity of human gastric and duodenal juice against medium and long chain triglycerides. *Gastroenterology,* **60,** 1.

Conrad, M. E. & Schade, S. G. (1968) Ascorbic acid chelates in iron absorption: a role for hydrochloric acid and bile. *Gastroenterology,* **55,** 35.

Cook, G. C. (1967) Lactase activity in newborn and infant Baganda. *British Medical Journal,* **1,** 527.

Cooke, A. R. (1975) Control of gastric emptying and motility. *Gastroenterology,* **68,** 804.

Crane, R. K. (1968) Absorption of sugars. In *Handbook of Physiology,* Section 6, Vol. IV, p. 1323, ed. Code, C. F. Washington, D.C.: American Physiological Society.

Creamer, B. (1967) The turnover of the epithelium of the small intestine. *British Medical Bulletin*, **23,** 226.
Cummings, J. H. (1975) Absorption and secretion by the colon. *Gut*, **16,** 323.
Dahlquist, A. & Lindquist, B. (1971) Lactose intolerance and protein malnutrition *Acta Paediatrica Scandinavica*, **60,** 488.
Donaldson, R. M., MacKenzie, I. L. & Trier, J. S. (1967) Intrinsic factor-mediated attachment of vitamin B_{12} to brush borders and microvillous membranes of hamster intestine. *Journal of Clinical Investigation*, **46,** 1215.
Drasar, B. S., Shiner, M. & McLeod, G. M. (1969) Studies on the intestinal flora. I. The bacterial flora of the gastrointestinal tract in healthy and achlorhydric persons. *Gastroenterology*, **56,** 71.
Duthie, H. L. (1971) Anal continence. *Gut*, **12,** 844.
Ebers, D. W., Smith, D. & Gibbs, G. E. (1956) Gastric acidity on the first day of life. *Pediatrics*, **18,** 800.
Edmonds, C. J. (1975) Electrical potential difference of colonic mucosa. *Gut*, **16,** 315.
Encrantz, J. C. & Sjovall, J. (1959) On the bile acids in duodenal contents of infants and children. *Clinica Chimica Acta*, **4,** 793.
Erlinger, S. (1972) Physiology of bile flow. *Progress in Liver Diseases*, **4,** 63.
Field, M. (1974) Intestinal secretion. *Gastroenterology*, **66,** 1063.
Fordtran, J. S. (1973) Diarrhea. In *Gastrointestinal Disease: Pathophysiology, Diagnosis and Management*, p. 291, ed. Sleisenger, M. H. & Fordtran, J. S. Philadelphia: Saunders.
Gotto, A. M., Levy, R. I., John, K. & Fredrickson, D. S. (1971) On the protein defect in abetalipoproteinaemia. *New England Journal of Medicine*, **284,** 813.
Grossman, M. I. and others (1974) Candidate hormones of the gut. *Gastroenterology*, **67,** 730.
Hadorn, B., Zoppi, G., Shmerling, D. H., Prader, A., McIntyre, I. & Anderson, C. M. (1968) Quantitative assessment of exocrine pancreatic function in infants and children. *Journal of Pediatrics*, **73,** 39.
Hadorn, B., Hess, J., Troesch, V., Verhaage, W., Gotze, H. & Bender, S. W. (1974) Role of bile acids in the activation of trypsinogen by enterokinase: disturbance of trypsinogen activation in patients with intrahepatic biliary atresia. *Gastroenterology*, **66,** 548.
Hamosh, M., Klaeveman, H. L., Wolf, R. O. & Scow, R. O. (1975) Pharyngeal lipase and digestion of dietary triglyceride in man. *Journal of Clinical Investigation*, **55,** 908.
Harvey, R. F. (1975) Hormonal control of gastrointestinal motility. *Digestive Diseases*, **20,** 523.
Hebs, J. J., Sunshine, P. & Kretchmer, N. (1969) Intestinal malabsorption in infancy and childhood. *Advanced Pediatrics*, **16,** 11.
Holmes, R. (1971) The intestinal brush border. *Gut*, **12,** 668.
Hunt, J. N. & Knox, M. T. (1968) Regulation of gastric emptying. In *Handbook of Physiology*, Section 6, Vol. IV, p. 1917, ed. Code, C. F. Washington D.C.: American Physiological Society.
Iyengar, L. & Selvaraj, R. J. (1972) Intestinal absorption of immunoglobulins by newborn infants. *Archives of Disease in Childhood*, **47,** 411.
Kimberg, D. V., Field, M., Johnson, J., Henderson, A. & Gershon, E. (1971) Stimulation of intestinal mucosal adenyl cyclase by cholera enterotoxin and prostaglandins. *Journal of Clinical Investigation*, **50,** 1218.
Koldovsky, O., Sunshine, P. & Kretchmer, N. (1966) Cellular migration of intestinal epithelia in suckling and weaned rats. *Nature* (London), **212,** 1389.
Koldovsky, O. (1969) In *Development of the Functions of the Small Intestine in Mammals and Man*, p. 153. Basel: Karger.
Laster, L. & Ingelfinger, F. J. (1961) Intestinal absorption—aspects of structure, function and disease of the small intestinal mucosa. *New England Journal of Medicine*, **264,** 1138.
Lewis, B. A., Gray, G. M., Coleman, R. & Michell, R. H. (1975) Differences in the enzymic, polypeptide, glycopeptide, glycolipid and phospholipid compositions of plasma membranes from the two surfaces of intestinal epithelial cells. *Biochemical Society Transactions*, **3,** 752.
Miller, R. A. (1941) Observations on the gastric acidity during the first month of life. *Archives of Disease in Childhood*, **16,** 22.
Misiewicz, J. J. (1975) Colonic motility. *Gut*, **16,** 311.
Muller, D. P. R., McCollum, J. P. K., Trompeter, R. S. & Harries, J. T. (1975) Studies on the mechanism of fat absorption in congenital isolated lipase deficiency. *Gut*, **17,** 838.
Muller, D. P. R., Manning, J. A., Mathias, P. M. & Harries, J. T. (1976) Studies on the intestinal hydrolysis of tocopheryl esters. *International Journal for Vitamin and Nutrition Research*, **46,** 207.
Murphy, G. M. & Signer, E. (1974) Bile acid metabolism in infants and children. *Gut*, **15,** 151.
Norman, A., Strandvik, B. & Ojamae, O. (1972) Bile acids and pancreatic enzymes during absorption in the newborn. *Acta Paediatrica Scandinavica*, **61,** 571.
Ockner, R. K. & Isselbacher, K. J. (1974) Recent concepts of intestinal fat absorption. *Reviews of Physiology, Biochemistry and Pharmacology*, **71,** 107.

O'Donnell, M. D., McGeeney, K. F. & Fitzgerald, O. (1975) Effect of free and conjugated bile salts on α-amylase activity. *Enzyme,* **19,** 129.

Palay, S. L. & Karlin, L. J. (1959) An electron microscopic study of the intestinal villus. I. The fasting animal. *Journal of Biophysical and Biochemical Cytology,* **5,** 363.

Parkinson, D. K., Ebel, H., Dibona, D. & Sharp, G. W. G. (1972) Localisation of the action of cholera toxin on adenyl cyclase in mucosal epithelial cells of rabbit intestine. *Journal of Clinical Investigation,* **51,** 731.

Peeters, T. & Vantrappen, G. (1975) The Paneth cell: a source of intestinal lysozyme. *Gut,* **16,** 553.

Poley, J. R., Dower, J. C., Owen, C. A. & Stickler, G. B. (1964) Bile acids in infants and children. *Journal of Laboratory and Clinical Medicine,* **63,** 838.

Quigley, J. P. & Gotterer, G. S. (1969) Distribution of ($Na^+ - K^+$)-stimulated ATPase activity in rat intestinal mucosa. *Biochimica et Biophysica Acta,* **173,** 456.

Rothberg, R. M. & Farr, R. S. (1965) Anti-bovine serum albumin and anti-alpha lactalbumin in the serum of children and adults. *Pediatrics,* **35,** 571.

Samloff, I. M. (1971) Pepsinogens, pepsins and pepsin inhibitors. *Gastroenterology,* **60,** 586.

Schultz, S. G., Frizzell, R. A. & Nellans, H. N. (1974) Ion transport by mammalian small intestine. *Annual Review of Physiology,* **36,** 51.

Schwartz, C. J., Kimberg, D. V., Sheerin, H. E., Field, M. & Said, S. I. (1974) Vasoactive intestinal peptide stimulation of adenylate cyclase and active electrolyte secretion in intestinal mucosa. *Journal of Clinical Investigation,* **54,** 536.

Sladen, G. E. G. (1972) A review of water and electrolyte transport. In *Transport Across the Intestine,* p. 14, ed. Burland, W. L. & Samuel, P. D. Edinburgh: Churchill Livingstone.

Trier, J. S. (1968) Morphology of the epithelium of the small intestine. In *Handbook of Physiology,* Section 6, Vol. III, p. 1125, ed. Code, C. F. Washington D.C.: American Physiological Society.

Trier, J. S. (1973) Anatomy of the small intestine. In *Gastrointestinal Disease : Pathophysiology, Diagnosis and Management,* p. 840, ed. Sleisenger, M. H. & Fordtran, J. S. Philadelphia: Saunders.

Ugolev, A. M. (1972) Membrane digestion. *Gut,* **13,** 735.

Walker, W. A. & Hong, R. (1973) Immunology of the gastrointestinal tract. *Journal of Pediatrics,* **83,** 517.

Walker, W. A. & Isselbacher, K. J. (1974) Uptake and transport of macromolecules by the intestine: possible role in clinical disorder. *Gastroenterology,* **67,** 531.

Walsh, J. H. & Grossman, M. I. (1975) Gastrin. *New England Journal of Medicine,* **292,** 1324.

Watkins, J. B., Ingall, D., Szczepanik, P., Klein, P. D. & Lester, R. (1973) Bile salt metabolism in the newborn. Measurement of pool size and synthesis by stable isotope technic. *New England Journal of Medicine,* **288,** 431.

Weber, A. M., Chartrand, L., Doyon, C., Gordon, S. & Roy, C. C. (1972) The quantitative determination of faecal bile acids in children by the enzymatic method. *Clinica Chimica Acta,* **39,** 524.

Weinstein, R. S. & McNutt, N. S. (1972) Cell junctions. *New England Journal of Medicine,* **286,** 521.

Wilson, F. A. & Dietschy, J. M. (1972) Characterization of bile acid absorption across the unstirred water layer and brush border of the rat jejunum. *Journal of Clinical Investigation,* **51,** 3015.

Youngs, G. (1972) Hormonal control of pancreatic endocrine and exocrine secretion. *Gut,* **13,** 154.

Zoppi, G., Andreotti, G., Pajno Ferrara, F., Njai, D. M. & Gaburro, D. (1972) Exocrine pancreas function in premature and full term neonates. *Pediatric Research,* **6,** 880.

3. Investigatory techniques

S. M. Packer, P. J. Milla and J. H. Tripp

Structural studies
Functional studies

Major advances have been made in the development and refinement of techniques for the investigation of gastrointestinal disease in childhood in the last decade, and this applies particularly to the younger age groups. These developments have had an important impact on the diagnosis and management of patients with a variety of disorders, as well as establishing paediatric gastroenterology as a major speciality branch of medicine. It should be emphasised that the primary approach to a patient must be an informed and skilled clinical one, and that the available investigatory techniques should be selected on the basis of a specific premeditated diagnosis whenever possible. This simple concept is sometimes ignored and replaced by a battery of tests, many of which are found to have been unnecessary in retrospect. A critical approach to the potential value of a particular investigation in diagnosis and management is essential in the planning of any investigatory programme for a patient. Tests should be the extension of informed logical thought in arriving at a diagnosis. It should also be remembered that the interpretation of the results of many investigations may be difficult even in expert hands, and close communication between the clinician and laboratory provides a team approach which can only enhance the standard of clinical care which can be offered to the sick child.

This chapter considers the more important investigatory techniques which are available for the study of gastroenterological problems in childhood and discusses their limitations where appropriate. For convenience sake and in keeping with the organisation of chapters 1 and 2, the techniques are broadly divided into those which delineate structure and those which assess function; a degree of overlap is unavoidable but it is hoped that this subdivision will prove to be helpful in clinical practice.

STRUCTURAL STUDIES

Radiological techniques

Good radiological facilities are essential for the investigation of gastroenterological problems but, in view of the potential hazards of exposure to radiation in childhood, the necessity for such procedures must be critically assessed. This is particularly important when sequential long-term radiological investigation is advisable such as in patients with chronic inflammatory bowel disease.

Plain radiology

Plain films of the abdomen can provide important information in both acute and chronic disease with regard to diagnosis and management.

Intestinal obstruction. In patients with acute obstruction a film taken in the erect position usually provides good supportive evidence to proceed to surgery; in addition, information regarding the level of the obstruction and any associated anomalies may also be obtained and may be helpful to the surgeons. Occasionally, suction via a nasogastric tube may mask the findings of distention and fluid levels, particularly in high obstructions such as with duodenal atresia. Introduction of air via the tube will usually produce a diagnostic film.

Although some information can be gained in patients with chronic obstruction (e.g. Hirschsprung's disease) further investigations such as mucosal biopsy and barium studies are almost invariably necessary.

Intestinal perforation. Classically the diagnosis rests on the presence of air between the diaphragm and liver on an erect film. In very sick children the same information can often be obtained from a decubitus film, thereby avoiding the manipulations which are necessary for an erect film.

Intra-abdominal calcification. The finding of calcification usually requires further studies, such as a cholecystogram and barium studies, to define the site of the lesions. Fetal peritonitis, meconium peritonitis, pancreatic disease, liver disease, gall-stones, neuroblastoma and renal calculi must be considered in any child with radiological evidence of abdominal calcification.

Pneumatosis. The detection of intramural gas and/or gas within the portal venous system is of grave prognostic significance and most commonly complicates enterocolitis in young infants.

Intra-abdominal masses. A plain film of the abdomen may reveal an abdominal mass and provide important information with regard to its nature. For example, the presence of gas, fluid, faeces or calcification within the mass; the site of the mass; any associated hepatosplenomegaly or bony metastases.

Foreign bodies. Many ingested foreign bodies such as fishbones, some plastic toys and lead-containing objects are radio-opaque, and a plain film of the abdomen may be helpful in the diagnosis of gastrointestinal symptoms in children in whom the ingestion of foreign bodies is suspected.

Contrast radiology

Alimentary tract. The contrast between the appearances of an intraluminal radio-opaque material (usually barium) and the mucosa and extramucosal tissues can provide very useful diagnostic information. The indications for a barium swallow are listed in Table 3.1.

Barium meal and follow-through studies of the small intestine are frequent investigations in paediatric practice but often provide limited information, as

Table 3.1 Indications for barium swallow

Recurrent vomiting and failure to thrive
Dysphagia
Suspicion of oesophageal varices
Mediastinal masses
Vascular rings
Persistent respiratory stridor
Foreign bodies
Assessment of oesophageal strictures

for example in children with suspected malabsorptive states such as coeliac disease; in these instances a peroral small intestinal biopsy should be the first investigation, and only if this is not diagnostic should barium studies be considered. Nevertheless a barium meal and follow-through can provide important information and the indications for this investigation are listed in Table 3.2.

The indications for a barium enema are shown in Table 3.3. This procedure is of great importance in newborns with clinical features of lower intestinal tract obstruction, as for example in Hirschsprung's disease. Rectal perforation may rarely complicate the procedure, particularly in the newborn, and in general self-retaining catheters should be avoided and contrast material run in very slowly. Gastrografin is sometimes used instead of barium and may be curative in conditions such as meconium ileus (see Ch. 4). A barium enema may also be curative as well as diagnostic in patients with intussusceptions (see Ch. 5). Barium enema does not always differentiate Crohn's disease from ulcerative colitis, and endoscopy and mucosal biopsy are usually necessary (see Ch. 6). Chronic constipation with or without overflow is not usually associated with any underlying organic disease in childhood, but an enema should be performed if there is any suspicion of Hirschsprung's disease.

Biliary tract. For technical details of the procedures available for cholecystography and cholangiography the reader is referred to Harris and Caffey (1953) and Hodgson (1970). Oral cholecystography or intravenous cholangiography is contraindicated in patients with active hepatocellular disease or when the serum level of bilirubin is greater than 85 μmol/l (5 mg/100 ml).

Oral cholecystography and intravenous cholangiography provide information on the structure and function of the gall bladder, the presence of gall-stones and the integrity of the extrahepatic biliary ducts. Both investigations have very limited application in childhood. Gall-stones, except for pigment stones in patients with chronic haemolytic anaemia, are extremely rare before puberty. Neither investigation has a place in the diagnosis of persistent neonatal jaundice.

Table 3.2 Indications for barium meal and follow-through

Congenital or postsurgical abnormalities
Hypertrophic pyloric stenosis when a tumour cannot be palpated
Suspected peptic ulcer
Gastrointestinal bleeding
Chronic inflammatory bowel disease
Intestinal malabsorption in association with a normal small intestinal biopsy

Table 3.3 Indications for barium enema

Neonatal intestinal obstruction
Intussusception
Chronic inflammatory bowel disease
Large bowel polyps
Chronic constipation

Operative cholangiography in infants with persistent jaundice is useful in assessing how much of the extrahepatic biliary duct system is patent, and it is an important aid in the decision on the type of surgical approach to be adopted in patients with extrahepatic biliary atresia.

Splenoportography (see Melhem and Rizk, 1970). This procedure should only be used in the final assessment of portal hypertension when all preliminary investigations have been completed. It provides excellent visualisation of the portal venous system, indicating the site of obstruction, the collateral circulation and its direction of flow, and it can be combined with splenic pulp pressure (i.e. portal vein pressure) measurements. It is not an emergency procedure and should be performed only when shunt surgery is being considered. In children under the age of 12 years it should be performed under general anaesthesia, and facilities for immediate surgery must be available if complications such as haemorrhage occur.

Selective angiography. Following retrograde introduction of a catheter via the brachial or femoral arteries, selective angiography may provide useful information in children with tumours, portal hypertension and circulatory abnormalities.

Radioisotopic scanning

The development of photoscanning techniques following the administration of radioisotopes represents an important advance in the diagnosis of hepatic, pancreatic and gastrointestinal disease.

Liver

Scanning has proved most useful in the detection of space-occupying lesions such as abscesses, cysts and primary or secondary tumours. In addition the technique can provide information on hepatocellular and reticuloendothelial function. The isotope most commonly used is ^{99}technetium sulphur colloid, which has a half life of six hours. Following an intravenous injection the isotope is taken up by normally functioning hepatocytes and Kupffer cells. Cells which are diseased or compressed by space-occupying lesions have an impaired capacity to take up the isotope and appear as 'cold' areas on the photoscan. A large abscess or tumour is easily visualised as a distinct cold area, whereas more diffuse disease presents a patchy pattern. Liver scanning is a complimentary diagnostic procedure and does not provide information for a definitive diagnosis (Rosenfield and Treves, 1974).

Pancreas

Pancreatic lesions often present diagnostic difficulties, and conventional techniques are frequently unhelpful. The pancreas can be well visualised by scanning using ^{75}Se-selenomethionine which is adequately concentrated by the gland within an hour of intravenous administration, and this technique is a useful diagnostic tool in selected patients (McCarthy, 1970). Interpretation, however, is complicated by the fact that the isotope is also taken up by the liver, but it is possible to eliminate this difficulty by applying the radiosubtract principle (Agnew, Youngs and Bouchier, 1973). Accurate interpretation of the results requires considerable experience, and it is critical to utilise the results of other clinical and laboratory investigations prior to arriving at a conclusion. Placed in its proper context pancreatic scanning is a useful adjunct in the diagnosis of conditions such as tumours, cysts and pancreatitis.

Gastrointestinal tract

Localisation of the site of occult or overt blood loss from the gastrointestinal tract can present an extremely difficult problem which may not be resolved even at laparotomy. Meckel's diverticulum is the most common congenital anomaly of the intestinal tract, and bleeding from ulcerated ileal mucosa adjacent to contained ectopic gastric mucosa is the commonest complication in children under the age of 2 years. Gastric mucosa takes up and secretes ^{99}technetium sodium pertechnate and scanning the abdomen following the administration of this isotope can be helpful in the diagnosis of bleeding from ectopic gastric mucosa (Leonidas and Germann, 1974).

Biopsy

Peroral small intestinal biopsy

The development of this technique has undoubtedly been an important advance in the rational diagnosis and management of a variety of disorders affecting the small intestine (Rubin and Dobbins, 1965; Trier, 1971). It can provide information on both the morphology and the function of the small gut. For example, characteristic morphological abnormalities are found in children with conditions such as coeliac disease, intestinal lymphangiectasia and abetalipoproteinaemia; assay of mucosal disaccharidase activities, coupled with morphological assessment, is important in differentiating primary from secondary sugar intolerance.

A variety of instruments are available but in our experience the Crosby and Watson capsules (Crosby and Kugler, 1957; Read *et al.*, 1962) are the ones of choice. Both capsules have a similar working mechanism, a spring-loaded knife block which fires by suction to cut off the mucosal biopsy specimen. Both are simple and straightforward to operate following the manufacturers' instructions, but their successful use is related to the experience of the operator. It is only by frequent practice that a reliable technique can be developed and maintained. Coupled with an experienced operator, a pathology department with the staff and facilities capable of utilising the biopsy material correctly is an essential prerequisite for the provision of a good clinical service. For example, the misinterpretation of poorly prepared sections is still responsible for incorrect diagnoses of coeliac disease. For these reasons biopsies are best performed in experienced centres. In addition to the conventional single port hole capsules, the Crosby capsule may be obtained with two ports enabling two biopsy samples to be obtained simultaneously in the same patient (Kilby, 1976). Instruments have also been developed to obtain multiple biopsy specimens from young infants (Carey, 1964; Ament and Rubin, 1973).

Preparation and technique. Platelet count, prothrombin and partial thromboplastin times, and clotting and bleeding times should precede biopsy. The prothrombin time is frequently prolonged in malabsorptive states and can be corrected within a few hours by intramuscular vitamin K (5 mg). A period of fasting, allowing only fluids, is necessary since solid food particles can obstruct the capsule and interfere with firing. This period varies from four hours in the infant to an overnight fast in the older child.

The necessity for sedation depends on the age of the patient, and how well-informed the child is of what the procedure entails. Sedation should be avoided whenever necessary since it tends to delay the passage of the capsule and is often unnecessary in young infants or children over the age of 5 years. In infants the biopsy tubing can be passed through a dummy allowing the baby to suck the dummy during the procedure; if sedation is necessary oral promazine hydrochloride (2 mg/kg) or diazepam (0·5–1·0 mg/kg) is usually satisfactory.

The passage of the capsule requires a quiet unflustered approach with frequent reassurance to the child. The patient should be seated at the edge of a chair or bed with an assistant steadying the forehead with one hand and holding both the child's hands with the other; infants and very young children can most conveniently be nursed in this position. The capsule is placed on the back of the tongue and then into the upper oesophagus with the first swallowing movement. The capsule tubing can be protected from teeth by a short length of firm outer tubing. Oesophageal passage of the capsule is encouraged by gently pushing on the tubing, and when it is judged to be in the distal oesophagus the patient lies on his right side and the capsule is slowly advanced. By placing the patient in this position before the capsule enters the stomach, the capsule almost invariably drops towards and reaches the pylorus. The position of the instrument is checked by fluoroscopic screening, and its passage through the pylorus can be observed as a sudden downward turn into the first part of the duodenum. Then, with the patient on his back, the capsule is seen to travel round the duodenal curve to the duodenojejunal flexure. Throughout these manoeuvres the minimum of excess tubing should be advanced into the stomach so as to prevent looping of the tubing. Delay in the capsule leaving the stomach may be reduced by metoclopramide (0·3 mg/kg to a maximum of 10 mg) which can be given carefully through the biopsy tube and flushed with saline. With the capsule in position just beyond the flexure it is flushed with a few millilitres of water and then with air in order to remove mucus or debris. It is then fired by suction using a 20 ml syringe; the movement of the knife block can usually be seen on fluoroscopy and confirms that the capsule has fired. The capsule is immediately withdrawn by steady traction; there may be a feeling of resistance initially, and then at the pylorus and cardia. The initial swallowing of the capsule and its subsequent withdrawal present the most distressful events of the whole procedure to the patient. If soft PVC tubing is used it may be necessary to advance the capsule to the pylorus with the aid of an introducer within the lumen of the tubing, but in our experience this is usually unnecessary. There are many advantages in performing the whole procedure from beginning to end in the screening room. After completion of the investigation the patient's pulse rate and blood pressure are recorded at frequent intervals for four to six hours, but no dietary restrictions are imposed.

Handling of the biopsy specimen. The laboratory requirements for each individual specimen should be determined beforehand and all the necessary equipment assembled. The tools for dismantling the capsule, a dissecting microscope and materials for fixing the specimen must be set out; dry ice should be available for snap-freezing a piece of the specimen if mucosal enzymes are to be assayed. Depending on the size of the port hole of the capsule the wet weight of the specimen varies from 10 to 30 mg; it should be promptly and carefully removed from the capsule, orientated mucosal side upwards in normal saline and examined under the dissecting microscope. Occasionally the dissecting microscopic appearances may be misleading and the parents should not be given a definitive diagnosis until stained sections of the biopsy have been carefully examined under the light microscope. A number of quantitative techniques have been developed and applied to biopsy sections in recent years; in clinical practice the most useful of these is that of Dunhill and Whitehead (1972) which determines the surface: volume ratio of the mucosa.

Complications. In experienced centres serious complications arising from an intestinal biopsy are now extremely rare. We have not encountered any serious complications using the Crosby capsule for the past 10 years, during which time several hundred biopsies have been performed.

Perforation and/or bleeding are most likely to occur in small marasmic infants weighing less than 4 kg, and biopsy should be avoided if at all possible in such patients. If coeliac disease is suspected in such patients it is probably wiser to institute a gluten-free diet without biopsy evidence and confirm the diagnosis at a later date by means of a formal gluten challenge. Occasionally the capsule can become firmly attached to the mucosa and cannot be withdrawn due to incomplete severing of the mucosa. Management is either to cut the tubing and await recovery of the capsule in the stools, or to leave the tubing loosely taped to the cheek allowing the child to eat, drink and move around normally. Attempts to dislodge the capsule by gentle traction should be made every six to eight hours; epigastric discomfort indicates that the capsule is still attached. The capsule usually becomes detached within 24 to 48 hours. Premature firing or failure to fire is almost invariably related to poor maintenance of the capsule.

Liver biopsy

This investigation should always be carried out in an experienced centre which has all the available facilities. The procedure can provide extremely valuable diagnostic information on the basis of applying a variety of laboratory techniques to the biopsy sample, e.g. light and electron microscopy, enzyme assays,

Table 3.4 Indications for liver biopsy

Hepatomegaly of unknown cause
Glycogen and lipid storage diseases
Prolonged jaundice particularly neonatal jaundice
Evaluation of chronic liver diseases such as chronic active hepatitis and Wilson's disease
Suspected liver disease without jaundice
Toxic hepatitis
Portal hypertension

histochemistry, determination of chemical contents, immunofluorescence, tissue culture and bacterial and viral culture. The clinical indications for liver biopsy in children are listed in Table 3.4.

Contraindications. Liver biopsy is contraindicated in the presence of (1) clotting defects (prothrombin index less than 60 per cent of control value; platelet count less than 50 000; prolonged bleeding time), (2) hydatid disease, because of the risk of dissemination and anaphylactoid shock, (3) vascular tumours of the liver, (4) infections of the pleura, lungs or peritoneum, and (5) suspected hepatic vein thrombosis. Moderate to severe ascites, a small impalpable liver and bile stasis (serum bilirubin greater than 425 μmol/l, i.e. 25 mg/100 ml) are relative contra-indications depending on the experience of the operator and the urgency of diagnosis.

Biopsy instruments. The two biopsy needles which are most suitable for use in children are the Menghini and Vim-Silverman needles, the former being almost invariably the instrument of choice (Menghini, 1970).

The major concern in children is the increased risk of liver trauma with bleeding or biliary peritonitis resulting from movement during the biopsy. The extremely short intrahepatic phase using the Menghini needle minimises this risk; its main disadvantage is the high failure rate in the presence of fibrosis. The needles are made with a variety of diameters (e.g. 1, 1·2, 1·4, 1·6, 1·9 and 2 mm), and generally speaking the larger the needle the greater the risk of bleeding. In children the 1·2 or 1·4 mm needles are most frequently used, and the 1 mm needle is confined to high-risk patients. The needle has a specially bevelled tip which allows for the tissue to be removed by aspiration alone, rotation within the liver being unnecessary.

The chief advantage of the Vim-Silverman needle is the higher yield of tissue in patients with cirrhosis. The intrahepatic phase is much longer (5–15 seconds) than with the Menghini needle (1 second), and consequently the risk of laceration is greater; moreover, the needle diameter is greater for an equivalent sized specimen. The apparatus consists of a cannula with an inner split cannula, the two sides of which tend to spring apart. The lumen is usually occluded with a trocar during insertion through the chest wall and, after advancing to the liver and removing the trocar, the longer inner split cannula is advanced into the liver. The outer cannula is then advanced to the lip of the split cannula, the whole instrument rotated through 360 degrees and then withdrawn; because of the necessary rotation the specimen is often distorted. This instrument should probably only be used in the investigation of cirrhosis when the Menghini technique may be unsuccessful.

Preparation and technique. The success and safety of liver biopsy depends on meticulous attention to detail. Since the Menghini needle is almost invariably used in children, details concerning the preparation of the patient and the biopsy technique will be described for this instrument.

The patient is admitted to hospital, a full blood count and clotting studies are performed, and blood is cross-matched and available; the child should fast for at least four hours prior to the biopsy. Young children should be premedicated with sleep-inducing drugs (e.g. pentobarbitone 4 mg/kg) or receive general anaesthesia. In older children a detailed explanation of the procedure together with pentobarbitone (2–3 mg/kg) is usually sufficient. Full surgical aseptic techniques should be employed throughout the procedure. The upper border of liver dullness is percussed in the midaxillary line and the site of needle penetration is marked one intercostal space below. Two to 3 ml of local anaesthesia (e.g. 1 per cent xylocaine) is injected to infiltrate the intercostal space down to the level of the pleura, and a 2 to 3 mm incision is made in the skin. Whilst an assistant presses firmly on the patient's chest the needle is inserted through the skin and continuous aspiration is applied to the attached syringe (10 ml Luer lock syringe containing 2–3 ml of saline); the needle is rapidly inserted into the liver and withdrawn in one movement with no rotation or lateral movement. The placement of the index finger of the left hand on the needle should limit the depth of penetration, and the whole manoeuvre should take no longer than one second. The core of liver tissue is gently flushed from the needle into a sterile container, and a satisfactory specimen should be longer than 1 cm. It is reasonable to repeat the biopsy if tissue is not obtained at the first attempt.

Following the biopsy the child should lie on his right side and remain in bed for 24 hours. The pulse rate is recorded at 15-minute intervals for the first hour and at hourly intervals for the ensuing four to six hours, and a full blood count should be performed 24 hours after the biopsy.

Complications. The incidence of complications is very variable and depends mainly on the general condition of the patient, the experience of the operator and the type and size of biopsy needle. The mortality rate varies from 0·02 to 0·1 per cent in experienced hands.

The major complications are (1) haemorrhage requiring transfusion and occasionally surgery, (2) biliary peritonitis, (3) pneumothorax, and (4) puncture of other viscera such as the gall bladder or kidney. Failure to obtain a biopsy specimen may be related to cirrhosis, a blunt needle or failure to maintain aspiration of the syringe during the passage of the needle through the chest cage into the liver. Local pain is not uncommon following biopsy and may require analgesia.

Rectal biopsy

As with other biopsy procedures examination of the rectal mucosa and submucosa can provide useful diagnostic information and, in experienced hands, there are no contraindications. Suspicion of the diagnosis of the following conditions is an indication for rectal biopsy: (1) Hirschsprung's disease, (2) ulcerative colitis and Crohn's disease, not only for diagnosis but also in reassessing the activity of the disease process and in the detection of pre-cancerous changes in the older child with long-standing disease, and (3) neural lipidoses.

The procedure may sometimes be worth considering in a wide variety of other conditions such as uraemic colitis, collagen diseases, pseudoxanthoma elasticum, Whipple's disease and histiocytosis X (Martin, Landing and Nakai, 1963).

Preparation and technique. The young child should be sedated with pento-barbitone (4 mg/kg) and the older child with a smaller dose (2–3 mg/kg); occasionally general anaesthesia may be necessary in young or unco-operative children.

Specimens can be obtained under direct vision through a proctoscope with an angled cutting forceps and are usually taken from the posterior wall of the rectum just below the peritoneal reflection. In the very rare event of perforation of the rectum, specimens obtained from this site will not lead to peritonitis. Bleeding can usually be rapidly controlled with direct pressure.

A suction biopsy can be obtained without the aid of a proctoscope or sigmoidoscope and, if carefully performed, causes no discomfort to the child. The principle by which the available instruments operate is identical to that for peroral small gut biopsy instruments. Multiple biopsy specimens can be obtained from varying intervals from the anus and may be helpful in defining the length of the aganglionic segment in Hirschsprung's disease. Suction biopsy has the disadvantage of sometimes obtaining superficial specimens which contain little or no submucosa and therefore preclude any comments on the presence or absence of ganglion cells. The recent development of histochemical staining of cholinesterase activity in mucosa, however, allows for a presumptive diagnosis of Hirschsprung's disease on such mucosal specimens in which ganglion cells are absent (Meier-Ruge, 1974). This technique should only be used in experienced centres since interpretation may be difficult. The histological appearances of the rectum in Crohn's disease and ulcerative colitis are described in Chapter 6.

Endoscopy

The aims of endoscopy are to visualise diseased areas of the gastrointestinal tract, to obtain biopsy samples and to perform the procedures with the minimal discomfort to the patient. Endoscopy of the lower and upper parts of the alimentary tract is established as an important diagnostic technique. The recent development of fibreoptic instruments represents a major advance in the field of endoscopy since it allows for a considerably more extensive examination of the alimentary tract than was previously possible. In addition, the technique may establish a diagnosis which was not apparent with conventional barium studies.

Proximal endoscopy

This enables the mucosa of the oesophagus, stomach and proximal duodenum to be visualised, as well as biopsy samples to be obtained from apparently diseased areas. In the younger unco-operative child general anaesthesia is advisable to avoid the possible complication of perforation (Gleason *et al.*, 1974). In the older child premedicatory drugs, as used for adults, are usually adequate. The indications for proximal endoscopy have not yet been clearly defined in children but include haematemesis, foreign bodies, suspected tumours, gastro-oesophageal reflux with or without hiatus hernia and suspected peptic ulcers.

Distal endoscopy

Sigmoidoscopy and proctoscopy. The conventional rigid sigmoidoscope allows for the examination of the rectum and sigmoid colon up to 12 cm in the infant and up to 20 to 25 cm in the older child. General anaesthesia is often necessary in the unco-operative patient, but with a sympathetic and informed approach the procedure can be performed under appropriate sedation. It should always be preceded by digital examination since this may provide valuable information with regard to sphincter tone, the presence of anal fissures, polyps or blood on the examining finger. The procedure is performed with the patient in the left lateral position. A well-lubricated warm sigmoidoscope with the obturator in place is gently pressed against the anus and passed into the rectum in a sacral direction. The obturator is removed and the instrument advanced under direct vision to the sigmoid; insufflation of air may aid advancement of the instrument but may be discomforting to the patient. The sigmoidoscope is then slowly withdrawn, the bowel mucosa carefully examined and appropriate mucosal biopsies obtained. Rare complications include perforation, bleeding and abdominal pain. Indications include occult or overt bleeding, chronic inflammatory bowel disease, persistent diarrhoea and suspected polyps or foreign bodies.

As with sigmoidoscopy digital examination should precede proctoscopy. Proctoscopy is performed at the bedside under sedation if necessary. Occasionally the procedure provides information which makes sigmoidoscopy unnecessary.

Colonoscopy. With the advent of fibreoptic paediatric colonoscopes, examination of the entire colon is now feasible in children. Experience with colonoscopy in children is, however, limited and the indications for this procedure have not been clearly defined. General anaesthesia is necessary in the young child whereas older patients may tolerate the procedure under heavy sedation and analgesia.

FUNCTIONAL STUDIES

Before embarking on investigatory techniques designed to assess specific aspects of gastrointestinal function, a careful clinical history and examination are essential in deciding which tests should be performed. As with all other investigations the critical and well-informed physician can minimise the number of tests which are necessary to arrive at a diagnosis, thereby reducing patient discomfort and financial costs. For example, sequential documentation of height and weight and inspection of stools can provide important information with regard to the presence of underlying organic disease.

Gastric acid secretion

The gastric parietal cells are functional and secrete acid within a few hours of birth (Avery, Randolph and Weaver, 1966a). In children maximal stimulation of gastric acid secretion by histamine or pentagastrin results in the secretion of juice of comparable hydrochloric acid concentration to that in adults, but the volume and total acid output are only about a third of adult values in the first decade and less than a tenth of adult values during the first year of life (Agunod *et al.*, 1969).

The measurement of basal gastric acid and maximally stimulated acid outputs is a particularly useful investigation in children with intractable peptic ulcers and/or those suspected of having the Zollinger-Ellison syndrome; it may also be a useful test in patients following small gut resections.

Procedure

Following an overnight fast a nasogastric tube is passed to the most dependent part of the stomach under fluoroscopic control. The stomach contents are aspirated and discarded, and four 15-minute aspirate collections are performed to establish basal secretory volume, pH and titratable acidity (i.e. basal acid output = mEq/hour or mEq/kg/hour). Maximal acid output is stimulated by intravenous histamine (1·0 to 1·5 mg/kg) or pentagastrin (6 mg/kg), gastric contents being collected at 15-minute intervals for two hours. Aliquots of each 15-minute collection pre- and poststimulation are titrated to pH 7 with 0·2N sodium hydroxide. Maximal acid output refers to the rate of acid secretion during the first hour after histamine or pentagastrin stimulation. Peak acid output refers to the two highest consecutive 15-minute acid secretory periods multiplied by two. Maximal and peak acid outputs are expressed as mEq of acid secreted per hour, or per kg per hour.

Results

In children with duodenal ulcers basal acid output is normal, whereas maximal and peak acid outputs are increased in a proportion of patients (Christie and Ament, 1976). In the Zollinger-Ellison syndrome basal acid output is increased, and there may be only a small and insignificant rise to peak output (Schwartz *et al.*, 1974). Hypersecretion of gastric acid and hypergastrinaemia may also occur following resections of the small bowel (Avery, Randolph and Weaver, 1966b; Strauss, Gerson and Yalow, 1974). Reduced acid output occurs in conditions such as pernicious anaemia, the Verner-Morrison syndrome (Verner and Morrison, 1958) and Menetrier's disease (Frank and Kern, 1967).

Small intestinal function

Carbohydrate absorption

Tests of carbohydrate absorption are indicated in children with chronic diarrhoea and in those who fail to thrive or have persistent diarrhoea following an episode of acute gastroenteritis.

Examination of faeces. The characteristic stools of patients with carbohydrate malabsorption are frothy, liquid and acid, and the perianal region is often excoriated; the pH of the stool is less than 5·5 but this is an unreliable test and its routine use should be discouraged. The most useful screening procedure is to test for reducing substances. Five drops of a freshly collected aliquot of liquid stool are diluted with 10 drops of water, and a Clinitest tablet added (Kerry and Anderson, 1964). The presence of more than half per cent reducing substances is taken as an indication of carbohydrate malabsorption. All carbohydrates consumed by children are reducing substances with the exception of sucrose. If sucrose intolerance is suspected an aliquot of stool should be boiled for a few minutes in the presence of hydrochloric acid (to hydrolyse the disaccharide to glucose and fructose) before testing for reducing substances. The application of thin layer chromatographic techniques enables the individual sugars to be identified and may be helpful in reaching a specific diagnosis (Soeparto, Stobo and Walker-Smith, 1972). Thus the presence of lactose and galactose in the absence of sucrose and fructose in a child consuming a diet which contains both disaccharides strongly suggests lactase deficiency.

Oral load tests. Oral loads of mono- or disaccharides can be performed in conjunction with the above tests. Following a fast, the duration of which will depend on the age and clinical state of the patient, the sugar under investigation is given in a dose of 1 to 2 g per kg body weight (maximum of 50 g) as a 10 per cent solution together with a carmine marker. Body weight, stool frequency and volume are carefully recorded prior to and throughout the test, and the stools containing the marker are tested for reducing substances and individual sugars. Urine may be simultaneously collected and tested for sugars. As an adjunct serial determination of blood glucose can be performed, as for a glucose tolerance test. Normally blood glucose concentrations increase by at least 1·7 mmol/l (30 mg/100 ml) during the test, whereas this increment is less than 1·1 mmol/l (20 mg/100 ml) in patients with sugar intolerance. A flat glucose tolerance curve may also be secondary to delayed gastric emptying.

The presence of sugars in the stool and/or urine may be a normal finding in newborns, particularly if breast fed. Lactulose (a non-reducing disaccharide composed of fructose and galactose) is formed from lactose during the commercial preparation and storage of milk; it cannot be hydrolysed by the human small gut and may be detected in the urine of normal infants.

Mucosal enzymes. The assay of disaccharidases in small intestinal mucosa obtained by peroral biopsy is usually an unnecessary procedure in the diagnosis and clinical management of patients with sugar intolerance. A diagnosis of clinical sugar intolerance is established by the other tests described above and appropriate dietetic treatment can be instituted; in these circumstances depression of mucosal disaccharidases can be predicted. The only firm indication for assaying mucosal disaccharidases is when a primary genetically determined defect in sugar absorption is suspected. A careful clinical history will almost invariably differentiate patients with primary sugar intolerance from those with the much commoner secondary form of intolerance.

The handling of biopsy material, the disaccharidase assays and the interpretation of results have been described in detail (Dahlqvist, 1970).

Breath tests. Unabsorbed carbohydrates are metabolised by colonic bacteria with the generation of hydrogen which is absorbed and then excreted by the lungs; there is a fairly good correlation between the amount of hydrogen produced and the amount excreted in breath. On this basis the quantification of hydrogen in breath following an oral load of sugar has been developed as a non-invasive test of sugar malabsorption in adults (Bond and Levitt, 1972). False negative results, however, are not uncommon, and its application to young infants poses certain technical problems.

D-xylose absorption. D-xylose is a relatively non-metabolisable pentose which is absorbed in the proximal small gut and excreted in the urine. The determination of five- or 24-hour urinary outputs, or one-hour blood levels following an oral load (0·4 g/kg up to a maximum dose of 7·5 g as a 3 per cent solution, or a standard 5 g dose), has been widely used as a screening test for suspected malabsorption, particularly coeliac disease. The difficulties of obtaining accurately timed collections of urine in childhood make the urinary xylose test extremely difficult to interpret and, on the basis of a carefully designed study, Lamabadusuriya, Packer and Harries (1975) recommended that it should be abandoned as an investigation in children. The finding of a one-hour blood xylose of less than 1·33 mmol/l (20 mg/100 ml) has been strongly recommended as a screening test for coeliac disease (Rolles *et al.*, 1973), but it should be emphasised that a normal one-hour level does not exclude this important diagnosis (Lamabadusuriya *et al.*, 1975) and is no substitute for the definitive investigation, an intestinal biopsy.

Fat absorption

The most reliable clinical test for assessing fat absorption is the quantification of faecal fat over a period of at least 72 hours. An adequate dietary intake of fat before and during stool collections is essential; in infants this should be at least 5 g per kg per day, in young children about 40 to 50 g and in older children 70 to 80 g per day. A red or blue carmine marker is given and collections begun from the appearance of the first coloured stool. Seventy-two hours (or five days) after administering the first marker the alternative coloured marker is given, and the collection of stools is completed by including the last stool before the appearance of the second marker. Infant stools may be collected using a polythene lining in the napkin, toddler stools using a potty or potty chair, and older children by careful co-operation with the child; if the stools are fluid a metabolic frame may be necessary. The stools are pooled and homogenised, and their fatty acid content analysed by the method of Van de Kamer (1949).

The results can be expressed either as absolute values of stool fat per day with an upper limit of normal of 5 g, or as a coefficient of absorption (i.e. per cent of fat absorbed). Fat excretion varies with age and the latter method is preferable in children. Normal values increase with age being greater than 60 per cent in premature infants, greater than 80 per cent in full-term ones, greater than 85 per cent up to six months, and greater than 90 per cent thereafter.

Lubrication of rectal thermometers or examining fingers, or certain creams applied to the perianal region, may result in spuriously high faecal fat values. If the diet contains medium chain triglycerides the method for measuring faecal fat must be modified (Jeejeebhoy, Ahmad and Kozak, 1970).

The collection of stools and their subsequent analysis is unpleasant for the ward and laboratory staff, and the test should be reserved for those instances where there is a real indication for its use. We believe it to be overused in paediatric practice, such as in patients suspected of having coeliac disease when an early peroral jejunal biopsy can avoid the necessity for any further investigations.

Screening tests. A variety of screening tests have been advocated for the assessment of fat absorption. These include measurement of serum turbidity following an oral load of fat, vitamin A absorption tests, ^{131}I-labelled triolein, oleic acid excretion and the measurement of fasting serum levels of carotene and cholesterol. All of these, however, are unreliable. Although no more reliable, microscopy of stool is a simple and rapid procedure for detecting excess fat globules; to the experienced eye this is probably the screening test of choice.

Protein absorption and loss

Total faecal nitrogen can be measured by the Kjeldahl method and can be combined with fat determinations. As for fat, the coefficient of absorption for nitrogen provides information on net absorption and does not discriminate between nitrogen loss into the lumen and malabsorption. Generally speaking faecal nitrogen is a much less useful investigation in clinical practice compared with faecal fat. Moreover, since faecal nitrogen and fat correlate well with each other, nitrogen losses can be assumed to be excessive in the presence of steatorrhoea.

Excessive loss of serum proteins into the gastrointestinal tract may occur in a wide variety of diseases affecting the stomach, small and large intestine (see Ch. 13). The most widely used test to assess protein loss is the determination of radioactive chromium (^{51}Cr) in stools following the intravenous administration of ^{51}Cr-tagged albumin (Waldmann, 1961). Twenty-five microcuries of ^{51}Cr-tagged albumin (or ^{51}CrCl) are given intravenously, and all stools are collected for a period of four days; particular care must be taken to ensure that faeces are not contaminated by urine since this will result in spuriously high values of protein loss. The stools are pooled, homogenised and an aliquot counted for radioactivity. Normally less than 1 per cent of the dose is excreted in the stools, more than 4 per cent being indicative of unequivocal protein loss.

Albumin labelled with ^{131}I, ^{14}C or ^{75}Se has been used to study albumin synthesis and turnover in association with the ^{51}Cr test (Walker, Lowman and Hong, 1973).

Fluid and electrolyte absorption

Abnormalities of fluid and electrolyte absorption in the small and/or large bowel result in diarrhoea in a variety of disease states, but the available investigatory techniques are complex and, at present, unsuitable for routine clinical use.

Simple measurement of stool volume, however, can provide important information in assessing the course and response to therapy of children with severe and protracted diarrhoeal states; similarly, determination of stool electrolytes may be useful in such patients. There is only one condition where measurement of stool electrolytes is diagnostic and that is congenital chloridorrhoea (see Ch. 11). The finding of a stool concentration of chloride which exceeds the sum of the concentrations of sodium and potassium is pathognomonic of this rare disorder.

Absorption of haematinics

Tests which assess the capacity of the small intestine to absorb haematinic substances such as iron, folic acid and vitamin B_{12} can provide important information with regard to the presence of disease as well as its site in the small gut. Defective iron and folate absorption occurs in proximal small gut diseases, whereas vitamin B_{12} malabsorption is associated with lesions of the terminal ileum; B_{12} malabsorption may also occur in proximal lesions which result in bacterial overgrowth, as well as in conditions in which gastric intrinsic factor secretion is impaired.

Malabsorption of iron is presumed in the presence of an iron deficiency anaemia, a low serum iron level with a normal or raised iron binding capacity, in the absence of evidence of blood loss. Similarly, folic acid malabsorption is presumed when the serum or red cell folate concentration is reduced in the absence of malignancy, or anticonvulsant or folic acid antagonist therapy.

Schilling test. After a two-hour fast 0·5 microcuries of radioactive vitamin B_{12} (^{57}Co B_{12}) is given orally. The fast is continued for a further two hours when 1 mg of non-radioactive B_{12} is administered intramuscularly to ensure saturation of body stores in order that an appreciable amount of the radioactive vitamin will be excreted in the urine following absorption. Normally more than 10 per cent of the labelled B_{12} will be excreted in the urine during the 24 hours following ingestion. If the value is less than 10 per cent the test should be repeated giving gastric intrinsic factor together with the labelled vitamin. This discriminates between B_{12} malabsorption secondary to intrinsic factor deficiency (e.g. pernicious anaemia) and malabsorption due to ileal disease. Bacterial overgrowth of the small gut may be associated with an abnormal Schilling test which is not corrected by the addition of intrinsic factor.

Bile salts and bacteria

The determination of total and individual bile salt concentrations, and the analysis of aerobic and anaerobic bacteria in the proximal small intestine, are considered together with tests of pancreatic function.

Pancreatic function

The assessment of pancreatic function involves the quantification of pancreatic enzymes, volume and bicarbonate in the proximal small intestine following stimulation of the gland. Enzyme activities reflect the function of the acinar cells, and volume and bicarbonate outputs are indicators of tubular function. The pancreas can be stimulated by the intravenous administration of cholecystokinin-pancreozymin and secretin, or by the administration of a test meal. The former method provides information on the secretory capacity of the pancreas to a systemic stimulus, whereas the latter technique gives more physiological information on the response of the gland to intraluminal substrates. The determination of faecal proteolytic enzymes has been advocated as a test of pancreatic function, but in our opinion this is a sufficiently unreliable test as to be discouraged in clinical practice.

Intravenous cholecystokinin-pancreozymin (CCK-PZ) and secretin

Following an overnight fast, or for young infants a four-hour fast, the patient is sedated one hour before the tube is passed into the fourth part of the duodenum under fluoroscopic control. Contamination by gastric secretions can be minimised by means of continuous suction with a second tube positioned in the pyloric antrum, or by a proximal occlusive balloon in the first part of the duodenum. Duodenal secretions are collected on ice by siphonage. Prior to the administration of CCK-PZ and secretin, the patients should be tested against any hypersensitivity to the hormones. CCK-PZ (2 iu/kg) is administered by slow intravenous infusion and juice collected for 20 minutes; secretin (2 iu/kg) is then given and juice collected for a further 30 minutes. The volume, bicarbonate concentration and activities of the pancreatic enzymes are determined and the expected normal values are shown in Table 3.5 (from Hadorn, 1972). The activity of pancreatic amylase does not reach adult levels until the age of 1 year or later, and thus only data from children over the age of 1 year are included in the table.

Test meal

In our opinion the stimulation of gall bladder contraction and pancreatic secretion by means of a test meal provides more meaningful information on intraluminal digestion compared with the intravenous administration of CCK-PZ and secretin.

McCollum, Muller and Harries (1977) have developed a test meal which is a modification of the Lundh meal (Lundh, 1962) and contains carbohydrate as glucose (4 per cent), protein as comminuted chicken (4 per cent) and fat as corn oil (4 per cent). Its composition enables it to be administered to children with

Table 3.5 Total output of duodenal juice volume, bicarbonate and enzymes (per kg body weight and per 50 min) in control children[a] following intravenous stimulation with cholecystokinin-pancreozymin and secretin (from Hadorn, 1972)

	Volume (ml)	Bicarbonate (mEq)	Chymotrypsin (μg)	Trypsin (μg)	Amylase[b] (iu)	Lipase
Mean	3·7	0·17	797	841	437	1381
Range	1·8–6·3	0·08–0·36	262–1862	300–2170	139–1000	305–3525

[a]Children with digestive complaints but no maldigestion or malabsorption, aged 3 months to 16 years (n = 36–50).
[b]Values refer only to children over the age of 1 year.

Table 3.6 Activities of pancreatic enzymes, and total and individual bile salt concentrations in control children[a] following a test meal

	Trypsin (μEq/min/ml)	Amylase (iu/ml)	Lipase (μEq/min/ml)	Esterase (μmol/min/ml)
Mean	46·4	34	860	1·6
Range	29·4–83·3	8·2–125	270–1920	0·57–3·30

	Total bile salt concentrations (mmol/l)	Ratio of glycine: taurine conjugated bile salts	Dihydroxy bile salts (% of total)
Mean	7·3	2·8:1	60
Range	3–16	1·3:1–4·0:1	53–70

[a]Children with suspected malabsorption who were proven to be normal following intensive investigation, aged 16 months to 16 years (n = 10)

suspected cows' milk protein or gluten intolerance, and to those with disaccharide intolerance, without precipitating gastrointestinal symptoms. Following an overnight fast, or for young infants a four-hour fast, the patient is sedated with intramuscular chlorpromazine (1 mg/kg) one hour before the procedure; a nasogastric tube is passed for administering the test meal (30 ml/kg to a maximum of 240 ml). The collecting tube, a single lumen PVC tube weighted at its end with a small mercury bag, is passed to the fourth part of the duodenum under fluoroscopic control. Postprandial juice is collected for two hours, and bicarbonate and pancreatic enzymes are quantified in aliquots from the collection. Normal values for the activities of pancreatic enzymes and total and individual bile salt concentrations are shown in Table 3.6. In patients in whom malabsorption is suspected of being secondary to bacterial overgrowth of the small gut, samples are collected into appropriate transport media for culture of anaerobic and aerobic bacteria.

Liver function

A variety of tests are available for the assessment of liver function, some reflecting hepatic damage and others providing information regarding the metabolic capacity of the organ.

Serum enzymes

Alterations in the activities of serum enzymes may reflect separate processes. For example, increased activity of the transaminases reflect tissue damage, whereas increased alkaline phosphatase activity indicates defective biliary secretion. These changes may not be tissue-specific and can reflect disease in more than one organ; in these circumstances differentiation of the isoenzymes will indicate which organ is involved.

Alkaline phosphatase. At an alkaline pH this enzyme catalyses the hydrolysis of organic phosphate esters and is primarily located in the liver, bone and intestinal mucosa. These tissues synthesise distinct isoenzymes which can be separated by electrophoretic techniques; normally the vast majority of the circulating alkaline phosphatases arise from bone and liver (Warnes, 1972). Thus elevations of enzyme activity may reflect abnormalities in any one of these tissues and, in childhood, allowances must be made during periods of rapid growth when there is a marked increase in osteoblastic activity. However, elevations are most commonly seen in cholestatic liver disease whatever its cause, the increased activity resulting from regurgitation of the enzyme from the liver into the circulation. Increased production of alkaline phosphatase by certain tumours of the liver may also cause increased circulating levels.

Normal values:

Age	(iu)
Birth	35–100
1 month	71–247
1 to 3 years	71–212
3 to 10 years	71–177
10 to 16 years	99–275

Transaminases. The transaminases catalyse the transfer of an α-amino group of an amino acid to an α-ketoacid, and there are two types which are of importance in clinical practice: glutamic oxaloacetic transaminase (GOT) which is synthesised in the heart, liver, muscle and kidney, and glutamic pyruvic transaminase (GPT) which is found primarily in the liver. The activity of both enzymes is increased in liver damage whatever its cause. Transaminase determinations are particularly useful in the early diagnosis of viral hepatitis and in the detection of non-icteric cases. Determination of transaminases may be helpful in other diseases affecting the liver such as Reye's syndrome and infectious mononucleosis. The normal values for GOT and GPT range from 6 iu/l to 17 iu/l, and 2 iu/l to 12 iu/l, respectively.

Other enzymes. Lactic acid dehydrogenase and isocitric dehydrogenase activities may be elevated in a variety of diseases other than those affecting the liver and probably offer no advantage over the transaminases.

Serum 5-nucleotidase and leucine-aminopeptidase are raised in ductal obstruction, but their elevation does not always parallel that of alkaline phosphatase. These three enzymes may be increased in the face of only a slightly raised concentration of bilirubin. Unfortunately they do not clearly differentiate jaundice due to intrahepatic cholestasis from that due to extrahepatic obstruction.

Serum bilirubin

Bilirubin is the end-product of haem metabolism, haem being derived from haemoglobin, myoglobin and certain cytochromes; these metabolic events take place in the reticuloendothelial cells of the liver and spleen. Serum bilirubin is present in conjugated and unconjugated forms, and the Van den Bergh reaction measures the conjugated water-soluble component. Differentiation of conjugated and unconjugated bilirubin, together with inspection of stools and estimation of urine urobilinogen, are useful tests in defining the origin of jaundice (see Ch. 16). The normal values for total and conjugated bilirubin range from 2 to 14, and 0 to 4 μmol/l, respectively.

Urine urobilinogen

Conjugated bilirubin is converted to urobilinogen by the endogenous bacterial flora of the bowel. The absorbed urobilinogen is recirculated through the liver, and a small proportion enters the systemic circulation to be excreted in urine. Increased amounts are excreted when liver function is inadequate to clear the absorbed bile pigment into bile and in conditions where synthesis of bilirubin is increased, such as in haemolytic states. Urobilinogen disappears from the urine in obstructive jaundice.

Serum proteins

Separation of the different plasma protein fractions by electrophoresis can provide important information regarding the liver's capacity to synthesise proteins, particularly albumin; in addition abnormalities in the globulin fractions may provide specific information on the aetiology of liver disease. Many disease entities alter serum protein patterns, and some examples are shown in Table 3.7.

Disturbances of coagulation

Factors I, II, V, VII, IX, X, XI and XIII are synthesised in the liver, and the synthesis of factors II, VII, IX and X are dependent on vitamin K. One or all of these factors may be deficient in patients with liver disease. Fibrinogen (factor I) is also synthesised by extrahepatic reticuloendothelial tissue and so may remain normal. Coagulation may also be disturbed as a result of thrombocytopenia, such as may occur in hypersplenism secondary to portal hypertension. Disturbances of coagulation in liver disease can be screened by estimating the prothrombin time, partial thromboplastin time, platelet count and by direct examination of a blood film for abnormally shaped red blood cells.

Table 3.7 Serum protein patterns in different disease states

	Serum concentrations in grams per litre					
	Albumin	Globulins				
		Total	$\alpha 1$	$\alpha 2$	β	γ
Normal	36–52	22–33	1–4	4–12	4–9	4–15
Cystic fibrosis	↓	↑	N	↑	N	↑↑
Biliary cirrhosis	↓	↑	↑	↑	↑↑↑	↑
Viral hepatitis	N or ↓	N or ↑	↓	↓	↑	N or ↑
Cirrhosis	↓↓	↑	N or ↑	N	↑	↑↑
$Alpha_1$-antitrypsin deficiency	N or ↑	N or ↑	absent	N	N	N or ↑

N = normal; ↑ and ↓ = increased and decreased concentrations, respectively.

Plasma ammonia

Ammonia is a toxic and key end-product of protein metabolism and, following conversion to urea in the liver, is excreted predominantly in the urine as urea. In patients with severe hepatic dysfunction the metabolism of ammonia is defective, and the resultant high circulating levels of ammonia have been implicated in the pathogenesis of hepatic coma. The determination of plasma ammonia concentrations is helpful in patients with impending hepatic failure and/or coma and in those with suspected primary enzymatic defects of the urea cycle. Normal plasma ammonia levels are less than 30 μmol/l.

Bromsulphalein (BSP) test

This is a sensitive test of the ability of the liver cells to excrete the anionic phthalein dye, bromsulphalein.

A 5 per cent solution of BSP (5 mg/kg) is administered intravenously following an overnight fast, and a venous sample of blood is collected 45 minutes later from a site other than that where the dye was injected; the concentration of BSP is then determined. It is an extremely irritant dye and great care should be taken not to inject it subcutaneously. The test should not be performed in jaundiced patients or within a week of the administration of halogen containing compounds or barbiturates. The results are expressed as per cent of retention at 45 minutes: the normal values for neonates and older infants are less than 15 and 5 per cent, respectively.

Rose Bengal ^{131}I test

Rose Bengal is a red dye which is taken up by the liver and rapidly excreted in bile. The rate of hepatic uptake and/or excretion is impaired when liver cells are damaged or when biliary flow is impaired. It is a useful test in conjunction with others (e.g. liver biopsy) in differentiating extrahepatic biliary atresia from the neonatal hepatitis syndrome (Sharp *et al.*, 1967).

The per cent of the administered dose in the faeces is normally 70 to 97; in infants with extrahepatic biliary atresia or the neonatal hepatitis syndrome the values are 8 or less, and 5 to 20 respectively. It should be stressed, however, that overlap values occur and that this test by itself does not always differentiate the two conditions referred to above.

Alpha$_1$-antitrypsin

Alpha$_1$-antitrypsin is a low molecular weight glycoprotein of the α_1-globulin fraction of serum proteins and accounts for 90 per cent of the tryptic-inhibitory capacity of human serum. Deficiency of this glycoprotein has been associated with two conditions, emphysema and cirrhosis (Cottrall, Cook and Mowat, 1974); both conditions, however, occur together only rarely in the same patient.

Serum caeruloplasmin

Wilson's disease (hepatolenticular degeneration) is associated with a deficiency of caeruloplasmin, an α_2 copper binding globulin which possesses copper oxidase activity; this oxidase activity is utilised in quantifying serum caeruloplasmin. Normal values range from 23 to 43 μg per 100 ml, and in Wilson's disease the concentration is less than 20 μg per 100 ml.

Alpha-1-fetoprotein

Fetal α-1-globulin is synthesised by embryonic liver cells and reaches maximum concentrations by about the thirteenth week of gestation after which it declines. It remains detectable in the newborn but disappears by about the age of 2 months.

This protein can be found in the serum of patients with hepatoblastoma, and in about a third of those with a teratoblastoma (Zeltzer *et al.*, 1974).

Examination of urine

The reducing sugars, galactose and fructose, are present in excessive amounts in the urine of patients with galactosaemia and hereditary fructose intolerance, respectively, and paper chromatographic analysis of urine is an important investigation in patients suspected of either of these two diagnoses. The diagnosis is confirmed by specific enzyme assays. A generalised aminoaciduria occurs in Wilson's disease and galactosaemia. In tyrosinosis and fructosaemia, phenolic acids are excreted in excessive quantities.

References

Agnew, J. E., Youngs, G. R., & Bouchier, A. D. (1973) Conventional subtraction scanning of the pancreas: an assessment based on blind reporting. *British Journal of Radiology,* **46,** 83.

Agunod, M., Yamaguchi, N., Lopez, R., Lubey, A. L. & Glass, G. B. J. (1969) Correlative study of hydrochloric acid, pepsin and intrinsic factor secretion in new borns and infants. *American Journal of Digestive Diseases,* **14,** 400.

Ament, M. E. & Rubin, C. E. (1973) An infant multipurpose biopsy tube. *Gastroenterology,* **65,** 205.

Avery, G. B., Randolph, J. G. & Weaver, T. (1966a) Gastric acidity on the first day of life. *Pediatrics,* **37,** 1005.

Avery, G. B., Randolph, J. G. & Weaver, T. (1966b) Gastric response to specific disease in infants. *Pediatrics,* **38,** 874.

Bond, J. H. & Levitt, M. D. (1972) Use of pulmonary hydrogen (H_2) measurements to quantitate carbohydrate absorption. *Journal of Clinical Investigation,* **51,** 1219.

Carey, J. B. (1964) A simplified gastrointestinal biopsy capsule. *Gastroenterology,* **46,** 550.

Christie, D. L. & Ament, M. E. (1976) Gastric acid hypersecretion in children with duodenal ulcer. *Gastroenterology,* **71,** 242.

Cottrall, K., Cook, P. J. L. & Mowat, A. P. (1974) Neonatal hepatitis syndrome and alpha-1-antitrypsin deficiency: an epidemiological study in South East England. *Postgraduate Medical Journal,* **50,** 376.

Crosby, W. H. & Kugler, H. W. (1957) Intraluminal biopsy of the small intestine: the intestinal biopsy capsule. *American Journal of Digestive Diseases,* **2,** 236.

Dahlqvist, A. (1970) Assay of intestinal disaccharidases. *Enzymologia Biologica et Clinica,* **11,** 52.

Dunhill, M. S. & Whitehead, R. (1972) A method for the quantitation of small intestinal biopsy specimens. *Journal of Clinical Pathology,* **25,** 243.

Frank, B. F. & Kern, F. (1967) Menetrier's disease. *Gastroenterology,* **53,** 953.

Gleason, W. A. Jnr., Tedesco, F. J., Keating, J. P. & Goldstein, D. P. (1974) Fibreoptic gastrointestinal endoscopy in infants and children. *Journal of Pediatrics,* **85,** 810.

Hadorn, B. (1972) Diseases of the pancreas in childhood. *Clinics of Gastroenterology,* **1,** 125.

Harris, R. & Caffey, J. (1953) Cholecystography in infants. *Journal of the American Medical Association,* **153,** 1333.

Hodgson, J. R. (1970) The technical aspects of cholecystography. *Radiology Clinics of North America,* **8,** 85.

Jeejeebhoy, K. N., Ahmad, S. & Kozak, G. (1970) Determination of faecal fats containing both medium and long chain triglycerides and fatty acids. *Clinical Biochemistry,* **3,** 157.

Kerry, K. R. & Anderson, C. M. (1964) A ward test for sugar in faeces. *Lancet,* **1,** 981.

Kilby, A. (1976) Paediatric small intestinal biopsy capsule with two ports. *Gut,* **17,** 158.

Lamabadusuriya, S. P., Packer, S. & Harries, J. T. (1975) Limitations of xylose tolerance test as a screening procedure in childhood coeliac disease. *Archives of Disease in Childhood,* **50,** 34.

Leonidas, J. C. & Germann, D. R. (1974) Technetium 99m pertechnate imaging in diagnosis of Meckel's diverticulum. *Archives of Disease in Childhood,* **49,** 21.

Lundh, G. (1962) Pancreatic exocrine function in neoplastic and inflammatory disease: a simple and reliable new test. *Gastroenterology,* **42,** 275.

Martin, L. W., Landing, B. H. & Nakai, H. (1963) Rectal biopsy as an aid in the diagnosis of diseases of infants and children. *Journal of Pediatrics,* **62,** 197.

McCarthy, D. M. (1970) *Pancreatic Scanning.* A thesis on the clinical use of the amino acid Se^{75}-I-selenomethionine in scintigraphic visualisation of the human pancreas in health and disease. Dublin, University College, National University of Ireland.

McCollum, J. P. K., Muller, D. P. R. & Harries, J. T. (1977) A test meal for assessing the intraluminal phase of absorption in childhood. *Archives of Disease in Childhood,* in press.

Meier-Ruge, W. (1974) Hirschsprung's disease: its aetiology, pathogenesis and differential diagnosis. In *Current Topics in Pathology,* Vol. 59. Berlin: Springer-Verlag.

Melhem, R. E. & Rizk, G. K. (1970) Splenoportographic evaluation of portal hypertension in children. *Journal of Pediatric Surgery,* **5,** 522.

Menghini, G. (1970) One second biopsy of liver—problems of its clinical application. *New England Journal of Medicine,* **283,** 582.

Read, A. E., Gough, K. R., Bones, J. A. & McCarthy, C. G. (1962) An improvement to the Crosby peroral intestinal biopsy capsule. *Lancet,* **1,** 894.

Rolles, C. J., Kendall, M. J., Nutter, S. & Anderson, C. M. (1973) One-hour blood xylose screening test for coeliac disease in infants and young children. *Lancet,* **2,** 1043.

Rosenfield, N. & Treves, S. (1974) Liver-spleen scanning in pediatrics. *Pediatrics,* **53,** 692.

Rubin, C. E. & Dobbins, W. O. (1965) Peroral biopsy of the small intestine. *Gastroenterology,* **49,** 676.

Schwartz, D. L., White, J. J., Saulsbury, F. & Haller, J. R., Jr. (1974) Gastrin response to calcium infusion: an aid to the improved diagnosis of Zollinger-Ellison syndrome in children. *Pediatrics,* **54,** 599.

Sharp, H. L., Krivit, W. & Lowman, J. T., (1967) The diagnosis of complete extra hepatic obstruction by Rose Bengal ^{131}I. *Journal of Pediatrics,* **70,** 46.

Soeparto, P., Stobo, E. A. & Walker-Smith, J. A. (1972) Role of chemical examination of the stool in the diagnosis of sugar malabsorption in children. *Archives of Disease in Childhood,* **47,** 56.

Strauss, E., Gerson, C. D. & Yalow, R. S. (1974) Hypersecretion of gastrin associated with short bowel syndrome. *Gastroenterology,* **66,** 175.

Trier, J. S. (1971) Diagnostic value of peroral biopsy of the proximal small intestine. *The New England Journal of Medicine,* **285,** 1470.

Van de Kamer, J. H., Ten Bokkel Huinink & Weijers, H. A. (1949) A rapid method for the determination of fat in faeces. *Journal of Biological Chemistry,* **177,** 347.

Verner, J. V. & Morrison, A. B. (1958) Islet cell tumour and a syndrome of refractory watery diarrhoea and hypokalaemia. *American Journal of Medicine,* **25,** 374.

Waldmann, T. A. (1961) Gastrointestinal protein loss demonstrated by ^{51}Cr-labelled albumin. *Lancet,* **2,** 121.

Walker, W. A., Lowman, J. T. & Hong, R. A. (1973) Measuring albumin turnover rates in patients with hypoproteinaemia. *American Journal of Diseases of Children,* **125,** 51.

Warnes, T. W. (1972) Alkaline Phosphatase. *Gut,* **13,** 926.

Zeltzer, P. M., Neerhout, R. C., Fonkalsrud, E. W. & Steihm, E. R. (1974) Differentiation between neonatal hepatitis and biliary atresia by measuring alpha fetoprotein. *Lancet,* **1,** 373.

PART 2

4. Surgical emergencies in the first few weeks of life

J. A. S. Dickson

Oesophagus
Pylorus
Duodenum
Jejunum and ileum
Large intestine
Duplications and megaileocolon
Diaphragmatic hernia
Exomphalos
Necrotising enterocolitis
Other lesions

The number and variety of abnormalities requiring urgent correction during the first few weeks of life precludes any completely satisfactory classification. The congenital obstructive lesions of the alimentary tract will be considered in anatomical order. The acquired and traumatic conditions, a miscellaneous group of rare congenital anomalies, and defects of the parietes affecting the gut, will also be discussed. Those conditions which may present later as well as in the neonatal period will also be considered.

OESOPHAGUS

Atresia and tracheo-oesophageal fistula

In the United Kingdom the incidence of oesophageal atresia and tracheo-oesophageal atresia is of the order of one per 3000 live births. There is no general agreement on a numerical classification, and simple descriptive terms are preferred, as shown in Figure 4.1.

In 85 per cent of cases there is a proximal oesophageal atresia associated with a fistula between the distal oesophagus and the trachea. In about 8 per cent the

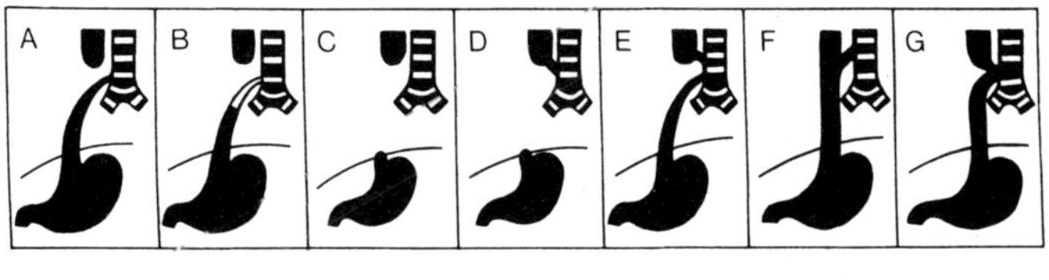

Fig. 4.1 The different varieties of oesophageal atresias and tracheo-oesophageal fistulae

Table 4.1 The incidence of other congenital anomalies associated with tracheo-oesophageal anomalies (from Holder *et al.*, 1964)

	Number of Patients
Total	1058
Congenital heart disease	201
Gastrointestinal	134
Genitourinary	109
Imperforate anus	99
Musculoskeletal	91
Central nervous system	63
Facial	53
Others	99

atresia is not associated with a fistula, and in this type there is a long gap between the proximal and distal oesophageal pouches. Fistula without atresia (H type) accounts for 5 per cent. The remaining 2 per cent covers a wide variety of anomalies including upper pouch fistulae, oesophageal diaphragms, multiple fistulae, bronchi arising from the oesophagus and laryngo-oesophageal clefts. Upper pouch fistulae may, however, be commoner; Dudgeon, Morrison and Woolley (1972) found it in 7 per cent of their cases, and this anomaly was present in 5 per cent of cases seen at The Hospital for Sick Children, Great Ormond Street. Associated anomalies are common, and in a survey of 1058 patients Holder *et al.* (1964) found that 505 (48 per cent) had other anomalies (see Table 4.1).

Clinical features and diagnosis

The essential feature is the inability to swallow which antenatally results in polyhydramnios in 20 to 25 per cent of affected pregnancies. After birth the babies drool saliva and froth at the mouth. The spill-over of saliva into the trachea produces choking attacks, cyanotic episodes and respiratory distress. In the common anomaly the tracheo-oesophageal fistula permits the regurgitation of gastric acid into the trachea, and this is aggravated by the gastric distension which results from air forced into the stomach by laboured breathing. It should be possible to make a diagnosis before the first feed is offered; if a feed is given there is choking and cyanosis. A high index of suspicion is necessary in all neonates with swallowing and respiratory problems, since the diagnosis can easily be established or excluded by passing a rubber catheter through the mouth; an adult female urethral catheter is suitable. Its progress will be arrested 10 to 12 cm from the gums in oesophageal atresia. This can be confirmed radiologically with a radio-opaque tube. A fine nasogastric tube may curl in the upper pouch and may even reach the stomach via the trachea and fistula. Radiography with contrast media is not recommended, since the risks of spill-over into the respiratory tract outweigh any advantages.

Management and prognosis

When the infant has to be transferred to a centre for surgery it is essential for the oesophagus and nasopharynx to be sucked out at least every 10 to 15 minutes and for the temperature to be maintained during the journey. Prior to surgery every effort must be made to improve the baby's general condition; intensive physiotherapy, correction of fluid and electrolyte imbalance and antibiotics may all be necessary. In the presence of acute abdominal distention, a preliminary gastrostomy may be helpful (Koop, Schnaufer and Broennie, 1974).

The aim of surgery is to achieve a primary anastomosis of the oesophagus, and this is possible in 75 per cent of cases. During the operation a fine feeding tube can be passed via the nose down the oesophagus and into the stomach (alternatively, a gastrostomy can be performed) to permit early postoperative feeding with milk. Postoperative complications include anastomotic leaks with empyema and tension pneumothorax, pneumonia, anastomotic strictures, recurrence of the fistula, inco-ordinate swallowing and hiatus hernia.

When a primary anastomosis is not possible or unsafe, the alternatives are a delayed primary anastomosis or late oesophageal replacement. In either instance division of any tracheo-oesophageal fistula is essential, and a gastrostomy is required for feeding. When a delayed anastomosis is planned, the upper oesophagus is kept clear of secretions by constant suction through a double lumen tube. The second thoracotomy can be performed when the baby weighs 3 kg and is thriving. Stretching of the oesophageal pouches has been recommended but its value is uncertain. The first step in a planned late oesophageal replacement is a left-sided cervical oesophagostomy. Any baby with troublesome spill-over problems whilst awaiting a delayed primary anastomosis should also have an oesophagostomy.

Following oesophagostomy and gastrostomy, these babies can be cared for at home as most mothers quickly learn the techniques of gastrostomy feeding and 'sham' oral feeding. Teaching the babies to swallow by oral 'sham' feeding is essential. There is no general agreement as to which oesophageal replacement procedure is best. Intrapleural colon, retrosternal colon and reversed gastric tubes have all been reported to give good results in special centres (Azar, Chrispin and Waterston, 1971; Singh and Rickham, 1971; Drainer, 1974). The timing of these procedures varies, but a reasonable time is at about the age of 1 year when the infant is thriving and weighs over 9 kg.

Overall the survival rates reflect the general condition of the patients, the nature of the defect and the presence of associated anomalies, as well as the skill of the surgical team. Reported survival rates have varied from 65 to 89 per cent (Myres, 1974), the former figure probably more accurately reflecting the general rate. Table 4.2 shows the factors which determine the risk to the patient (from Waterston, Bonham-Carter and Aberdeen, 1962).

Tracheo-oesophageal fistula without atresia (H type)

The clinical features of this lesion, and those of a persistent upper pouch or recurrent lower pouch fistula after repair of an atresia, are due to escape of fluid into the trachea and air into the oesophagus (Eckstein *et al.*, 1970). Typically cyanosis and choking occur with the first feed, and there is persistent abdominal

Table 4.2 Factors determining the risk to patients with oesophageal atresia and tracheo-oesophageal fistula (from Waterston, Bonham-Carter and Aberdeen, 1962)

Group A	Good risk	Birth weight 2·5 kg No significant pneumonia No other major anomaly
Group B	Moderate risk	Birth weight 1·8–2·5 kg or A + pneumonia or anomaly
Group C	High risk	Birth weight 1·8 kg or A + pneumonia and anomaly or B + pneumonia or anomaly

distention. Recurrent chest infections, particularly involving the right upper lobe, are common.

The diagnostic problem is to differentiate overspill into the larynx due to incoordinated swallowing from a direct leak into the trachea via a fistula, and to localise the fistula accurately before surgery. This can best be achieved by the technique of cine-swallow using dionosil as a contrast medium. Division of the fistula through a neck incision or through the chest cage is usually straightforward and relieves the immediate problems; there may be temporary residual symptoms secondary to disordered oesophageal function.

Congenital oesophageal stricture

Congenital strictures of the oesophagus are rare. Congenital narrowing of the mid or upper oesophagus can be due to webs, diaphragms, cartilaginous rings or ectopic mucosa, but narrowing of the distal oesophagus is more likely to be acquired from acid reflux and ulceration. Whatever the site of the stricture, difficulty in swallowing with or without vomiting is the presenting feature. When possible, dilatation of the stricture gives immediate relief, and repeated dilatation is all that is required in a few patients. Others require a gastrostomy followed by resection of the stricture (Holinger *et al.*, 1954).

Duplications of the oesophagus

These are discussed later under duplications and megaileocolon.

PYLORUS

Pyloric atresia

This rare abnormality presents as a complete pyloric obstruction with persistent vomiting from birth. Plain films of the abdomen show only a gastric air bubble. When this is the sole anomaly the results of a modified pyloroplasty are excellent. Occasionally a solid segment requires excision and a Bilroth 1 anastomosis. An association with epidermolysis bullosa has been observed (J. Plaschkes, personal communication).

Hypertrophic pyloric stenosis (see Dodge, 1974)

Congenital hypertrophic pyloric stenosis is one of those conditions which bridge the immediate neonatal period and early infancy. The pyloric hypertrophy is not present at birth; symptoms may start in the first week of life but more usually between the second and third weeks. Untreated the natural history of the disease is for the vomiting to continue into the third month of life, survivors recovering spontaneously soon after this.

The condition is commoner in first-born children from the higher socio-economic classes, and males are affected about five times as frequently as females. The pattern of inheritance is polygenic, and there is therefore an increased risk in siblings and the offspring of affected children; this is highest (20 per cent) for the first-born male child of a mother who herself was affected. The aetiology is obscure. The increasingly recognised association with other congenital gut obstructions, oesophageal atresia, anorectal anomalies, meconium ileus and duodenal atresia is also unexplained.

Clinical features

The patients present with vomiting which is never bile-stained and usually starts in the second or third weeks of life, but may present from very soon after birth or much later. Vomiting becomes increasingly copious and forceful and eventually projectile. Initially the infant is irritable and hungry, but with increasing failure to thrive the baby becomes miserable and lethargic and the vomiting less forceful. When the stomach is full, visible peristalsis is easily seen and the palpation of a pyloric tumour, either during a test feed or immediately after a vomit, clinches the diagnosis. The other features of constipation, starvation stools, dehydration and metabolic alkalosis, are the inevitable consequences of pyloric obstruction and loss of gastric secretions. A useful diagnostic rule of thumb is that the tumour should have been felt by two experienced observers at separate times, one of whom should, but not necessarily, be the surgeon. When there is any doubt about the diagnosis radiological studies should be performed. A plain film will often show pyloric hold up and dilation of the stomach, with absent gas distal to the pylorus; barium studies are confirmatory and outline the long narrow pyloric canal. The presence or absence of gastro-oesophageal reflux should be noted since it will influence postoperative progress and management.

Management and prognosis

There is now almost universal agreement in the United Kingdom that pyloromyotomy (Ramstedt's operation) is the treatment of choice. The only exceptions are infants of about 3 months who are continuing to thrive since they are likely to recover spontaneously. Most infants are now referred before any appreciable biochemical disturbances have developed, and require no special preparation for surgery apart from a single gastric washout two to three hours before the operation. When present, dehydration and metabolic alkalosis must be corrected and surgery postponed for 24 to 48 hours. Where a skilled paediatric anaesthetist is available general anaesthesia is preferable, otherwise local anaesthesia is adequate. The variety of incisions in use to approach the pylorus indicates that no single one is preferable to another. The technique of pyloromyotomy has not changed since its original description. Postoperatively oral feeds should be resumed as soon as the baby accepts them, and there is

Table 4.3 Associated anomalies and per cent mortality rates in 503 infants with duodenal atresia (From Fonkalsrud, de Lorimer and Hays, 1969)

Anomalies	Number of patients	Mortality rate (%)
Down's syndrome	150	30
Congenital heart disease	86	17
Tracheo-oesophageal fistula	34	7
Renal anomalies	26	5
Imperforate anus	17	
Skeletal anomalies	14	
Meckel's diverticulum	12	
Omphalocele	4	
Miscellaneous	75	15

little benefit in slow reintroduction of feeds. There are two well-recognised postoperative problems. An incomplete myotomy may result in continuing signs of obstruction; most infants, however, will settle with conservative management and several days should elapse before surgical re-exploring of the abdomen. The abdominal wound has a deservedly bad reputation for dehiscence and herniation, which is probably due to preoperative malnutrition rather than the surgical technique employed.

Medical management, is probably only indicated in well-nourished infants whose symptoms are mild and of late onset (i.e. after the age of 2 months).

The only acceptable survival rate for the treatment of hypertrophic pyloric stenosis is 100 per cent.

DUODENUM

Obstructive lesions of the duodenum may be broadly classified as intrinsic or extrinsic. Intrinsic obstructions may be due to atresia, stenosis or a diaphragm which may be complete or contain a pin-hole opening. An annular pancreas is only of significance if it is associated with an intrinsic duodenal obstruction. The second part of the duodenum near the ampulla of Vater is the commonest site for intrinsic obstructions, but any part can be involved. Extrinsic obstructions are most commonly associated with malrotation, Ladd's bands and volvulus neonatorum. The relationship of the obstruction to the ampulla of Vater will determine whether the vomit is bile-stained, which it usually is; occasionally the obstructive duodenal lesion is associated with obstruction of the common bile duct and ascending cholangitis. Uncommonly the common bile duct has two openings into the duodenum, one on each side of the obstruction.

Duodenal atresia is less common than oesophageal atresia, occurring in about one out of every 5000 live births. Associated anomalies are very common, and an appreciable proportion of affected cases also have Down's syndrome, as shown in Table 4.3 (Fonkalsrud, de Lorimer and Hays, 1969).

Clinical features and diagnosis

Maternal polyhydramnios is common and the baby presents with vomiting during the first day of life, which frequently precedes the first feed; the vomit is bile-stained in over half the patients and the absence of bile has led to serious delay in diagnosis. The characteristic 'double bubble' on plain films of the abdomen is diagnostic. This sign may be absent if gastric aspiration or vomiting has immediately preceded the film; the injection of 10 ml of air down a nasogastric tube provides adequate contrast in these circumstances.

Management and prognosis

When the patient has to be transferred to a centre for surgery, a freely draining nasogastric tube aspirated frequently is essential to prevent inhalation of vomit. Delay in diagnosis will result in dehydration and metabolic alkalosis, which must be corrected before surgery.

Surgery involves bypassing the obstruction either directly by a duodeno-duodenostomy or by utilising the first free loop of jejunum in a duodeno-jejunostomy (Young and Wilkinson, 1966). The dilated hypertrophied proximal duodenum takes some time to function normally and reflux of duodenal contents into the stomach may persist for some time following surgical relief of the obstruction. A temporary gastrostomy is therefore usually performed in order to maintain an empty stomach and duodenum and so to prevent vomiting. The placement of a fine tube alongside the gastrostomy tube and across the anastomosis allows for early feeding within 24 hours of surgery. If the gastric aspirate is filtered through gauze and returned via the transanastomotic tube, the need for intravenous fluid replacement therapy is minimised; this facilitates postoperative management and survival, particularly in the very small newborn. The transanastomotic tube should be thin-walled silicone rubber; the more rigid standard infant feeding vinyl tubes and thick silicone rubber tubes can result in perforation of the gut. Reduction in the volume of gastric aspirate is an indication of improved gastric emptying and, after six to eight days, oral feeding is usually possible; when oral feeds are fully tolerated the transanastomotic tube can be removed. Removal of the gastrostomy tube should be delayed until about 12 days postoperatively or later, depending on when normal oral feeding is established. The gastrostomy wound usually closes spontaneously.

Applying a risk-grading similar to that for oesophageal atresia (see Table 4.2), the risk pattern is similar with an overall survival rate of just over 70 per cent, most deaths being related to the associated anomalies (Perrelli and Wilkinson, 1975).

JEJUNUM AND ILEUM

Atresia

Atresias may occur at all levels of the small bowel. They vary from simple occluding diaphragms to widely separated bowel ends with defects in the mesentery, and they can be single or multiple. The bowel proximal to the atresia which is very dilated and hypertrophied may outgrow its blood supply or undergo a secondary volvulus. The distal bowel is narrow and contains white mucous plugs some of which may be bile-stained. The theory that atresias result from intrauterine accidents (e.g. volvulus, vascular insufficiency, intussusception or strangulation in a hernial orifice) rather than defects in embryological development (Louw, 1966) is supported by the presence of bile pigment in the distal bowel, the occasional occurrence of a localised meconium peritonitis and the loss of long segments of gut which may occur (Tawes and Nixon, 1971). Atresia and meconium peritonitis may also be complications of meconium ileus. Except in the rare variant known as the 'apple peel anomaly' (Dickson, 1970), where the dorsal mesentery and the superior mesenteric arterial supply to the small bowel is absent with a resultant loss of most or all of the jejunum, other associated anomalies are less common than with duodenal and anorectal anomalies (de Lorimer, Fonkalsrud and Hays, 1969).

The overall incidence of jejunal and ileal atresias is slightly lower than that of duodenal atresia and is of the order of one in every 6000 live births.

Clinical features and diagnosis

Hydramnios occurs only in association with the most proximal obstructions. Bile-stained vomiting usually starts during the first day of life. Except in the most proximal obstructions, abdominal distention develops rapidly and is greatest in the more distal lesions; the very dilated segment immediately proximal to the atresia may be visible through abdominal wall. Normal meconium is not passed, and a rectal washout will produce white mucous plugs from the microcolon.

Supine and erect films of the abdomen are usually adequate for diagnosis. Increasing dilatation of a reduced number of small bowel loops with fluid levels ending in one very dilated loop are the characteristic findings. Speckled areas of calcification indicate an old perforation and meconium peritonitis. There is no gas in the distal bowel or rectum unless it has been introduced by a rectal examination or washout. Contrast studies are usually not necessary, but an enema will show a normally placed microcolon.

Management and prognosis

With early diagnosis fluid and electrolyte replacement is unnecessary, but if the diagnosis has been delayed, replacement therapy should precede surgery. The dilated distal blind segment of gut is frequently damaged and slow to regain function, even in uncomplicated cases, and should therefore be resected except in infants with a very short gut. Continuity is restored by an oblique end-to-end technique. Any remaining blind ends will subsequently form a pouch or loop which can later cause malabsorption and bleeding. The Bishop–Koop operation, which is the procedure of choice in patients with meconium ileus, has been used but is seldom necessary (Louw, 1966). Multiple atresias or diaphragms present a difficult problem. When the total length of remaining normal small bowel exceeds 70 cm (measured along the antimesenteric border of the gut) simple resection of all the abnormal gut is probably best. When less gut remains simple diaphragms should be perforated internally and left with an in-dwelling splint; multiple atresias require multiple anastomoses. Post-operatively bowel function usually returns within 48 hours and subsequent progress depends on the length of remaining bowel, particularly on the length of terminal ileum. The minimum length of remaining small bowel which is compatible with long-term survival is between 20 and 25 cm, and children with more than 80 to 100 cm remaining usually present few problems.

The overall survival rate should be around 75 to 80 per cent (Louw, 1966; Tawes and Nixon, 1971). Unavoidable deaths are caused by meconium peritonitis, a very short gut, prematurity and associated anomalies.

Malrotation and volvulus

Malrotation may occur as an isolated abnormality or be associated with a large omphalocele, gastroschisis or a diaphragmatic hernia. It is only of importance if it is associated with Ladd's bands across the second part of the duodenum or an unstable narrow mesenteric isthmus, which predisposes the neonate to a volvulus. Complete situs inversus is less common and usually of no surgical significance. In the clinically important malrotations the duodenum does not cross the midline and runs into the jejunum on the right side of the vertebral column; the small bowel lies on the right side of the abdomen and the caecum is near the midline. Peritoneal bands (Ladd's bands) run from the caecum to the posterior abdominal wall and gall bladder area, crossing the second part of the duodenum. They may obstruct the duodenum in their own right, but more commonly a volvulus occurs just distal to the bands. The volvulus results in duodenal obstruction initially, but with increasing twisting and tightening the whole midgut strangulates and the prognosis rapidly becomes hopeless. Since the diagnosis can only be made by direct inspection, early surgery is essential in all newborns presenting with duodenal obstruction.

Clinical features and diagnosis

The initial postnatal progress is usually normal, and gastrointestinal symptoms may be even delayed for months or years. As milk feeding is established the first twist develops, presumably due to the increased activity of the gut and the weight of its contents. The infant refuses feeds and vomits, the vomit becoming bile-stained. The volvulus may be intermittent and result in recurrent symptoms, which may extend over several months. Strangulation must be suspected if the infant's general condition suddenly deteriorates, if blood is passed per rectum or if the examining finger is blood-stained on rectal examination; the abdomen rapidly becomes distended and the obstructed loops of bowel may be palpable on abdominal examination.

Malrotation and volvulus should be suspected in any infant who develops intestinal obstruction after an uneventful postnatal period or when symptoms of obstruction are intermittent. Plain films of the abdomen may show the presence of gastric and duodenal gas bubbles with absence of gas distal to the duodenum. More commonly successive films show progressive emptying of the distal gut or dilated closed loops in the centre of the abdomen. If the obstruction is acute these radiological changes are an indication for surgery. When the obstruction is subacute or intermittent, the diagnosis can be confirmed by barium studies. A barium meal will show either the duodenal obstruction or the non-rotated duodenum, whereas an enema demonstrates the caecum to be positioned in the left hypochondrium or central abdomen and the whole large bowel to be on the left side of the abdomen.

Management and prognosis
Because of the risk of strangulation the need for surgery is urgent. The volvulus is untwisted, all adhesions are divided, Ladd's bands are divided and the gut is freed until it is possible to lay the small bowel to the right and the large bowel to the left of the abdomen. No attempt should be made to restore the normal arrangement of the gut but the mesenteric isthmus must be widened to prevent recurrences. The gut may be sutured in its new position (Bill and Grauman, 1966). Some surgeons perform an appendicectomy whereas others prefer not to open the gut lumen.

If strangulation has already occurred simple resection of the infarcted gut is performed when there is an adequate length of healthy gut remaining. When there is insufficient obviously viable bowel remaining a 'second look' policy is worth adopting. The bowel is arranged in its optimum position and the abdomen closed. Twenty-four hours later the abdomen is re-explored in the hope that some of the previously non-viable appearing gut may have recovered. This policy can sometimes offer the chance of survival in an otherwise hopeless situation.

In the absence of strangulation and infarction of the bowel, the results of surgery are excellent and recurrence of the volvulus is unusual. When resection is necessary, the prospects and quality of survival depend on the length of surviving gut.

Early management following resection. The average length of the small intestine in the newborn is 250 cm, and the minimum length compatible with survival is about 20 to 25 cm assuming that the ileocaecal valve is left intact (Wilmore, 1972). Postoperative problems, however, should be anticipated even when there is a greater length of small gut remaining. The immediate problems are the body losses of fluid and electrolytes and malabsorption, and intravenous feeding is essential until an adequate oral intake has been achieved. Disaccharide and cows' milk protein intolerance not infrequently follows resection, and these two dietary constituents should be initially excluded from the feeding regime, particularly if a long length of gut has been removed. Feeds can be given by a continuous nasogastric drip at first, and later as small frequent feeds. Unabsorbed bile salts may exacerbate diarrhoea by their toxic effects on the colonic mucosa, and the oral administration of binding resins such as cholestyramine is sometimes helpful. When it has been necessary to remove the ileocaecal valve, bacterial overgrowth of the remaining small gut may contribute to the malabsorption and an appropriate antibiotic should be given. Even after an oral feeding regime has been established there is a tendency to recurrent episodes of diarrhoea, which may require fluid and electrolyte replacement. Adaptation of the remaining small bowel occurs gradually during the two to three months following surgery. The long-term effects of small intestinal resection are considered in Chapter 7.

Meconium ileus

Meconium ileus is the earliest and most acute of the intestinal problems complicating cystic fibrosis, and occurs in about 15 per cent of affected cases (Dickson and Mearns, 1975). The mechanism which results in the formation of meconium, which is so viscid that it forms a bolus obstruction in lower small gut, is not known. Pancreatic insufficiency, an increased albumin content of the meconium and other abnormalities of the intestinal secretions may all play a part.

Clinical features and diagnosis

The clinical picture is that of complete antenatal small bowel obstruction. The outstanding sign is abdominal distention which, in contrast to other obstructions, is present from birth. The distended meconium-filled loops of bowel may be visible and are often palpable in the abdomen. Bile-stained vomiting from the first day of life is almost invariable, and only in incomplete cases is any meconium passed rectally.

Plain abdominal films are of less diagnostic help than in atresias. The 'ground glass' appearance (Neuhauser, 1946) is an inconstant finding, but the appearance of abdominal distention with only a few fluid levels should suggest the diagnosis (White, 1956). The presence of a high obstruction with multiple fluid levels suggests other complications. In apparently uncomplicated cases or when the diagnosis is in doubt a gastrografin enema is diagnostic and will often relieve the obstruction (Lillie and Chrispin, 1972).

Management and prognosis

As discussed above, in uncomplicated cases a gastrografin enema often is all that is required. Gastrografin may result in marked losses of fluid into the gut lumen and the baby's state of hydration must be carefully monitored during and after the enema. Excessive pressure or volume changes should be avoided during the enema, since a perforation may be caused or demonstrated. If the obstruction is not completely relieved, the enema is repeated 24 hours later.

Surgery is necessary in complicated cases as well as in uncomplicated cases not relieved by the gastrografin enema. The procedure of choice is the Bishop–Koop operation (Bishop and Koop, 1957) in which, after resection of the obstructed loop, continuity is restored by an end-to-side anastomosis. The free end of the distal bowel is brought out on to the abdominal wall and functions as a safety valve ileostomy during the few days required for the passage of normal intestinal contents to clear the terminal ileum and colon of mucous plugs. Closure of the ileostomy can be performed prior to discharging the infant from hospital, but it is probably wiser to delay closure for a few months until the infant is thriving. Neonatal meconium obstruction has been reported in the absence of cystic fibrosis (Rickham and Boeckman, 1965) and confirmation of the diagnosis by means of a sweat test is essential. Early survival rates of over 80 per cent are now possible in uncomplicated cases.

LARGE INTESTINE

Hirschsprung's disease (see Fig. 4.2 for modes of presentation)
Hirschsprung in 1887 first described this condition as a lethal disease of infancy characterised by intractable constipation, gross dilatation of the colon and an empty rectum. It was not until over 50 years later that it became recognised that the disease was associated with an absence of ganglion cells from lengths of bowel varying from the distal rectum to the entire large and small intestine. In intestinal hypoganglionosis ganglion cells are present but in reduced numbers, and the term pseudo-Hirschsprung's disease has been used to describe delayed maturation of ganglion cells.

Clinical features and diagnosis
The majority of cases present in the neonatal period, and the severity of the symptoms and signs do not necessarily correlate with the length of affected gut; necrotising enterocolitis is a potentially fatal complication (Nixon, 1964; Fraser and Wilkinson, 1967). The first sign is usually a delay in the newborn passing meconium. Delayed passage of meconium is common in premature babies, but the majority of babies with Hirschsprung's disease are born at term. Abdominal distention, which can be so severe as to cause respiratory embarrassment, and vomiting are early features. Typically rectal examination reveals a normal but empty rectum, and if the affected segment is short a finger can be passed into the dilated proximal bowel. On withdrawing the examining finger there is an explosive decompression as meconium is expelled through the passively stretched narrow segment. Meconium is nearly always present in the colon even when the whole colon is aganglionic.

Radiology, anorectal manometry and mucosal suction biopsy are the available diagnostic methods. With distal obstructions a plain abdominal film will show gross distention of the large and small bowel; the colon may be particularly

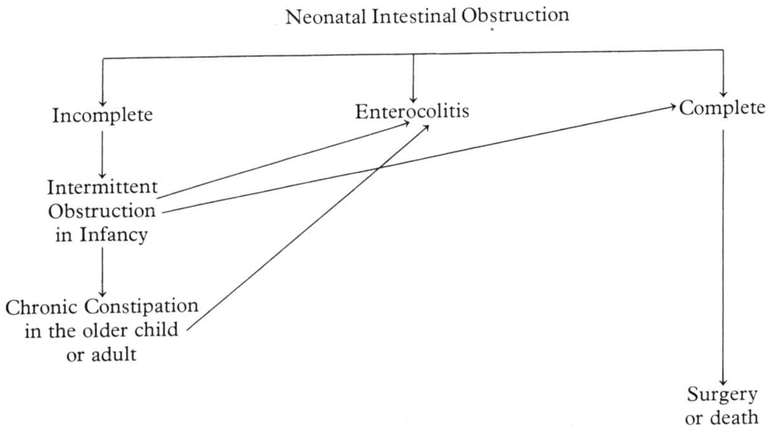

Fig. 4.2 The presentation of Hirschsprung's disease

distended and the rectum empty. In experienced hands a barium enema is diagnostic in 80 to 90 per cent of cases, even in the neonatal period (Lillie, 1969).

The examination should not be immediately preceded by digital rectal examination or washouts since these procedures may stretch the distal bowel and deflate the proximal gut.

Anorectal manometry. Normally the inflation of a balloon placed in the rectum inhibits the internal anal sphincter. In Hirschsprung's disease this inhibitory effect is absent, and should the balloon be in aganglionic gut abnormal rectal waves can be identified (Aaronson and Nixon, 1972). This simple test has not yet fulfilled its early promise, and both false positive and false negative results may be obtained in the neonatal period.

Mucosal biopsy. Suction mucosal biopsies of the rectum can be taken at 2 and 4 cm from the anal verge and, if frozen sections are treated with a cholinesterase stain, a histological report can be obtained within three to four hours. In Hirschsprung's disease there is a striking increase in the number of nerve fibres and overall cholinesterase activity in the mucosa and submucosa, and ganglion cells are absent (Meier-Ruge, 1974); in our experience, however, cholinesterase activity is not always reliable and a full thickness biopsy examined by a frozen section technique should precede the definitive surgical procedure.

Management and prognosis

There is no general agreement on an optimum plan of management. In short-segment disease, treatment varies from daily rectal washouts for six weeks followed by one of the modifications of the Duhamel operation (Ehrenpreis, 1970), to an immediate right transverse colostomy with a pull-through procedure at the age of 1 year followed by closure of the colostomy a few weeks later. It is agreed, however, that two principles are important in the management of Hirschsprung's disease: immediate relief of obstruction, and excision of the aganglionic segment followed by anastomosis of ganglionic bowel to the anal canal.

Relief of obstruction. An immediate colostomy is the safest procedure, the siting of the colostomy depending on the length of aganglionic gut. In short-segment disease a transverse colostomy is a relatively simple procedure which allows the definitive operation to be performed in totally defunctioned bowel. It is, however, the view of many surgeons that in both short- and long-segment disease the colostomy should be situated in the most distal ganglionic segment. When the aganglionosis extends proximal to the hepatic flexure, an ileostomy should be performed. When the disease extends into the terminal small bowel, frozen sections are essential at the time of laparotomy for accurate placing of the stoma.

Definitive surgery. Three surgical procedures are currently in use:

1. The original Swenson pull-through operation, in which a low anastomosis is achieved by intussuscepting the anal canal and performing the anastomosis outside the anus (Swenson, 1957),

2. The Duhamel technique where the lower aganglionic bowel is left *in situ* and the ganglionic bowel pulled through behind it (Duhamel, 1956); a blind side-to-side anastomosis between these can then be achieved by one of a variety of manoeuvres,
3. The third technique was described by Soave (1966) but was performed by other surgeons around the same time. The rectum is transected above the pelvic floor and its mucosa cored out. After resection of the remaining aganglionic bowel the ganglionic colon is pulled through to the anus in the raw tunnel.

Each of these three operations gives good results in experienced hands. The Swenson procedure is technically the most difficult but, this apart, there is insufficient evidence to choose between them.

Complications and prognosis. The most important complication of Hirschsprung's disease is enterocolitis which may occur at any stage of the disease, even following an apparently successful operation. It accounts for the majority of deaths (Boley and Kleinhaus, 1974) and adds urgency to the management of this condition in the neonatal period. Although the aetiology of enterocolitis has not been clearly defined, it appears to be related to the obstructive element of the disease and the relief of obstruction is therefore an urgent matter. In long-segment disease immediate colostomy is mandatory. In short-segment disease it is sometimes safer to relieve the obstruction gradually by means of colonic saline washouts once or twice daily and passing a flatus tube every six hours, followed by a colostomy when the infant's condition improves. General management is similar to that for non-specific enterocolitis, as outlined later.

In the newborn the mortality rate is about 20 to 25 per cent, most deaths being due to enterocolitis (Freeman, 1971). Following successful surgery the children usually become continent of faeces at a somewhat later age than normal, but the subsequent control of defaecation is satisfactory in 70 to 90 per cent of patients (Ehrenpreis, 1970). Some children have persistent and troublesome constipation which may require an internal sphincterotomy (Lawson, 1972). A minority of patients fail to achieve bowel continence and require a permanent colostomy.

Late onset Hirschsprung's disease

Although 60 to 70 per cent of patients present in the neonatal period, some children present later with intractable constipation which may alternate with episodes of diarrhoea; the diagnosis may even be delayed to early adult life.

Clinical features and diagnosis

Once the condition has been suspected the diagnosis is much simpler than in the newborn and involves the same investigatory techniques. The disease is predominantly of the short-segment type. The only difficulty arises with very-short-segment disease, and this is considered separately.

Clinical differentiation from other causes of constipation is usually clear. Symptoms precede potty training, there may be failure to thrive and intermittent diarrhoea may be a feature. On rectal examination the anal canal and lower rectum are empty. This empty segment, with faecal loading in the proximal dilated gut which may be within reach of the examining finger, distinguishes Hirschsprung's disease from the loaded rectum and anal canal of 'rectal inertia'. Digital assessment of anal sphincter tone is too subjective to be generally useful. A barium enema must be performed without bowel preparation. The appearances of an empty and narrow or relatively normal rectum suddenly expanding into the dilated proximal bowel are diagnostic. Histological diagnosis by suction biopsy is simple, but should be confirmed by examining frozen sections at the time of the pull-through surgical procedure. Anorectal pressure studies show the typical failure of relaxation of the internal sphincter.

Management

The same principles of treatment apply as in the newborn. Some surgeons prefer, if the bowel can be emptied by regular washouts and the child's general condition improves sufficiently, to proceed to a pull-through operation without a preliminary colostomy. Others consider that a preliminary colostomy, to rest and permit complete clearance of contents from the dilated colon and rectum, is safer. All the procedures described in the newborn are used in the older child and are technically easier to perform; postoperative problems with bowel training and control seem to be fewer in the older child.

Very-short- and ultra-short-segment Hirschsprung's disease

The term very-short- and ultra-short-segment disease has been applied to a group of patients in whom there is an abnormal sphincter response but in whom ganglion cells are present down to the level of the anal canal. As there is neither absence of ganglion cells nor any abnormality of the cholinsterase-staining reaction, 'internal sphincter spasm' is probably a better description of this entity.

Clinical features and diagnosis

The two conditions present in a very similar fashion with severe chronic constipation; overflow faecal soiling is a common feature but failure to thrive is uncommon. On rectal examination the rectum is usually loaded with faeces down to the anal verge. In very short segment disease this is due to a packing effect, the hypertrophied proximal bowel forcing the faecal bolus into the aganglionic segment, dilating it and moving the apparent cone distally. A barium enema will not differentiate these conditions from 'rectal inertia' and the diagnosis can only be established by biopsy and anorectal manometry. A series of suction biopsies should be taken at 1 cm intervals so that a complete picture of the innervation of the anal canal and lower rectum can be obtained. Anorectal pressure studies will identify isolated internal sphincter spasm.

Management

Many patients can be managed along the lines established for 'rectal inertia'; and the short length of affected bowel precludes any form of pull-through procedure. An extended internal sphincterotomy appears to be the logical operation, and good results have been reported (Lynn, 1966); it is important, however, that the secondary rectal inertia be treated. A full anal sphincter stretch performed under general anaesthesia should probably precede an internal sphincterotomy since it is sometimes curative and avoids the permanent impairment of faecal control which may follow sphincterotomy.

Anorectal anomalies

There is no universally agreed classification of these anomalies which are frequently grouped together under the blanket term of 'imperforate anus'. The international classification proposed at Melbourne in 1970 (Santulli, Kiesewetter and Bill, 1970) has failed to achieve the agreement hoped for and is very complicated for general use. Similarly, modifications of the original classification of Ladd and Gross have proved unsatisfactory (Wilkinson, 1972).

For the purposes of general discussion anorectal anomalies will be divided into four main groups (Nixon, 1972):

1. Low anomalies (see Fig. 4.3)
   Infralevator; the bowel ends blindly or by a fistula below the pelvic floor (Ladd and Gross, I, II and IIIa; International Classification, male 1–5, female 12–16).
2. Intermediate anomalies
   (Ladd and Gross, IIIa; International Classification, male 6, female 17–21)
3. High anomalies (see Fig. 4.2)
   Supralevator; the bowel ends blindly or by a fistula above the pelvic floor. (Ladd and Gross, IIIb; International Classification, male 8–10, female 23–26)
4. Atresia or stenosis of the middle third of the rectum (Ladd and Gross IV; International Classification male 7 and 11, female 22 and 27).

The overlaps reflect the difficulties in terminology and description.

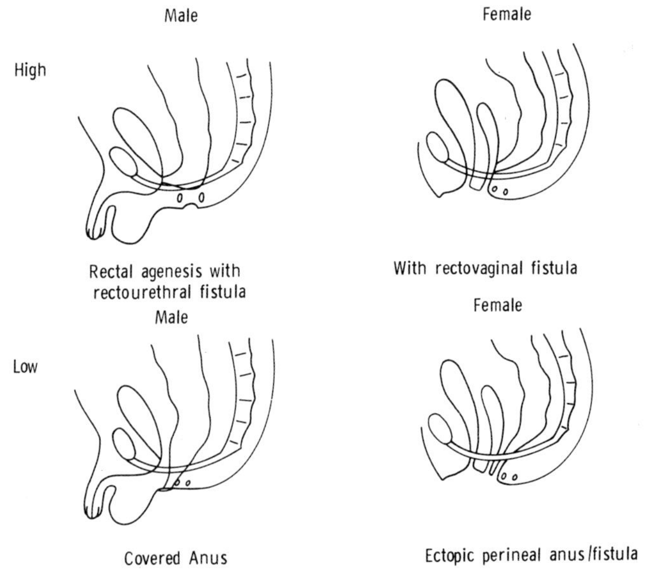

Fig. 4.3 Schematic representation of high and low anorectal anomalies

Clinical features

With the exception of the fourth group the diagnosis of an anorectal anomaly is obvious on routine examination of the newborn. Atresia or stenosis of the middle third of the rectum presents as low large bowel obstruction.

Diagnosis and management

Low anomalies. In the male, anal stenosis or an ectopic perineal anus should be recognised early and treated by dilatation.

A 'covered anus' can be recognised by the appearance of a triangular skin tag pointing anteriorly over the site of the anus. Meconium staining may be seen in pits on either side of the skin tag or as a streak leading anteriorly from the apex. Simple excision of the 'cover' overlying the anal canal followed by regular dilatation of the slightly anteriorly placed anus gives excellent results.

In the female these anomalies include anal stenosis, an anterior perineal anus and anovulvar fistula. Provided a skin bridge is left between the 'anus' and vagina, these lesions also respond well to dilatation with, in some instances, a small cut-back procedure to enlarge the opening posteriorly.

Intermediate anomalies. In the male anorectal atresia or agenesis with a recto-bulbar fistula is a very rare anomaly. The external appearances of the anus are similar to those in the high anomalies. The emergency treatment is a colostomy.

In the female intermediate anomalies include anorectal atresia or agenesis, with rectovestibular or low rectovaginal fistulae. Management is controversial and includes enlarging the opening backwards, transposing the anus from a perineal approach to its normal site, or a formal abdominoperineal operation. The nature and timing of the operative procedure depends on the anatomy of the lesion and the preference of the surgeon. Transposition can be performed in the neonatal period but is best deferred until before starting school, between the age of 4 and 5 years, or until puberty. When an abdominoperineal operation is planned, a colostomy in the neonatal period is essential.

High anomalies. In males with anorectal atresia or agenesis, with or without a rectourethral fistula, there is no evidence of an anus in the perineum; and meconium may be passed in the urine. The immediate treatment of choice is a right transverse colostomy, but definitive treatment should be delayed until a complete anatomical diagnosis has been established.

In the female high lesions include rectal atresia or agenesis, with a high retrovaginal fistula or a rectocloacal fistula. There is no anus, vaginal and urethral openings are usually present, and more rarely there is a single perineal opening (i.e. cloaca); meconium is passed from the vagina or cloaca. A recto-cloacal fistula may be associated with urinary tract obstruction. The immediate treatment is a right transverse colostomy. An abdominoperineal pull-through procedure is best delayed until the age of 6 months to 1 year when the infant is thriving. The colostomy can usually be closed two weeks following surgery.

Investigations

The investigations which are necessary in children with anorectal anomalies fall into two broad groups: those required to define the exact anatomy of the anomaly prior to definitive treatment, and those required to identify any associated lesions, particularly those involving the renal tract. These investigations should generally be deferred until the infant is thriving and, in babies with a colostomy, until this has been washed clear of meconium.

A water-soluble contrast loopogram through the distal limb of the colostomy will demonstrate the termination of the rectum and the presence and position of a fistula; this technique is preferable to the commonly recommended inverted plain radiograph. An intravenous pyelogram is essential since 40 to 50 per cent of infants with an anorectal anomaly have an associated anomaly of the renal tract. A cystogram is also required in most of the affected males and in many of the females.

Prognosis

The proportion of children who survive (80 per cent) is similar to that for other congenital obstructive lesions of the alimentary tract, and most deaths are due to associated anomalies particularly those affecting the renal tract and heart. In the survivors the results with regard to bowel control are disappointing: control is adequate in 75 to 90 per cent, near normal in only 50 per cent and 10 to 25 per cent fail to achieve any control of bowel function (Puri and Nixon, personal communication). Thus, up to a quarter of children are left with what, in effect, is a perineal colostomy, and a terminal abdominal colostomy may be the best final solution for this group of patients.

DUPLICATIONS AND MEGAILEOCOLON

Duplications are of two types, tubular and cystic (Forshall, 1961). Both tubular duplications and the localised areas of dilatation of the gut which occur in megaileocolon are associated with vertebral anomalies. These and the rare patent neurenteric canal have been attributed to an embryological splitting of the notochord (Bentley and Smith, 1960). All duplications are anatomically closely related to the normal gut, lie on its mesenteric border, share the same blood supply and often the same outer muscle coat. Tubular duplications follow a variety of tracks, running parallel to long lengths of colon or small bowel, ending blindly at both ends or communicating with the adjoining bowel; they often track posteriorly to end on the vertebral column. In the thoracic cage duplications may form cysts which adhere to the oesophagus and aorta, and these can track through the diaphragm to communicate with intra-abdominal cysts or the duodenum and jejunum.

Clinical features and diagnosis

Closed duplications usually present as palpable abdominal masses or as cystic swellings on radiology of the chest; large cystic abdominal duplications can present with gross abdominal distention, which may be clinically indistinguishable from ascites. As they enlarge thoracic cysts cause respiratory distress. Cysts localised in critical parts of the alimentary tract such as the duodenum may obstruct the lumen, whereas those in more mobile parts such as the jejunum or ileum can initiate a volvulus. Communicating duplications may cause bleeding from ulceration due to heterotopic gastric mucosa or from stagnation of the contents of the loop. Communications through a vertebral defect can lead to meningitis or spinal cord compression.

The diagnosis is established by barium studies which may show stretching of the gut over the cyst, areas of dilatation or a diverticulum. Hemivertebrae or round defects in the vertebral column are useful diagnostic markers.

Management

Simple abdominal cystic duplications can be excised together with the adjacent gut, as can be short tubular duplications. In the case of long tubular duplications it is preferable to shell out the mucosa from the duplication, leaving the seromuscular layer to adhere and fibrose; this avoids the necessity of removing long lengths of normal intestine. Thoracic lesions are best treated by a combination of cyst resection and shelling out of mucosa over the oesophagus and aorta. Occasionally (e.g. tubular duplications of the colon), the construction of a series of large openings between the duplication and the normal bowel lumen is the simplest solution.

DIAPHRAGMATIC HERNIA (see Bonham-Carter, Waterston and Aberdeen, 1962)

Of the three types of diaphragmatic hernia which present in infancy (i.e. Bochdalek, Morgagni and hiatus) a postero-lateral hernia through a large diaphragmatic defect (Bochdalek) presents the most urgent of all surgical emergencies in the newborn. Eighty per cent of these are left-sided and contain small bowel, stomach, spleen, part of the colon and often a lobe of liver; right-sided hernias are frequently smaller but nevertheless may contain the same abdominal viscera with the exception of the spleen. The entry of air into the alimentary tract leads to increasing compression of the lungs and respiratory distress. The combination of increasing respiratory distress, cyanosis, dextrocardia and a scaphoid abdomen is almost diagnostic. The diagnosis is easily confirmed by plain films of the chest and abdomen. Survival depends on early diagnosis and the amount of functioning lung, and long-term gastroenterological problems are uncommon (Johnson, Deaner and Koop, 1967).

The foramen of Morgagni is a retrosternal defect in the diaphragm, and usually only a single loop of small or large bowel or an abnormal lobe of liver enters the thoracic cage; this lesion seldom results in symptoms in the neonatal period. The patient may remain symptomless and the hernia detected as an incidental finding on a chest film or, more rarely, intestinal obstruction may result from incarceration of the bowel (Baran *et al.*, 1967).

Diaphragmatic hernias should be approached and repaired from the abdomen. This permits early closure of the diaphragm, correction of any associated malrotation and occasionally a 'skin only' closure to prevent increased intra-abdominal pressure.

EXOMPHALOS (see Young, 1969)

The term exomphalos can be applied to all hernias located at the umbilicus, and these can be classified as follows: (1) hernia into the umbilical cord, (2) omphalocele, and (3) gastroschisis.

The severity of the first two lesions depends on the size of the defect. A hernia into the umbilical cord reflects the persistence of a physiological umbilical hernia; the abdominal muscles are intact, and the sac may contain large and small bowel but not liver. Since the abdominal wall is intact, returning the gut to the abdomen presents few problems, even with large sacs. Manipulative reduction followed by strapping of the hernia has been recommended. Intestine, however, may be adherent to the apex of the sac and surgical repair is generally preferable since it is a safe and simple procedure.

Omphalocele

This term refers to a group of anomalies in which there is an intact sac with a wide base and a defect of the abdominal wall muscle. The defect may extend proximally to involve the sternum and anterior diaphragm, or caudally with an extroversion of the bladder; the sac always contains liver. With relatively minor defects, simple closure is possible. Very large defects, particularly in small babies or when they are associated with cardiac anomalies, are best treated by simple painting of the sac with an antibacterial agent. In these circumstances the sac epithelialises over a period of three or more months, after which an abdominal wall repair is required. Intermediate-sized defects can be treated in this way but surgery is preferable; this involves either a simple skin cover achieved by mobilising skin flaps over the sac, or a temporary repair with reinforced silastic membrane. With the latter procedure the sac is gradually reduced in size over a period of two weeks, after which the abdomen can be completely closed avoiding the need for a late repair.

Gastroschisis

This refers to an anomaly in which the gut herniates through a small transverse defect in the abdominal wall, usually to the right of the umbilicus. There is no sac, the gut is grossly thickened, with loops matted together, and appears shorter than normal. The abdominal cavity is frequently too small to permit the gut to be returned without splinting the diaphragm. In these severe cases the procedure of choice is to stretch the abdominal wall followed by returning as much gut as will go easily back into the abdominal cavity and covering the remainder with a pocket of reinforced silastic membrane sutured to the edge of the defect. This pocket is then gradually reduced in size and can usually be closed after about two weeks (Gilbert *et al.*, 1968). The major postoperative complications are sepsis and intestinal obstruction. Sepsis can be minimised by maintaining the skin-membrane junction dry and by the application of topical antibacterial and antifungal agents. Intravenous feeding should be started in the immediate postoperative period since gut function takes from 10 days to two months to return to normal.

Associated anomalies

All major umbilical defects are associated with malrotation of the midgut. There is a 10 to 20 per cent incidence of Meckel's diverticulum, and intrinsic gut obstructions such as duodenal obstructions and small gut atresias occur in less than 5 per cent of patients. Exomphalos is one of the features of Beckwith's syndrome (Irving, 1967); the other major features are macroglossia, gigantism, hepatosplenomegaly and neonatal hypoglycaemia.

NECROTISING ENTEROCOLITIS (see Dickson, 1975; Santulli *et al.*, 1975)

Most frequently idiopathic necrotising enterocolitis occurs in premature babies weighing less than 1500 g who, in the first two weeks of life after a normal immediate postnatal period, become lethargic and pale, develop gastric retention, abdominal distention and bile-stained vomiting, and who either pass no stools or develop bloody diarrhoea. The infant's temperature may be high or low, and the respiratory and pulse rates are raised. Disseminated intravascular coagulation and sclerema may occur and are bad prognostic signs. The extent of the mucosal lesions may vary from a few centimetres to the whole gut from duodenum to rectum, and the lesions may extend transmurally and lead to perforation. In infants who survive, healing of the lesion may be complete or result in strictures or even total obstruction; intestinal malabsorption is a common sequel.

The aetiology of necrotising enterocolitis has not been clearly defined. Not all affected babies are premature or small or have been subjected to perinatal asphyxia. There is an association with congenital cyanotic heart disease, exchange transfusions, hyperosmolar feeds and Hirschsprung's disease. Bacterial infection generally appears to be secondary rather than primary, though epidemics of Salmonella and Klebsiella infections in premature baby nurseries may apparently cause necrotising enterocolitis. Breast-feeding is probably protective, but if given as expressed milk it must be fresh and collected in plastic containers to preserve the protective constituents.

Diagnosis

The radiological appearances of pneumatosis intestinalis are diagnostic. There is gas in the submucosal plane of the bowel and, in severe cases, also in the portal venous system. The bowel wall is oedematous and there is evidence of free fluid and inflammatory changes in the parietal peritoneum. Obstruction is characterised by dilated loops with fluid levels and perforation by free gas.

Management

The earlier that treatment is instituted, the greater are the chances of survival. The principles of management are: (1) cessation of oral feeding, (2) maintenance of fluid and nutritional requirements by intravenous feeding, (3) intravenous antimicrobial therapy with a combination of gentamycin and penicillin or cloxacillin, and (4) 12 hourly plain films of the abdomen to assess progress and to identify perforation at an early stage. Surgery is indicated only if the bowel perforates, and possibly for persistent obstruction. All non-viable gut should be excised and the free ends exteriorised since anastomoses frequently break down. Following recovery further surgery will be required to close the enterostomies, and sometimes to relieve any strictures which may have developed. Survival rates depend on the type of patient being treated and the speed and efficacy of treatment, and vary from 12 to over 90 per cent.

OTHER LESIONS

Retropharyngeal intubation (Astley and Roberts, 1970)
During either endotracheal intubation or less commonly whilst passing an oral catheter to exclude oesophageal atresia, the tube may perforate the posterior wall of the pharynx and be passed down the wall of the oesophagus sometimes as far as the diaphragm. Management involves gastric feeding via a fine nasogastric tube for seven to 10 days until healing has occurred; continuous aspiration of upper pharyngeal secretions is necessary during this period.

Swallowed endotracheal tube (Dickson and Fraser, 1967)
This complication results from dislodgement of tubes used for resuscitative intubation of the newborn. The tube usually comes to rest with its upper end in the oesophagus and its lower end on the greater curvature of the stomach, and can easily be removed by oesophagoscopy.

Perforations of the stomach and rectum (Robarts, 1968)
Whether perforation of the stomach is due to trauma from rigid nasogastric tubes, congenital muscle defects or areas of vascular necrosis in the wall is usually difficult to determine. Plain abdominal films reveal a gross pneumoperitoneum. Severe respiratory embarrassment can be temporarily relieved by abdominal aspiration. The results of closure of the perforation are directly proportional to the speed with which this is achieved following the perforation.

The rectum may be perforated by clumsy insertion of a rectal thermometer or from saline washouts, particularly in babies with enterocolitis due to Hirschsprung's disease and in those with stercoral ulceration over a faecal plug. Intraperitoneal perforations result in abscess formation, and sometimes a lethal peritonitis. Closure of the defect and the treatment of any underlying cause are urgently required.

Meconium peritonitis (Rickham, 1955)
Meconium peritonitis results from antenatal perforation of the bowel, usually due to one of the causes already discussed; meconium ileus should not be confused with meconium peritonitis. Minor degrees can sometimes be recognised on microscopic examination of resected length of atretic small bowel. More severe leaks of meconium show up as speckled or diffuse intraperitoneal calcification on plain films of the abdomen, and this appearance may occasionally be seen in the absence of any signs of intestinal obstruction or perforation. The most severe form, giant cystic meconium peritonitis, presents a major problem. The abdominal cavity is divided into two compartments: a meconium- and pus-filled anterior compartment into which air enters after birth; posterior to this lies the intestine, matted together by adhesions and covered by a thick inflammatory membrane and communicating with the cavity through a perforation.

The infant usually presents with gross abdominal distention and intestinal obstruction at birth. A plain film of the abdomen shows a large cavity containing fluid and air in the anterior abdomen, and intra-abdominal calcification. Surgery is mandatory for survival. The cavity should be emptied of its contents, the bowel freed and the perforation exteriorised; this procedure is technically usually difficult and often accompanied by severe bleeding.

Milk bolus obstruction (Cook and Rickham, 1969)
The milk plug, inspissated milk curd, or milk bolus obstruction is usually a clearly defined entity, although certain features overlap with those seen in necrotising enterocolitis and functional intestinal obstruction. The condition appears to be related to feeding infants with cows' milk, particularly when they are fed from birth with reconstituted full-cream powder preparations.

Typically, a previously normal baby develops signs of obstruction around the end of the first week of life. An unusual and confusing feature is that about half the affected infants have blood in their stools, or following rectal examination the finger is blood-stained. Plain films of the abdomen show small bowel obstruction with dilated loops and fluid levels; in the right iliac fossa bowel is replaced by an amorphous appearance suggesting a faecal bolus containing crescents of gas. The diagnosis is best confirmed by a gastrografin enema which may, in itself, relieve the obstruction. If the diagnosis is in doubt or the enema fails to relieve the obstruction, a laparotomy should be performed; the milk bolus can be manually broken up without opening the lumen and the fragments milked down into the colon.

Meconium plug syndrome (Clatworthy *et al.*, 1956; Ellis and Clatworthy, 1966)
In this syndrome the bowel lumen becomes obstructed by a plug of normal meconium. The clinical features are those of an apparently low obstruction which are relieved by the passage of a bolus of meconium following a saline washout or a gastrografin enema. A similar appearance may be seen in short-segment Hirschsprung's disease, the functional intestinal obstruction being associated with a premature or traumatic delivery, and in mild cases of meconium ileus. The long-term prognosis in uncomplicated cases is excellent.

The small left colon syndrome
By providing a name for the apparent obstructions at the splenic flexure of the colon in the neonatal period, Davis, Allen and Favara (1974) made an important contribution to paediatric surgery. Philippart, Reed and Georgeson (1975) further defined the condition in eight cases, all children of diabetic mothers.

The clinical presentation is identical to that of Hirschsprung's disease with failure to pass meconium and abdominal distention. The characteristic finding on a contrast enema is a narrow left colon which is less distensible than normal and relatively aperistaltic with an apparent 'cone' at the splenic flexure; this appearance has been confirmed at laparotomy. The distal colon is ganglionic, and in the majority of cases the obstruction recovers spontaneously with conservative management; rarely caecal perforation has been recorded. The aetiology of the condition and its occurrence in infants of diabetic mothers is unexplained. The greater likelihood of a neonatal obstruction at the splenic flexure being of this nature rather than due to Hirschsprung's disease suggests that when facilities are available for the rapid exclusion of Hirschsprung's disease, the early management should be conservative.

Functional intestinal obstruction (Howat and Wilkinson, 1970)
Idiopathic and functional intestinal obstruction has been alluded to above. It occurs in premature infants, when it may be associated with immaturity of the ganglion cells and reflex arcs. It may also occur following traumatic deliveries in association with neonatal asphyxia, and occasionally for no obvious reason. The clinical features are those of subacute obstruction of the bowel. The baby fails to pass meconium in the first 24 hours of life. Plain films of the abdomen show uniform dilatation of the bowel with gas in the rectum and an absence of fluid levels. Complete recovery is the rule, and the only treatment required is withdrawal of feeds for a short period followed by their gradual resumption.

References

Aaronson, I. & Nixon, H. H. (1972) A clinical evaluation of anorectal pressure studies in the diagnosis of Hirschsprung's disease. *Gut,* **13,** 138.

Astley, R. & Roberts, K. D. (1970) Intubation perforation of the oesophagus in the newborn baby. *British Journal of Radiology,* **43,** 219.

Azar, H., Chrispin, A. R. & Waterston, D. J. (1971) Esophageal replacement with transverse colon in infants and children. *Journal of Pediatric Surgery,* **6,** 3.

Baran, E. M., Houston, H. E., Lynn, H. B. & O'Connell, E. J. (1967) Foramen of Morgagni hernias in children. *Pediatric Surgery,* **62,** 1076.

Bentley, J. F. R. & Smith, J. R. (1960) Developmental posterior enteric remnants and spinal malformations. The split notochord syndrome. *Archives of Disease in Childhood,* **35,** 76.

Bill, A. H. & Grauman, D. (1966) Rationale and technique for stabilisation of the mesentery in cases of non-rotation of the midgut. *Journal of Pediatric Surgery,* **1,** 127.

Bishop, H. C. & Koop, C. E. (1957) Management of meconium ileus, resection, Roux-en-Y anastomosis and ileostomy, irrigation with pancreatic enzymes. *Annals of Surgery,* **145,** 410.

Boley, S. J. & Kleinhaus, S. (1974) Hirschsprung's disease: choice of operation. In *Abdominal Operations,* Vol. 2, 6th edition. London: Butterworths.

Bonham-Carter, R. E., Waterston, D. J. & Aberdeen, E. (1962) Hernia and eventration of the diaphragm in childhood. *Lancet,* **1,** 656.

Clatworthy, H. W., Jr. *et al.* (1956) The meconium plug syndrome. *Surgery,* **39,** 131.

Cook, R. C. M. & Rickham, P. P. (1969) Neonatal intestinal obstruction due to milk curds. *Journal of Pediatric Surgery,* **4,** 599.

Davis, W. S., Allen, R. P. & Favara, B. E. (1974) Neonatal small left colon syndrome. *American Journal of Roentgenology Radium Therapy and Nuclear Medicine,* **120,** 322.

de Lorimer, A. A., Fonkalsrud, E. W. & Hays, D. M. (1969) Congenital atresia and stenosis of the jejunum and ileum. *Surgery,* **65,** 819.

Dickson, J. A. S. (1970) Apple peel small bowel: an uncommon variant of duodenal and jejunal atresia. *Journal of Pediatric Surgery,* **5,** 595.

Dickson, J. A. S. (1975) Keynote address: Necrotising enterocolitis in the newborn infant. *Report of the Sixty-eighth Ross Conference on Pediatric Research.* Columbus, Ohio: Ross Laboratories.

Dickson, J. A. S. & Fraser, G. C. (1967) 'Swallowed' endotracheal tube: a new neonatal emergency. *British Medical Journal,* **2,** 811.

Dickson, J. A. S. & Mearns, M. B. (1975) Meconium ileus. In *Recent Advances in Paediatric Surgery,* 3rd edition, p. 143, ed. Wilkinson, A. W. Edinburgh: Churchill Livingstone.

Dodge, J. A. (1974) A fresh look at pyloric stenosis. In *Modern Trends in Paediatrics,* ed. Apley, J., p. 229. London: Butterworth.

Drainer, I. K. (1974) Gastric oesophagoplasty in the treatment of oesophageal atresia. *Journal of the Royal College of Surgeons of Edinburgh,* **19,** 282.

Dudgeon, D. L., Morrison, C. W. & Woolley, M. (1972) Congenital proximal tracheoesophageal fistula. *Journal of Pediatric Surgery,* **7,** 614.

Duhamel, B. (1956) Une nouvelle operation pour le megacolon congenital: L'abaissement retro-rectal et transanal du colon et son application au traitment de quelques autres malformations. *Presse Medicale,* **64,** 2249.
Eckstein, H. B., Aberdeen, E., Chrispin, A., Nixon, H. H., Waterston, D. J. & Wilkinson, A. (1970) Tracheo-oesophageal fistula without oesophageal atresia. *Zeitschrift fur Kinderchirurgie und Grenzgebiete,* **9,** 43.
Ehrenpreis, T. (1970) Hirschsprung's disease. In *Surgical Conditions in Infancy and Childhood.* Chicago: Year Book Medical Publishers.
Ellis, D. G. & Clatworthy, H. W., Jr. (1966) The meconium plug syndrome revisited. *Journal of Pediatric Surgery,* **1,** 54.
Fonkalsrud, E. W., de Lorimer, A. A. & Hays, D. M. (1969) Congenital atresia and stenosis of the duodenum. A review compiled from the members of the surgical section of the American Academy of Pediatrics. *Pediatrics,* **43,** 79.
Forshall, I. (1961) Duplication of the intestinal tract. *Postgraduate Medical Journal,* **37,** 570.
Fraser, G. C. & Wilkinson, A. W. (1967) Neonatal Hirschsprung's disease. *British Journal of Surgery,* **3,** 7.
Freeman, N. W. (1971) Long-segment Hirschsprung's disease. Proceedings of the Royal Society of Medicine, **64,** 30.
Gilbert, M. G., Menicia, L. F., Brown, W. T. & Linn, B. S. (1968) Staged surgical repair of large omphaloceles and gastroschisis. *Journal of Paediatric Surgery,* **3,** 702.
Hirschsprung, H. (1887) *Jahrbuch Kinderheilkunde,* **27,** 1.
Holder, M., Cloud, D. T., Lewis, J. E. & Pilling, G. P. (1964) Esophageal atresia and tracheo-oesophageal fistula: a survey of its members by the Surgical Section of the American Academy of Pediatrics. *Pediatrics,* **34,** 542.
Holinger, P. H., Johnston, K. C., Potts, W. J. & da Cunha, F. (1954) Conservative and surgical management of benign strictures of the oesophagus. *Journal of Thoracic Surgery,* **28,** 345.
Howat, J. M. & Wilkinson, A. W. (1970) Functional intestinal obstruction in the neonate. *Archives of Disease in Childhood,* **45,** 800.
Irving, I. M. (1967) Exomphalos with macroglossia: a study of eleven cases. *Journal of Paediatric Surgery,* **2,** 499.
Johnson, D. G., Deaner, R. M. & Koop, C. E. (1967) Diaphragmatic hernia in infancy: factors affecting the mortality rate. *Surgery,* **62,** 1082.
Koop, C. E., Schnaufer, L. & Broennie, M. (1974) Esophageal atresia and tracheoesophageal fistula: supportive measures that affect survival. *Pediatrics,* **54,** 558.
Lawson, J. O. N. (1972) Observations on residual segment obstruction in treated Hirschsprung's disease. In *Progress in Pediatric Surgery,* Vol. 4, ed. Rickham, P. P., Hecker, W. & Prevot, J. Munich: Urban and Schwarzenberg.
Lillie, J. G. (1969) The radiology of Hirschsprung's disease in infancy. In *Recent Advances in Paediatric Surgery,* 2nd edition, p. 88, ed. Wilkinson, A. W. London: Churchill.
Lillie, J. G. & Chrispin, A. R. (1972) Investigations and management of neonatal obstruction by gastrografin enema. *Annals of Radiology,* **15,** 237.
Louw, J. H. (1966) Jejunoileal atresia and stenosis. *Journal of Pediatric Surgery,* **1,** 8.
Lynn, H. (1966) Rectal myectomy for aganglionic megacolon. *Mayo Clinic Proceedings,* **41,** 289.
Meier-Ruge, W. (1974) Hirschsprung's disease: its aetiology pathogenesis and differential diagnosis In *Current Topics in Pathology,* **59,** 132. Berlin: Springer-Verlag.
Myres, N. A. (1974) Oesophageal atresia: the epitome of modern surgery. *Annals of the Royal College of Surgeons of England,* **54,** 277.
Neuhauser, E. B. D. (1946) Roentgen changes associated with pancreatic insufficiency in early life. *Radiology,* **46,** 319.
Nixon, H. H. (1964) Review article: Hirschsprung's disease. *Archives of Disease in Childhood,* **39,** 109.
Nixon, H. H. (1972) Anorectal anomalies: with an international proposed classification. *Postgraduate Medical Journal,* **48,** 465.
Perrelli, L. & Wilkinson, A. W. (1975) Mortality in neonatal duodenal obstruction. A review of 76 cases compared with a previous review of 142 cases. *Journal of the Royal College of Surgeons of Edinburgh,* **20,** 365.
Philippart, A. I., Reed, J. O. & Georgeson, K. E. (1975) Neonatal small left colon syndrome: intramural not intraluminal obstruction. *Journal of Pediatric Surgery,* **10,** 733.
Rickham, P. P. (1955) Peritonitis in the neonatal period. *Archives of Disease in Childhood,* **30,** 23.
Rickham, P. P. & Boeckman, C. R. (1965) Neonatal meconium obstruction in the absence of mucoviscidosis. *American Journal of Surgery,* **109,** 173.
Robarts, F. H. (1968) Neonatal perforation of the stomach. *Zeitschrift fur Kinderchirurgie,* Suppl. Zu Bd, **5,** 62.

Santulli, T. V., Kiesewetter, W. B. & Bill, A. H., Jr. (1970) Anorectal anomalies: a suggested international classification. *Journal of Pediatric Surgery,* **5,** 281.
Santulli, T. V., Schullinger, J. N., Heird, W. C., Gongaware, R. G., Wigger, J., Barlow, B., Blanc, W. A. & Berdon, W. E. (1975) Acute necrotising enterocolitis in infancy: a review of 64 cases. *Pediatrics,* **55,** 376.
Singh, A. & Rickham, P. P. (1971) Subtotal colonic replacement of the oesophagus in infancy. *British Journal of Surgery,* **58,** 377.
Soave, F. (1966) Hirschsprung's disease: technique and results of Soave's operation. *British Journal of Surgery,* **53,** 1023.
Swenson, O. (1957) Follow-up on 200 patients treated for Hirschsprung's disease during a ten year period. *Annals of Surgery,* **146,** 706.
Tawes, R. & Nixon, H. H. (1971) Etiology and treatment of small intestinal atresia: analysis of a series of 127 jejuno-ileal atresias and comparison with 62 duodenal atresias. *Surgery,* **69,** 41.
Waterston, D. J., Bonham-Carter, R. E. & Aberdeen, E. A. (1962) Oesophageal atresia: tracheo-oesophageal fistula. A study of survival in 218 infants. *Lancet,* **1,** 819.
White, H. (1956) Meconium ileus. New roentgen sign. *Radiology,* **66,** 567.
Wilkinson, A. W. (1972) Congenital anomalies of the anus and rectum. *Archives of Disease in Childhood,* **47,** 960.
Wilmore, D. W. (1972) Factors correlating with a successful outcome following extensive intestinal resection in newborn infants. *Journal of Pediatrics,* **80,** 88.
Young, D. G. (1969) Anterior abdominal wall defects. In *Recent Advances in Paediatric Surgery,* 2nd edition, Chap. 12, ed. Wilkinson, A. W. London: Churchill.
Young, D. G. & Wilkinson, A. W. (1966) Mortality in neonatal duodenal obstruction. *Lancet,* **2,** 18.

5. Surgical conditions in the infant and older child

J. A. S. Dickson

Appendicitis
Carcinoid syndrome
Intussusception
Remnants of the vitello-intestinal duct
Hiatus hernia and gastro-oesophageal reflux
Caustic strictures of the oesophagus
Achalasia of the cardia
Teratoma of the stomach
Peptic ulcer
Small bowel lymphosarcoma
Polyps
Anal lesions
Abdominal hernias
Swallowed foreign bodies
Abdominal trauma
Peritonitis

As in the neonatal period, the multiplicity and protean nature of the gastrointestinal disorders which require surgical treatment in infancy and later in childhood prevent a clinically useful classification. The sequelae of surgical procedures performed in the newborn may require further surgical intervention in infancy and childhood (e.g. intra-abdominal adhesions or anastamotic stenoses resulting in intestinal obstruction), but these are not discussed in this chapter. The common problems and a miscellaneous group of relatively rare conditions will be considered.

APPENDICITIS

Acute appendicitis is the commonest acute surgical emergency affecting the abdomen and must always be considered in the differential diagnosis of any child presenting with acute abdominal symptoms (Brown, 1956). Although commonest in the older child and young adult, appendicitis occurs at all ages from the first few weeks of life to extreme old age; it is least common and most lethal at these extremes of life. Excluding the first week of life no child is too young to have appendicitis.

Aetiology and pathology

Studies in the experimental animal have demonstrated that obstruction with secondary infection results in acute inflammation of the appendix (Wagensteen and Bowers, 1937), and in man obstruction may be the most important factor in the genesis of the disease. It is probable that obstruction and the resultant increase in intraluminal pressure interferes with venous flow and that these events lead to thrombosis, haemorrhage and oedema, and bacterial invasion of the wall of the appendix. Faecoliths, adhesions, lymphoid hyperplasia and functional factors have all been implicated as causes of obstruction. Alternative hypotheses propose that mucosal ulceration of the mucosa results from viral infections and that the process is perpetuated by secondary bacterial infection. The aetiology of acute appendicitis has not been clearly defined, and it is probable that a variety of factors may act singly or in concert in the development of this common condition.

The pathological process is the same at all ages. An acute inflammatory process progresses to a closed loop obstruction with transmural infection of the wall of the appendix followed by necrosis and perforation. In the older child the appendix becomes wrapped in omentum; in the younger child the omentum is short and tenuous, but the frequently retrocaecal placed appendix is in a naturally walled-off position, and even a free appendix may be sealed off from the general peritoneal cavity by the adherence of loops of bowel. An appendix abscess usually takes a few days to develop from the onset of symptoms. Only in their faster progression do the symptoms and signs in the younger child differ from those in the older.

Clinical features and diagnosis

The triad of abdominal pain, vomiting and a low grade fever with tenderness and guarding in the right iliac fossa are the typical clinical features of appendicitis in the older child. In the younger patient, particularly those under the age of 2 years, the presenting features are fever, vomiting and crying, and the correct diagnosis is often delayed.

In the early stages body temperature is usually raised only up to 38°C but continues to increase with the onset of peritonitis; in young children higher temperatures may occur in the early stages of appendicitis.

The most important single physical signs are persistent tenderness and guarding over the appendix in the right iliac fossa; rebound tenderness is not a helpful sign in childhood. Similarly rectal examination is usually unhelpful under the age of 5 years; in the older child, particularly when diarrhoea is a presenting feature, rectal examination is important in the diagnosis of pelvic appendicitis. A tender mass in the right iliac fossa or one arising from the pelvis is indicative of an appendix abscess.

In the early stages of the disease distinguishing appendicitis from simple colic can be difficult, and a short period of careful clinical observation usually resolves the dilemma. A diagnosis of appendicitis should be suspected in any child with abdominal pain, but the differential diagnosis is formidable. Among the conditions which should be considered are simple colic, possibly related to dietary indiscretions or constipation, mesenteric adenitis, abdominal migraine, viral or bacterial infections of the bowel, urinary tract infections, intussusception, basal pneumonia, torsion of an ovarian cyst or testis, occult abdominal trauma, primary peritonitis, infective hepatitis, deep iliac adenitis and less frequently diabetes mellitus, porphyria and the Henoch Schonlein syndrome. In children of ethnic groups in which sickle-cell disease is prevalent (e.g. those of West African origin), abdominal pain may result from small infarcts on the bowel wall and is best treated conservatively. Appendicitis in these children may be complicated by progressive sickling and vascular obstruction in the mesentery of the terminal ileum and ascending colon.

Appendicitis may occur in association with upper respiratory infections and with measles.

Management, complications and prognosis

In the early or uncomplicated case appendicectomy is simple and satisfactory. After perforation, however, with local or generalised peritonitis intravenous correction of fluid and electrolyte losses and control of the infection by antibiotics should precede removal of the appendix. There is no clear evidence on which antibiotic regimes are best. Either ampicillin or cephaloridine can be used alone, or ampicillin can be combined with cloxacillin or gentamycin; a combination of lincomycin and gentamycin can also be used. An appreciable proportion of intra-abdominal infections following perforation of the appendix are caused by non-sporing anaerobes, particularly by strains of bacteroides. A recent controlled study provides evidence that metronidazole is highly effective in the prevention and treatment of bacteroides infections after appendicectomy; therapeutically effective serum levels of metronidazole were achieved when the drug was administered rectally as suppositories (Willis *et al.*, 1976).

An appendix abscess should usually be drained surgically and the appendix removed during the operation only if this can be performed without disseminating infection within the abdominal cavity.

Conservative management is rarely indicated in children in whom the infection progresses rapidly and unpredictably. A child with a history of longer than two days who has a palpable, clearly defined mass and who is improving should probably be treated conservatively with antibiotics and a fluid diet. Any child who requires intravenous fluids and gastric suction also requires an operation.

Whether an appendix abscess is treated conservatively or by surgical drainage an appendicectomy should be performed after about two to three months since recurrence of the appendicitis is common.

Complications include abscess formation in the wound, in the right and left iliac fossa, in the pelvis and in the subphrenic spaces. Intestinal obstruction secondary to sepsis may be an early complication or may develop later, secondary to adhesions. Incisional hernias occasionally occur.

The overall mortality rate in appendicitis is less than 1 per cent, and most deaths are secondary to infection or to problems in fluid management following delayed diagnosis (Pledger and Buchan, 1969).

CARCINOID SYNDROME

Very rarely in children a carcinoid tumour will be found in an appendix removed for suspected appendicitis. These tumours have the same low potential to metastasise as they do in adults, but the full carcinoid syndrome with diarrhoea, tachycardia, and flushing is very rare in children (Ryden, Drake and Franciosis, 1974). The biochemical hallmark of metastatic carcinoids is the increased urinary output of 5-hydroxyindoleacetic acid.

INTUSSUSCEPTION (see Ravitch, 1959; Dennison and Shaker, 1970)

An intussusception is an invagination of a segment of bowel into an adjoining and usually lower segment. It is an uncommon condition with an incidence of between one and two cases per 1000 live births. In the commonest form, the idiopathic intussusception of childhood, the apex and origin of the intussusception is usually in the terminal ileum or at the ileocaecal valve.

Aetiology and pathology

Children between the ages of 3 months and 2 years are most frequently affected, with a peak incidence between 6 and 9 months. Of all affected patients an obvious precipitating cause (e.g. Meckel's diverticulum, ileal polyps and enteric cysts) is present in only 2 to 7 per cent. Although one of these lesions is more likely to be a precipitating cause in children over the age of 2 years, the idiopathic form is still the commonest. Acute intussusception in the neonatal period is rare but may result in atresias. A seasonal incidence with peaks related to winter upper respiratory tract infections and summer enteritis, combined with a frequent association with mesenteric adenitis, suggests the possibility of a viral aetiology; there is some supportive evidence for this theory (Bell and Steyn, 1962). The occurrence of intussusception in the Henoch Schonlein syndrome and following abdominal surgery, particularly if much retroperitoneal dissection is necessary, suggests that disordered peristalsis may play an aetiological role.

The intussuscepted bowel progresses round the colon and, if the diagnosis is delayed, it can reach and prolapse from the rectum. Strangulation of the gut and irreducibility of the intussusception are most likely when the apex is in the narrow small bowel. In tropical countries, particularly Africa, a form of intussusception in which the apex is in the anterior wall of the caecum is seen in children of all ages (Olumide, Adedeji and Adesola, 1976); strangulation and irreducibility are much less likely in this form.

Clinical features and diagnosis

The signs and symptoms are closely related to the progression of the disease, initial symptoms being colic and vomiting. The spasms of pain are associated with pallor which persists between them, and the patient remains restless and irritable. After the passage of a normal stool the typical red currant jelly stool consisting of blood and mucus is seen. Later the abdomen becomes distended and the vomiting copious and bile-stained. Dehydration and infection spreading through the bowel wall lead to fever and tachycardia. On examining the abdomen the characteristic finding is a sausage-shaped mass with its curve and position following the line of the gut from the ascending colon round to the sigmoid and rectum. Any of the typical clinical features may be missing. The onset of vomiting may be delayed, colic is occasionally absent and an abdominal mass may not be palpable because of positioning behind the liver, muscle guarding or abdominal distention.

Erect and supine plain films of the abdomen are very helpful in confirming the diagnosis. The caecal gas shadow is absent, and there are dilated loops of small bowel leading into the site of the intussusception, which may appear as a soft tissue mass with a crescent of gas outlining its distal margin. If there is any doubt a barium enema will outline the mass in the bowel lumen, as well as often reducing the intussusception.

Management and prognosis

An intussusception is an acute surgical emergency and, as in appendicitis, most deaths are related to dehydration and infection, and when necessary these must be treated prior to any surgery.

The place of a therapeutic barium enema to reduce the intussusception, which can be successful in about 75 per cent of cases, is controversial. In many parts of the world this is the initial treatment of choice, whereas in the United Kingdom most centres prefer the speed and certainty of surgical reduction. When there is a history of less than 24 hours in a child who is in good condition, or when an enema is required for diagnosis, an attempt at reduction is safe and reasonable. Free reflux of barium into the terminal loop of small bowel is the essential sign of a successful reduction, and in its absence the abdomen should be explored. Operative reduction is most easily performed through a transverse supraumbilical incision with most of the procedure under direct vision. There is often a sudden increase in pulse rate and a fall in blood pressure immediately following the reduction. This should be anticipated and treated by an infusion of blood or plasma. An irreducible intussusception should be resected through healthy gut and end-to-end anastomosis performed. In uncomplicated cases with a healthy caecal wall there is no contraindication to appendicectomy.

Recurrences occur in about 5 per cent of cases after both operative and barium enema reduction. The mortality rate is about 1 per cent, and deaths are usually associated with delays in diagnosis and treatment.

REMNANTS OF THE VITELLO-INTESTINAL DUCT

During early intrauterine development the vitello-intestinal duct leads from the midpoint of the developing gut through the umbilicus to the yolk sac. Normally it atrophies and completely disappears, but remnants persist in about 2 per cent of individuals. Most commonly this is at the ileal end as a Meckel's diverticulum which is present in 1 to 2 per cent of all children. Persistence of the umbilical end produces a small everted umbilical polyp which is covered by mucosa; of the midportion an umbilical cyst; and of the whole tract a vitello-intestinal fistula. Occasionally incomplete atrophy leaves a fibrous cord attaching the ileum to the umbilicus, which may form the apex for a volvulus or the trapping band for an internal hernia. The umbilical polyp can be distinguished from the commoner umbilical granuloma by its velvety secreting surface which may cause excoriation of adjacent skin. Both lesions are treated by simple diathermy excision. A patent vitello-intestinal duct allows bowel contents to escape at the umbilicus; the duct is often associated with narrowing of the ileum at its origin. Rarely the gut may intussuscept through the umbilicus. Excision of the track and correction of any ileal narrowing is simple and effective. The rare cyst formed by persistence of the middle region of the duct presents either as an infected abscess or a symptomless mass behind the umbilicus; it should be excised.

Meckel's diverticulum

A Meckel's diverticulum arises from the antimesenteric border of the gut and is usually symptomless. It can contain pancreatic tissue or acid-secreting gastric mucosa; in the latter event there is a risk of peptic ulceration at the junction of the diverticulum with the normal ileum. The commonest presenting feature of peptic ulceration is bleeding, often exanguinating, in the first two years of life. Perforation of the ulcer is very uncommon. A Meckel's diverticulum must be suspected in any young child with severe rectal bleeding. The diagnosis is difficult to confirm using conventional contrast radiology. The acid-secreting mucosa takes up pertechnate and this can be identified as a 'hot spot' on a technetium scan in about 70 per cent of cases (Jewett, Duszynski and Allen, 1970).

Surgical treatment involves excision of the diverticulum together with a segment of ileum to include the ulcer. An inverted diverticulum may form the apex of an intussusception and must be excised following reduction of the intussusception. Diverticulitis of these usually wide-necked diverticulae is very uncommon and clinically indistinguishable from appendicitis. They are easily identified and removed through a standard grid-iron incision. It is usual to excise a Meckel's diverticulum found incidentally at laparotomy in order to prevent later complications.

HIATUS HERNIA AND GASTRO-OESOPHAGEAL REFLUX (see Waterston, 1954; Carré, 1959)

The junction of the oesophagus and stomach is normally situated below the hiatus of the diaphragm leaving a short length of oesophagus within the abdominal cavity. The term hiatus hernia implies that part of the stomach protrudes through the oesophageal hiatus into the chest. Gastro-oesophageal reflux is not synonymous with a hiatus hernia and frequently occurs in babies who have a normally situated gastro-oesophageal junction.

Reflux of gastric contents into the lower oesophagus is common in young infants, particularly during crying or winding; this may result in regurgitation or vomiting of feeds. More severe reflux may result in frequent vomiting and is associated with a range of abnormalities variously referred to as achalasia of the cardia, congenital short oesophagus, partial thoracic stomach and hiatus hernia. It is likely that most of these lesions represent greater or lesser degrees of severity of the same basic anomaly (i.e. a sliding oesophageal hiatus hernia) and they should therefore be classified together.

Clinical features, diagnosis and prognosis

The outstanding symptom is regurgitation and/or vomiting starting in the first week of life occurring after and between feeds. The vomit does not contain bile but may be blood-stained. At this age the differential diagnosis rests between hiatus hernia, hypertrophic pyloric stenosis, simple feeding mismanagement and infections. Minor degrees of reflux recover spontaneously, and in the majority of infants the vomiting resolves by 12 months of age. More severe reflux can be associated with failure to thrive, aspiration of gastric contents and chronic recurrent pulmonary infections, ulceration of the lower oesophagus leading to acute or chronic bleeding, dysphagia from spasm and finally stricture formation. A hiatus hernia and reflux can be associated with hypertrophic pyloric stenosis and an oesophageal hernia following its surgical repair.

A barium swallow and meal by an experienced paediatric radiologist is the essential diagnostic procedure. This will demonstrate the reflux, the presence of spasm or a stricture at the lower oesophagus and define the position of the cardia relative to the diaphragmatic hiatus. Oesophagoscopy is essential to assess the degree of oesophagitis and stricture formation.

Management

The initial management involves thickening the feeds and nursing in an upright sitting position. Specially constructed sitting boxes are necessary for infants with severe vomiting and failure to thrive; these must be used with care since babies are at risk of developing a radial palsy from an arm hanging over the edge and scoliosis from the hunched up position of a hypotonic infant sitting in the box. In many instances it is possible for the baby to sleep in the prone position during the night.

Surgery is only indicated for those infants in whom medical measures fail to control the reflux and who fail to thrive, become anaemic, or develop a stricture. Under the age of 12 months gastropexy, provided this produces an adequate length of oesophagus within the abdominal cavity, combined with tightening of the hiatus is a simple and effective procedure for reflux in the absence of stenosis (Boerema and Germs, 1955). In the presence of stenosis or in children over the age of 12 months, a more major procedure is required. The oesophagus is mobilised to ensure an adequate length within the abdomen and then is retained by a Nissen fundoplication, in which the body of the stomach is wrapped around and sutured in front of the oesophagus (Nissen, 1964). A thoracic approach, which permits better mobilisation of the oesophagus, is preferable. At the time of operation the pylorus should be inspected and, if it is narrowed, a pyloroplasty or pyloromyotomy should be performed. Having controlled the reflux, oesophagitis and spasm will be relieved and residual strictures can be dilated. Rarely severe strictures with destruction of much of the lower oesophagus require resection and colonic replacement.

CAUSTIC STRICTURES OF THE OESOPHAGUS

The accidental ingestion of corrosives (most commonly liquid caustic soda preparations) can result in ulceration of the mouth, extensive destruction of the oesophagus and less commonly the stomach and duodenum; the end-result may be one or more oesophageal strictures. Spill-over into the upper respiratory tract can produce scarring and strictures in and around the larynx.

Emergency treatment consists of corticosteroids (e.g. prednisone 2 mg/kg/day for three weeks), and antibiotics to control infection and to reduce the degree of scarring during the healing process. Early oesophagoscopy and the passage of a nasogastric tube permits early feeding and maintains a dilatable channel. Impenetrable strictures must be excised and replaced by colon.

ACHALASIA OF THE CARDIA (see Ellis and Olsen, 1969)

Achalasia of the cardia refers to a failure of the lower end of the oesophagus to relax and, although predominantly a disease of adult life, it may occur in older children. The typical clinical features are dysphagia and retrosternal discomfort relieved by regurgitation of food and weight loss. Differential diagnoses include oesophageal stricture and anorexia nervosa in older children. The appearances of a barium swallow are diagnostic: the oesophagus is dilated and terminates in a distal 'rat tail', the barium moving slowly into the stomach. Balloon pressure studies will confirm the disordered oesophageal motility. Treatment is either by balloon dilatation or Heller's oesophageal myotomy. The immediate results are excellent, but the long-term prognosis is less certain.

TERATOMA OF THE STOMACH (see Atwell, Claireaux and Nixon, 1967; de Angelis, 1969)

Teratomas of the stomach are very rare, and in children they are nearly always benign. Presenting symptoms include upper abdominal pain, vomiting and an epigastric mass which often shows calcification on a plain film of the abdomen. As with other rare tumours of the stomach (e.g. adenoma, lipoma, leiomyoma) treatment involves excision of the tumour and the involved part of the stomach.

PEPTIC ULCER (see Tudor, 1972)

The incidence of peptic ulcer disease in childhood has not been clearly established. In some parts of the world it is probably overdiagnosed whereas in other parts the reverse is true.

Clinical features and diagnosis

Acute ulcers

Acute gastric or duodenal ulcers may occur in the neonatal period and infancy following acute stresses such as severe respiratory distress. They can present with bleeding, perforation or obstruction.

In later childhood acute peptic ulcers may occur in association with severe stress situations such as severe burns (Curling's ulcer), meningitis (Cushing's ulcer) or the administration of corticosteroids. They are more likely to occur in children with previously proven ulcers or with conditions which are known to be associated with peptic ulceration (e.g. cirrhosis, chronic lung disease, hypertrophic pyloric stenosis and following small intestinal resection). These stress ulcers are equally distributed between the stomach and duodenum, and there is no sex predilection.

Severe bleeding with haematemesis or melaena is usually the presenting feature of acute stress ulcers irrespective of the age of the child. The bleeding does not often resolve with conservative measures, and surgery may be necessary.

Chronic ulcers

Chronic peptic ulcers are seen predominantly in children from school age upwards. The symptom of abdominal pain relieved by alkali, food or vomiting is similar to that seen in adults; there is frequently a strong family history of peptic ulcer disease. Generally speaking males are affected more frequently than females (3:2), and duodenal ulcers are commoner than gastric ulcers (8:1).

The Zollinger–Ellison syndrome (Wilson, Schulte and Meade, 1971) should be considered in older children when symptoms are resistant to convential therapy, who have multiple or past bulbar ulcers, or who develop recurrent ulceration after operation.

The diagnosis of acute or chronic peptic ulceration in childhood is based on the clinical features, radiology and endoscopy. Barium studies should be interpreted by an experienced paediatric radiologist, since fear and anxiety may considerably influence the appearance of the duodenum during such studies. Gastric acid studies are of little help in diagnosis. The recent development of fibre endoscopy may well prove to be a very useful diagnostic technique, particularly in those children in whom there is an impressive history of peptic ulcer disease but in whom radiological investigations are inconclusive.

Management

Acute stress ulcers require emergency treatment when associated with bleeding, perforation or obstruction. Treatment and control of any precipitating cause is as important as management of the complications of the ulcer.

In the chronic adult type of peptic ulcer, medical treatment is aimed at neutralisation of gastric acidity by food or antacid preparations. Frequent snacks are just as effective as antacids and easily become a part of a child's routine. In very anxious patients a tranquillizer such as diazepam may be helpful. For the ulcer not responding to medical treatment, surgery should be considered. Gastroenterostomy, partial gastrectomy and vagotomy with a drainage procedure have all been performed, but it seems likely that a highly selective vagotomy will prove to be the operation of choice. In patients with the Zollinger–Ellison syndrome total gastrectomy with removal of accessible adenomas and their secondaries has been the procedure of choice. If removal of a tumour restores the serum gastrin level to normal and it remains normal, however, total gastrectomy can be avoided. Children of any age thrive remarkably well after total gastrectomy (Rosenlund, 1967).

SMALL BOWEL LYMPHOSARCOMA

Lymphosarcoma arises from the lymphoid tissue in the wall of the gut or from the lymph nodes in the mesentery, the commonest sites being the distal jejunum and ileum. Although rare it is about the fifth commonest malignant disease of childhood. The clinical presentations are variable and include intussusception, progressive chronic intestinal obstruction with malabsorption and general malaise with a palpable abdominal mass. It is seldom possible to achieve a complete surgical excision of the tumour, but the obstruction can usually be relieved either by a bypass or by excision of the strictured area. The lesion is radiosensitive and radiotherapy can be combined with chemotherapeutic regimes similar to those used in acute leukaemia.

Although a complete remission can be expected, recurrence occurs in most cases and is then resistant to further therapy.

POLYPS

Peutz–Jeghers syndrome (See Dormandy, 1957)

This rare syndrome is characterised by mucocutaneous pigmentation of the lips, face and fingers, and is associated with gastrointestinal polyposis. The polyps may cause intussusceptions and gastrointestinal bleeding leading to anaemia. The polyps are usually benign though malignant changes may occasionally develop. The condition is inherited in an autosomal dominant fashion. Treatment is chiefly supportive, surgery being reserved for the relief of complications since excision of all the polyps is not possible.

Familial polyposis coli (see Sachatello, Pickren and Grace, 1970; Calabro, 1962)

Although commoner than the Peutz–Jeghers syndrome, familial polyposis is still a rare disease with an incidence of about one in every 8300 births; it is transmitted as an autosomal dominant. Multiple adenomatous polyps develop insidiously throughout the large intestine and, if left, invariably undergo malignant change. Symptoms rarely develop before the age of 10 years, although cases have been identified as early as 2 years of age and malignant changes have been reported by the age of 13 years.

The presenting clinical features are usually diarrhoea and the passage of blood and mucus in the stools. Sigmoidoscopy and barium enema show the unmistakable appearance of the colon carpeted by polyps. Treatment is surgical and excision of the colon is essential. Initially this was combined with an ileostomy and proctectomy. More recently an ileoproctostomy followed by regular inspection of the rectum and diathermy destruction of the polyps has been advocated. It is possible, however, that stripping of the mucosa from the rectum down to the anal canal, followed by an endorectal pull-through of the ileum into the rectum, will prove to be the best procedure.

Generalised juvenile polyposis

It has been suggested that generalised juvenile polyposis represents an hereditary syndrome distinct from the Peutz-Jeghers syndrome, familial polyposis coli, juvenile polyposis coli and isolated juvenile retention polyps (Sachatello *et al.*, 1970). Numerous polyps develop in the stomach, small bowel, colon and rectum. The polyps are smooth or lobulated and contain multiple mucin-containing cysts, which accounts for the term 'retention polyps'. They vary in diameter from a few millimetres to a few centimetres and, in contrast to the adenomatous polyps of adult life, are benign lesions. They may show features of haemorrhage secondary to infarction from torsion of the polyp on its pedicle, inflammation and hamartomatous malformation. Children present with recurrent episodes of abdominal pain secondary to repeated intussusceptions, they may pass the polyps rectally and patients may also have chronic gastrointestinal bleeding. The extensive gastrointestinal involvement precludes surgical treatment, except for relief of episodes of intussusception and obstruction.

Juvenile polyps

This entity is distinct from generalised juvenile polyposis (Veale *et al.*, 1966). There is usually a family history of polyps, the polyps appear during the first decade of life and may be solitary or multiple. Histologically they are identical to the polyps seen in generalised juvenile polyposis and they are not premalignant. They cause rectal bleeding, recurrent episodes of abdominal pain and frequently prolapse through the rectum. Some polyps are palpable on rectal examination, and others can be visualised on sigmoidoscopy. A double contrast barium enema will usually identify polyps from the proximal colon. Those polyps which are not accessible via sigmoidoscopy can be visualised and removed using a fibrendoscopy instrument.

Adenomatous polyps

Adenomatous polyps present in a similar way to those described above but are premalignant. They should be removed together with their basal mucus membrane.

ANAL LESIONS

Anal fissure

Anal fissures are common lesions in childhood, particularly in infants and young children. In the infant fissures may be multiple and secondary to oedema and inflammation of the perianal skin, as well as to passage of hard stools. Treatment should be directed to the underlying cause (e.g. ammoniacal dermatitis or candidiasis).

In the older child fissures nearly always result from the passage of hard stools. The fissure is a submucosal split which may be associated with a sentinel pile from the tearing down of one of the anal valves. The lesion is initially very painful and accompanied by bleeding. This pain is usually of short duration, and problems chiefly arise from the pain of defaecation leading to a deliberate holding back of stool with further stretching of the fissure when it is passed. Crohn's disease and ulcerative colitis should be considered in children with chronic fissures.

Most fissures probably heal spontaneously. Treatment is aimed at maintaining soft stools until the fissure has healed; topical anaesthetic creams, so helpful in adults, are of little value in children since they must be applied immediately before the passage of a stool to be effective. Fissures which do not heal within a few weeks should be biopsied and examined histologically, and at the same time the anus should be dilated (Watts, Bennett and Goligher, 1965).

Perianal sepsis

Perianal abscess

Perianal abscesses are common and present with a painful swelling in the anal region. They arise from subcutaneous bleeding, secondary to an acute thrombotic pile, from cracks or fissures, or with no apparent precipitating cause. Early incision and unroofing of the abscess is essential to avoid extension and fistula formation.

Ischiorectal abscesses are less common and require early incision and free drainage; occasionally these may be secondary to foreign bodies perforating the rectum.

Fistula in ano

A fistula *in ano* can arise secondary to an abscess or as a complication of inflammatory bowel disease. Fistulae usually present as abscesses which recur after apparent healing following incision and drainage. Superficial fistulae are easily treated by excision and laying open of the track. Histological examination of the specimen for evidence of chronic inflammatory bowel disease is essential. High level fistulae with an internal opening above the puborectalis are more difficult to manage but are fortunately rare.

Rectal prolapse

Prolapse of the rectum may be due to herniation of the rectal wall in association with paralysis or defects of the pelvic floor muscles, as in children with spina bifida. Rectal prolapse may also be associated with chronic diarrhoea, as in cystic fibrosis, or with constipation. The first essential in treatment is correction of the underlying cause. Manual reduction of the prolapse is usually simple but recurrence with the next bowel action is common. Prolapses are most easily reduced immediately after they occur, and this is usually necessary with decreasing frequency. Occasionally strapping together of the buttocks is necessary to maintain the prolapsed rectum reduced. When these measures are unsuccessful submucosal injection of phenol in almond oil, as for haemorrhoids in adults, is often effective. Only rarely is it necessary to resort to a circumferential perianal stitch or more complicated repair procedures.

Haemorrhoids

Internal haemorrhoids are rare in childhood and seldom require any treatment. They may not be apparent in patients examined under general anaesthesia, since they are best seen in the conscious child who is voluntarily straining during examination with an anal speculum.

ABDOMINAL HERNIAS

External abdominal hernias in children may occur in the inguinal region through a persistent processus vaginalis, at the umbilicus through an incompletely closed umbilical ring, through defects in the supraumbilical linea alba (i.e. supraumbilical and epigastric hernias) or down the femoral canal. Incisional hernias may arise following the repair of difficult diaphragmatic hernias and congenital umbilical defects or may result from sepsis and faulty healing of abdominal wounds. Rare hernias, like gluteal and obturator hernias, are only diagnosed at laparotomy for intestinal obstruction. Direct inguinal hernias and false hernias secondary to muscle paralysis are rare and seldom seen apart from children with spina bifida. The importance of all hernias lies in the risk of irreducibility with obstruction and possible strangulation of loops of gut.

Inguinal hernia

Indirect inguinal hernias occur in 1 per cent of children with a male to female sex ratio of 10:1. A swelling in the inguinal region and/or scrotum may be noticed at any age, and irreducible hernias are most likely at the time of their initial appearance and during the first six months of life. True strangulation with infarction of gut is rare, but pressure on the testicular vessels can result in thrombosis and infarction of the testis. There is usually no difficulty in identifying an inguinal hernia as the cause of an intestinal obstruction; small hernias may, however, be missed or the hernia may have spontaneously reduced itself before the child is seen, when the only clues will be thickening and oedema of the cord and oedema of the testis.

In the differential diagnosis other inguinal swellings such as a communicating hydrocele, particularly when associated with ascites, a hydrocele of the cord, an undescended testis and enlarged lymph nodes, should be considered. When there is a history of recurrent inguinal swelling and there is no obvious hernia apparent at the time of examination, gentle rolling of the spermatic cord over the pubic bone will enable the experienced examiner to identify the presence of a sac. Girls with bilateral indirect inguinal hernias should have buccal scrape studies for sex chromatin to exclude the testicular feminisation syndrome.

Management

Management depends on whether the hernia is irreducible or not. Strangulation rarely complicates an irreducible inguinal hernia, and surgery can be technically very difficult. Most hernias can be reduced by sedating the child and nursing in a head down position; gentle manual pressure may be necessary to complete reduction. An elective herniotomy should be performed two days later. If these conservative measures fail to reduce the hernia, emergency surgery is necessary.

An elective herniotomy for children with reducible hernias is a simple procedure in all except very small babies. It should be performed as soon as possible following diagnosis so that the risks of irreducibility and strangulation are avoided.

Umbilical hernia

Umbilical hernias result from a circular defect at the umbilical cicatrix and are particularly common in negroid children. Strangulation and rupture of the sac may occur but is very rare. Most umbilical hernias remain asymptomatic and close spontaneously. Surgery is only very occasionally performed before the age of 5, and hardly ever before the age of 2 years. A short period of strapping, not exceeding six weeks, should be considered in infants less than 3 months of age who have repeated episodes of crying with swelling of the hernia. In the older child omentum may become trapped in an almost closed hernia causing obscure abdominal pain which is completely relieved by herniotomy.

Supraumbilical and epigastric hernias

These are usually merely protrusions of extraperitoneal fat through defects in the linea alba. A supraumbilical hernia is distinguished from a true umbilical hernia not by its relation to the umbilicus but by its eliptical or transverse slit shape. Both supraumbilical and epigastric hernias may cause pain as a result of trapping of their contents. Surgical repair is simple and relieves any symptoms.

Femoral hernia

Femoral hernias are only occasionally seen in children. The swelling is below the inguinal ligament and lateral to the pubic tubercle.

SWALLOWED FOREIGN BODIES

Children have a notorious tendency to swallow foreign bodies of all types. Objects such as coins or pebbles may become lodged in the upper oesophagus, when they may cause dysphagia and, if left for any length of time, lead to ulceration and stricture formation; alternatively they may be held up at the site of an already existing stricture. They must be removed as soon as possible under direct vision through an oesophagoscope. Most foreign bodies which reach the stomach will pass through the remaining gut spontaneously. With blunt objects such as coins and marbles, considerable patience may be required. Sharp objects may arrest at any part of the gut and result in perforation; long objects may arrest in the tight bends of the duodenum and ulcerate through the bowel wall. If objects such as these have failed to progress over a period of 24 hours or the child develops abdominal pain and tenderness, surgical exploration and removal is indicated.

Most objects, even those not normally considered radio-opaque, will be visible on a soft tissue exposure of the abdomen and their progress can be easily followed. This is fortunate since searching the stools for foreign bodies, though always recommended, is often unsuccessful.

Trichobezoar

This term refers to a collection of hair as a ball in the stomach and results from a child swallowing his own hair, and wool and fluff from garments and blankets. It is usually associated with underlying psychopathology. The clinical features are abdominal pain, anorexia and a mobile mass in the epigastrium. A barium meal shows the barium to be trapped in the interstices of the hair ball. Laparotomy is necessary to remove hair balls.

ABDOMINAL TRAUMA

The diagnosis is easy when there is a clear-cut history of a fall or a road traffic accident, but it may be more difficult in children who deny injuries incurred in forbidden activities or in young children with non-accidental injuries inflicted by adults. The most frequently affected organs are the spleen, kidney, liver, gut and mesentery, and pancreas. Gut lesions include rupture and haematomata of the duodenum and tears of the mesentery. Rupture of a hollow viscus is rapidly followed by peritonitis, and rupture of solid organs is accompanied by the signs of acute blood loss.

Duodenal haematomas are caused by blunt trauma from falls, such as on to the back of a chair or over the handlebars of a bicycle. The clinical features are those of duodenal obstruction, and barium studies show narrowing and obstruction usually in the second part of the duodenum. If the diagnosis is in doubt a laparotomy should be performed and the haematoma evacuated. If the diagnosis is certain most cases will recover spontaneously after a week to 10 days with conservative management.

PERITONITIS

Peritonitis may be primary or secondary to another focus within the peritoneal cavity. Primary infections of the peritoniteum, which are becoming increasingly less common, are due to the pneumococcus or streptococcus or occasionally viruses. Patients with the nephrotic syndrome, immune deficiency states and pneumococcal pneumonia are particularly likely to develop primary peritonitis. Secondary peritonitis may complicate appendicitis, intussusception, Meckel's diverticulum, peptic ulcer and intra-abdominal surgery.

Clinically there is abdominal pain, distention, generalised tenderness and guarding, vomiting and often diarrhoea; there is associated general malaise, a high fever and sometimes shock. The white cell count is strikingly increased to 20 000 to 50 000 cells per cubic millimetre and, although the diagnosis can be confirmed by needle aspiration of the peritoneum, it is more usually made at laparotomy. Appropriate intravenous antibiotics should be administered in large doses for at least 10 days.

Tuberculous peritonitis (see Singh, Bhargava and Jain, 1969; Borhanmanesh *et al.*, 1972)

Tuberculous peritonitis remains a relatively common disease in the developing parts of the world but is very rare in industrialised countries. The peritoneum becomes infected secondary to small bowel and/or mesenteric lymph node involvement. The diagnosis is confirmed by histology and culture, and treatment is with the conventional antituberculous drugs.

References

Atwell, J. D., Claireaux, A. E. & Nixon, H. H. (1967) Teratoma of the stomach in the newborn. *Journal of Pediatric Surgery,* **2,** 197.

Bell, T. M. & Steyn, J. H. (1962) Viruses in lymph nodes of children with mesenteric adenitis and intussusception. *British Medical Journal,* **2,** 700.

Boerema, I. & Germs, R. (1955) Fixation of the lesser curvature of the stomach to the anterior abdominal wall after reposition of the hernia through the oesophageal hiatus. *Archives of Chirurgie,* **7,** 351.

Borhanmanesh, F., Hekmat, K., Vaezzadeh, K. & Rezai, H. (1972) Tuberculous peritonitis: prospective study of 32 cases in Iran. *Annals of Internal Medicine,* **76,** 567.

Brown, J. J. M. (1956) Acute appendicitis in infancy and childhood. *Journal of the Royal College of Surgeons of Edinburgh,* **1,** 268.

Calabro, J. J. (1962) Hereditable multiple polyposis syndromes of the gastrointestinal tract. *American Journal of Medicine,* **33,** 276.

Carre, I. J. (1959) The natural hitory of partial thoracic stomach (hiatus hernia) in children. *Archives of Disease in Childhood,* **34,** 344.

de Angelis, V. R. (1969) Gastric teratoma in a newborn infant. Total gastrectomy with survival. *Surgery,* **66,** 794.

Dennison, W. M. & Shaker, M. (1970) Intussusception in infancy and childhood. *The British Journal of Surgery,* **57,** 679.

Dormandy, T. L. (1957) Gastrointestinal polyposis with mucocutaneous pigmentation. Peutz–Jeghers syndrome. *New England Journal of Medicine,* **256,** 1093, 1141, 1186.

Ellis, F. H. & Olsen, A. M. (1969) *Achalasia of the Esophagus.* Philadelphia: Saunders.

Jewett, T. C., Duszynski, D. O. & Allen, J. E. (1970) The visualisation of Meckel's diverticulum with ^{99}mTc-pertechnetate. *Surgery,* **68,** 567.

Nissen, R. (1964) The treatment of hiatal hernia and esophageal reflux by fundoplication. In *Hernia,* ed. Nyhus, L. M. & Harkins, H. M., p. 488. Philadelphia: Lippincott.

Olumide, F., Adedeji, A. & Adesola, A. O. (1976) Intestinal obstruction in Nigerian children. *Journal of Pediatric Surgery,* **11,** 195.

Pledger, H. G. & Buchan, R. (1969) Deaths in children with acute appendicitis. *British Medical Journal,* **2,** 466.

Ravitch, M. M. (1959) *Intussusception in Children.* Springfield, Illinois: Thomas.

Rosenlund, M. L. (1967) The Zollinger–Ellison syndrome in children: a review. *American Journal of Medical Science,* **254,** 884.

Ryden, S. E., Drake, R. M. & Franciosis, R. (1974) Carcinoid neoplasms of the appendix in children. *American Journal of Pathology,* **74,** 149.

Sachatello, C. R., Pickren, J. W. & Grace, J. T. (1970) Generalized juvenile gastrointestinal polyposis. *Gastroenterology,* **58,** 699.

Singh, M., Bhargava, A. & Jain, K. (1969) Tuberculous peritonitis. *New England Journal of Medicine,* **281,** 1091.

Tudor, R. B. (1972) Gastric and duodenal ulcers in children. *Gastroenterology,* **62,** 823.

Veale, A. M., McCole, I., Bussey, H. J. & Morson, B. C. (1966) Juvenile polyposis coli. *Journal of Medical Genetics,* **3,** 5.

Wagensteen, O. H. & Bowers, W. F. (1937) Significance of the obstructive factor in the genesis of acute appendicitis. *Archives of Surgery,* **34,** 496.

Waterston, D. J. (1954) Hiatus hernia. In *Recent Advances in Paediatrics.* London: Churchill.

Watts, J. M., Bennett, R. C. & Goligher, J. C. (1965) Stretching of anal sphincters in the treatment of fissure-in-ano. *British Medical Journal,* **2,** 342.

Willis, A. T., Ferguson, I. R., Jones, P. H., Phillips, K. D., Tearle, P. V., Berry, R. B., Fiddian, R. V., Graham, D. F., Harland, D. H. C., Innes, D. B., Mee, W. M., Rothwell-Jackson, R. L., Sutch, I., Kilbey, C. & Edwards, D. (1976) Metronidazole in prevention and treatment of bacteroides infections after appendicectomy. *British Medical Journal,* **1,** 318.

Wilson, S. D., Schulte, W. J. & Meade, R. C. (1971) Longevity studies following total gastrectomy in children with the Zollinger–Ellison syndrome. *Archives of Surgery,* **103,** 108.

6. Chronic inflammatory bowel disease

J. A. S. Dickson

Ulcerative colitis
Crohn's disease (regional enteritis)
Acute terminal ileitis and its relation to Crohn's disease

On a worldwide basis the commonest causes of chronic inflammatory bowel disease are schistosomiasis, amoebiasis and tuberculosis. These conditions are all rare in the developed parts of the world, and in this chapter chronic inflammatory bowel disease refers to ulcerative colitis and Crohn's disease. The clinical features of both diseases overlap, diagnostic difficulties occur in up to 20 to 25 per cent of cases and in a small proportion of patients certain differentiation may not be possible (Kirsner, 1975).

ULCERATIVE COLITIS

Ulcerative colitis is a chronic disease affecting the large bowel characterised by ulceration and inflammation of the mucosa; in contrast, in Crohn's disease the lesions are transmural. The disease pursues a chronic subacute course, or one with alternation between acute relapses and quiescent remissions, or any mixture of these. The following general accounts of ulcerative colitis are suggested for further reading: Edwards and Truelove, 1963; Davidson, Bloom and Kugler, 1965; Broberger and Lagercrantz, 1966; Davidson, 1967; Wright, 1970; de Dombal, 1971.

Epidemiology

The overall incidence of the disease appears to be increasing. The age distribution in childhood is shown in Figure 6.1. The decline in numbers seen after the peak is probably accounted for by children over the ages of 8 to 10 years being referred to adult clinics where the incidence is greatest between the third and sixth decades of life. The high incidence of the disease during the first year of life is as yet unexplained. The overall annual incidence rate of all ages varies between 3 and 6 per 100 000, and in childhood this is below 4 per 100 000. In contrast to adults, both sexes are equally affected in childhood. The disease is commoner in white compared with non-white races and Jews appear to be particularly susceptible; it also appears to be commoner in people from the higher socioeconomic groups of society.

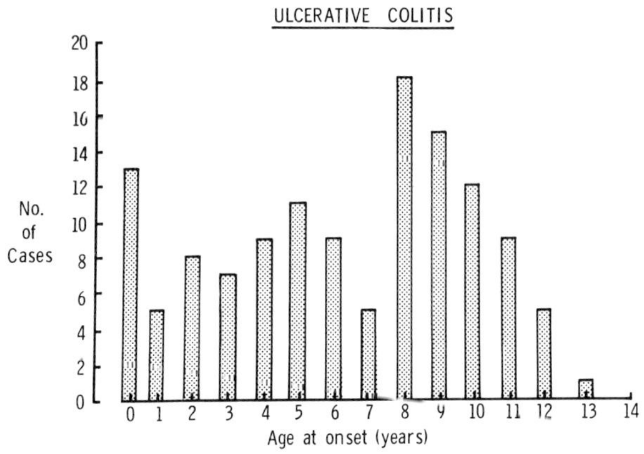

Fig. 6.1 Age distribution of ulcerative colitis in childhood

Aetiology

The aetiology of ulcerative colitis is not known but a variety of explanations have been proposed, including infective, genetic, psychosomatic and immunological causes.

Four of the 33 children described in Table 6.1 had close relatives with inflammatory bowel disease (ulcerative colitis in three and Crohn's disease in one), and other studies indicate that 10 to 15 per cent of the members of a family with ulcerative colitis also have the disease. Psychological trauma in some patients may influence the onset and course of the disease, but this is probably not of major aetiological importance. Immunological abnormalities have been described, but their significance is not yet clear.

Clinical features

Gastrointestinal

With the rare exception of fulminating toxic colitis the presenting symptoms are related to the chronic mucosal ulceration, and the symptoms in 33 patients presenting at the Hospital for Sick Children are listed in Table 6.1. Bloody diarrhoea is the presenting symptom in the vast majority of children, although

Table 6.1 Symptoms in 33 patients with ulcerative colitis presenting at The Hospital for Sick Children, Great Ormond Street

Symptom	Number of patients with Symptom
Diarrhoea	33
Blood in stools	32
Slime in stools	18
Joint pain	2
Listlessness	1

macroscopic blood may rarely be absent from the stools throughout the course of the disease. The blood coats the surface of the stool as well as being mixed within it; some of the stools, which are associated with urgency, consist only of slime, mucus and pus with shreds of mucosa. Thus bleeding and diarrhoea are closely related though not all stools will be blood-stained. The diarrhoea is often most troublesome on rising in the morning, tending to improve during the day; when present nocturnal diarrhoea is particularly wearing for the patient and family. Abdominal pain may be vague, generalised and persistent, but cramping, lower abdominal pain preceding defaecation is more usual. Anorexia, listlessness, nausea, weight loss and an intermittent low grade fever are common. Growth failure may occasionally be a feature, as may delayed puberty be in older children.

The signs on clinical examination are usually nonspecific. There is often evidence of weight loss and a hypochromic anaemia with a raised erythrocyte sedimentation rate. Only in the presence of toxic megacolon is there abdominal distention, and tenderness over a spastic colon is more common. Anal fissures and/or fistulae and perianal or ischiorectal abscesses are much less frequent than in Crohn's disease.

Extraintestinal

Extraintestinal manifestations of ulcerative colitis include erythema nodosum and pyoderma gangrenosum, recurrent mouth ulcers, arthritis and ankylosing spondylitis (McEwen, Lingg and Kirsner, 1962; Jayson, Salmon and Harrison, 1970), ocular lesions (Wright *et al.*, 1965), and liver disease (Eode, 1970; Perrett *et al.*, 1971).

Diagnosis

Bacterial (i.e. Salmonella, Shigella and certain strains of *E. coli*) and amoebic dysentery must be excluded by cultures of fresh specimens of stool.

Radiology

A plain abdominal film may show an abnormal colonic gas pattern with oedema of the bowel wall and a loss of the normal haustral pattern. Spastic regions will be devoid of gas; the absence of gas from the rectum indicates rectal involvement, and mucosal islands (pseudopolypi) may be present in the bowel wall. A double contrast barium enema will confirm the abnormal mucosal pattern with ulceration, loss of haustration and disordered motility. Submucosal abscess cavities may be clearly seen in advanced disease when the whole mucosal pattern is lost. On the lateral view of the pelvis widening of the space between the rectum and sacrum is a sign of proctitis.

Endoscopy

Direct inspection and biopsy of the rectal and colonic mucosa with the conventional rigid sigmoidoscope or a fibre optic colonoscope is the method of choice for establishing the diagnosis. The endoscopic appearances may be abnormal even in the presence of a normal barium enema and should be performed in children who present with clinical features suggestive of ulcerative colitis in whom radiological investigations are normal. In young children endoscopy is more safely performed under general anaesthesia, but in older co-operative children the procedure can be performed under heavy sedation (e.g. intravenous diazepam). The gross and microscopic features are the same as those seen in adults. In early disease the appearances are those of a red velvety mucosa with loss of the vascular pattern and multiple mucosal haemorrhages; contact bleeding is easily produced. In more advanced disease there are patchy superficial ulcers, which are variable in extent, and residual islands of mucosa (pseudopolypi) surrounded by a raw granulating surface. Following successful medical treatment all these mucosal abnormalities can resolve completely. Biopsies confirm the diagnosis and may reveal inflammatory changes even in the absence of ulceration. Differentiation from Crohn's disease is not possible in 10 to 20 per cent of cases. The histological appearances under light microscopy are: (1) diffuse infiltration of the mucosa with chronic inflammatory cells, mainly lymphocytes and plasma cells but also eosinophils, (2) vascular congestion and mucosal haemorrhages, and (3) goblet cell depletion and reactive hyperplasia, and some of the tubules contain an accumulation of polymorphonuclear leucocytes forming crypt abscesses. In active chronic disease there is an increase in mucosal lymphoid tissue. Initially remissions are accompanied by complete resolution of the mucosal abnormalities, but with recurrent attacks the mucosa becomes permanently atrophic and ultimately shows metaplasia of the Paneth cells.

Fibre optic colonoscopy makes it possible to define the extent of the large bowel disease and to differentiate between granular proctitis and proctocolitis. Total colonic involvement is commoner in children compared with adults and was present in 19 of the series of 33 patients seen at The Hospital for Sick Children.

Management

In the management of a child with confirmed ulcerative colitis it is essential to acknowledge that (1) the disease is usually life-long, (2) interference with growth and schooling may leave a permanent legacy to carry into adult life, (3) an ileostomy may cause severe emotional disturbances around puberty, and (4) the long-term risks of carcinoma of the colon.

Medical

General measures. Faecal losses of water, sodium, chloride, potassium and bicarbonate may result in dehydration, hypokalaemia and metabolic acidosis, and these abnormalities must be corrected. Blood loss may lead to an iron deficiency anaemia which, in mild to moderate disease, can be corrected with oral or parenteral iron. In severe disease anaemia may be accompanied by hypoalbuminaemia, and in these circumstances blood transfusion serves a dual purpose. There is no good evidence that a low-residue diet is beneficial, but some patients may benefit from a milk-free diet possibly due to an allergy to cows' milk protein. The diet should be appetising and contain adequate protein and calories. Opiates and anticholinergic agents should be avoided since they may predispose to the development of toxic megacolon. There is no good evidence that psychotherapy is beneficial, but it may be helpful for some children.

Specific measures. Cortisone or its analogues are the agents of choice for inducing a remission, and sulphasalazine (Salazopyrin) is the drug of choice for maintaining the remission (Truelove and Witts, 1954, 1955; Dissanayake and Truelove, 1973). Azathioprine in combination with steroids may be of value in some patients with relapse of established disease and may permit a reduction in steroid dosage (Rosenberg *et al.*, 1975). Steroids can be administered intravenously, orally or rectally according to the severity and extent of the disease. Their side-effects can be minimised by an alternate day regime. The side-effects of sulphasalazine include haematological abnormalities such as haemolytic anaemia, methaemoglobinaemia, macrocytosis, leukopenia, thrombocytopenia and aplastic anaemia, and hypersensitivity reactions such as the Stevens–Johnson syndrome, exfoliative dermatitis and photosensitisation.

In children with moderate to severe disease (excluding toxic megacolon) treatment is started with a combination of prednisolone (2 mg/kg/day) and sulphasalazine (1–3 g/day depending on age of patient). If a remission is achieved the dose of prednisolone is reduced after two to three weeks in a slow step-wise fashion and withdrawn after a further period of four to eight weeks. Sulphasalazine is continued indefinitely at the same dosage unless side-effects supervene. If this regime is unsuccessful intravenous steroids or ACTH are considered. In mild distal disease remission can be induced with steroid suppositories, or fluid or foam retention enemas, and the remission maintained with oral sulphasalazine.

Surgery

Most children with moderate to severe disease will come to surgery but often not until early adult life. Because of the risk of carcinoma elective surgery should be considered in all children with a 10-year history of disease, particularly when there is total colonic involvement. The indications for surgery are:

1. Toxic megacolon not responding to medical treatment within 48 to 72 hours (see below), or severe acute disease not responding to intensive medical treatment within four to eight days.
2. Chronic disease leading to growth failure, delayed puberty or serious interference with schooling.
3. Colonic perforation.
4. Severe local (e.g. perianal fistulae or abscesses) or systemic (e.g. arthritis, eye lesions or liver disease) complications.

Choice of operation. In acute disease with or without perforation colectomy with an ileostomy and the formation of a distal sigmoid colostomy or proctotomy is accepted as the procedure of choice. In the very ill child Turnbull's procedure (Turnbull *et al.*, 1970) of an ileostomy combined with a transverse and possibly a sigmoid colostomy may be a safer procedure.

In chronic disease the debate of whether total proctocolectomy with ileostomy

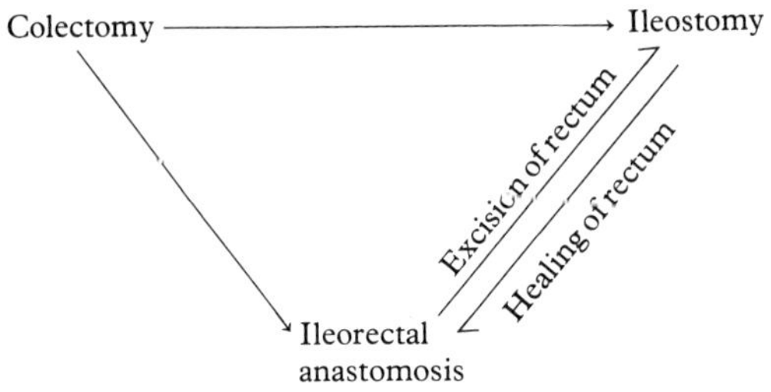

Fig. 6.2 Surgical management of ulcerative colitis in childhood.

is preferable to colectomy with an ileorectal anastomosis is as applicable to children as it is to adults (Aylett, 1971; Goligher, 1971). Many paediatric surgeons consider that, when possible, an ileorectal anastomosis is preferable in the prepubertal patient. Parents not prepared to commit their children to a permanent ileostomy can accept a colectomy and ileostomy with retention of the rectum in the hope that an ileorectal anastomosis will be possible at a later date. A plan of surgical management is suggested in Figure 6.2.

Following an ileorectal anastomosis an inspection and biopsy of the residual rectum should be performed yearly for the first five years, even in the absence of symptoms, and every six months thereafter so that histological changes suggestive of early carcinoma can be detected.

Complications

The most immediately life-threatening complication of ulcerative colitis is toxic megacolon.

Toxic megacolon

There is acute dilatation of all or part of the colon associated with signs of marked systemic toxicity. It is an acute emergency which usually occurs during a relapse of chronic intermittent disease but may be the presenting feature. It is particularly likely to complicate total colonic disease. The inflammatory process usually involves the whole thickness of the bowel wall and may extend to the serosa, and the loss of muscular tone accounts for the dilatation.

Clinical features and diagnosis. The child is usually acutely ill with anorexia, fever (38–40°C), tachycardia, abdominal pain, and often diarrhoea and dehydration. The abdomen is distended, diffusely tender and bowel sounds are often absent. There is anaemia and leucocytosis. Shock may be present particularly if the colon has perforated.

A plain film of the abdomen reveals gaseous distention of the colon with oedema of the bowel wall. Air is present under the diaphragm in plain erect radiographs if the colon has perforated. A barium enema carries the risk of perforating the unhealthy mucosa and should if possible be avoided. When toxic megacolon is the presenting feature, confirmation of a diagnosis of ulcerative colitis by sigmoidoscopy is necessary, although this also carries a risk of perforation.

Management. Dehydration and electrolyte imbalance (particularly hypokalaemia) must be corrected with appropriate intravenous solutions, and anaemia and hypoalbuminaemia with blood transfusions. Nasogastric suction should be started and a broad spectrum antibiotic given intravenously. If the child has been receiving opiates or anticholinergic drugs, they must be stopped. In the older child large daily intravenous doses of hydrocortisone (300–400 mg) or ACTH (40–80 u) should be started immediately. Apart from a slightly more rapid response to ACTH there is little difference between the action of the two drugs (Kaplan *et al.*, 1975). The response to treatment must be followed closely and plain films of the abdomen taken at least once daily. Toxic megacolon should be managed jointly by a physician and a surgeon from the outset. Perforation is an indication for immediate surgery.

The criteria for clinical remission are a reduction in bowel actions to two stools per day without blood, cessation of fever and tachycardia, the haemoglobin returning to normal and a weight gain (Kaplan *et al.*, 1975; modified from Truelove and Witts, 1955). The absence of progressive improvement within 48 to 72 hours of starting treatment is an indication for surgery, and in adults this policy has reduced the mortality from an average rate of 23 per cent to 5·6 per cent (Binder, Patterson and Glotzer, 1974).

Outcome. The overall mortality figures in both medically and surgically treated patients has varied between 12 and 30 per cent. In patients who respond to medical treatment recurrence is frequent, and an appreciable proportion will require early surgery.

Carcinoma

Carcinoma of the colon is much commoner (7 to 11 times commoner) in adults with ulcerative colitis than in the general population. The risk of cancer is related to the duration and extent of disease and is more likely to occur in patients who have had severe initial attacks. In children approximately 3 per cent will have developed colonic cancer after 10 years of disease (Devrode *et al.*, 1971). After 10 years about 20 per cent of patients whose disease started in childhood will develop cancer each decade. The risk of cancer is also greater when the whole colon is diseased and may be one of the reasons why children are at greater risk.

Overall results

Approximately 70 per cent of children with total colitis will eventually require surgery, whereas less than 10 per cent of those with partial involvement of the colon will. In those requiring surgery an ileorectal anastomosis is possible in about half. The end-results of these procedures in terms of resumption of growth and improvement in general health and relief of related symptoms are excellent. Ulcerative colitis is a chronic debilitating disease which can be cured at the cost of removal of the colon; the disadvantage for many children will be a permanent ileostomy.

Granular proctitis (non-specific ulcerative proctitis)

Granular proctitis is limited to the rectum; the sigmoidoscopic and histological features are identical to those seen in the more extensive disease, as are the age and pattern of onset (Farmer and Brown, 1966). Rectal bleeding, which is rarely severe, is a common presenting symptom, and there is a change in bowel habit, either diarrhoea or constipation. Tenesmus and lower abdominal cramping pain often accompany the diarrhoea. Extra colonic manifestations and systemic symptoms are rare, and the disease usually pursues a benign course. It extends proximally and develops into frank ulcerative colitis in less than 15 per cent of patients, and the risk of carcinoma is negligible. Treatment is with topical steroids and systemic steroids are rarely indicated.

CROHN'S DISEASE (REGIONAL ENTERITIS)

Crohn's disease was established as a clinical and pathological entity in 1932 (Crohn, Ginzburg and Oppenheimer, 1932), and the reader is referred to an interesting historical review of the condition by Dr Crohn (1967).

Since this original description it has become apparent that any part of the alimentary tract, from mouth to anus, can be affected. The condition may be defined as a chronic granulomatous disease of the gut of unknown aetiology which progresses with acute episodes and periods of remission.

Epidemiology

Crohn's disease can occur at any age but most commonly presents during the third decade. Children are more likely to have diffuse involvement of the jejunum and ileum than adults. The incidence appears to be increasing in both the United States and Europe, an increase which is only partly due to re-classification of some cases following the recognition that the colon can be involved without small intestinal disease. The sex incidence has varied in different series, but in the United Kingdom the disease is slightly commoner in females.

Aetiology

As with ulcerative colitis the aetiology of Crohn's disease is not known. Genetic, immunological, infective and psychological factors have all been implicated. That genetic and environmental factors are important is suggested by 3 to 11 per cent of patients with Crohn's disease having close relatives affected by chronic granulomatous disease, and the increased incidence of arthritis, ankylosing spondylitis, eczema and hayfever in the relatives of patients with Crohn's disease supports this possibility (Hammer, Ashurst and Naish, 1968). Immunological abnormalities have been reported but it is not clear whether these are primary or secondary in the pathogenesis of the disease. The histological abnormalities found in Crohn's disease are similar to those seen in other granulomatous diseases, such as sarcoidosis and tuberculosis. Some reports have shown the Kveim test to be positive in up to 50 per cent of patients with Crohn's disease, suggesting a possible relationship to sarcoidosis. The finding that bowel or lymph node homogenates from patients with Crohn's disease produce sarcoid-like granulomata when injected into the footpads of mice provides support for a transmissible agent playing a role in the pathogenesis of the disease (Mitchell and Rees, 1970). The evidence that psychological factors contribute to pathogenesis is even less impressive than for ulcerative colitis.

Pathology (see Morson, 1968)

Ulcerative colitis is a disease which affects the mucosa predominantly, whereas Crohn's disease affects the whole thickness of the bowel wall. Also, in contrast to ulcerative colitis, the disease affects the bowel in a discontinuous fashion with diseased segments separated by normal bowel.

The microscopic lesion is a chronic non-caseating sarcoid-like granuloma (epitheloid granuloma) surrounded by oedema, which breaks through into the lumen to form fissures and submucosal ulcers or through to the serosa leading to superficial tubercles or more commonly adhesions and fistulae into adjacent organs. The affected bowel is thickened and immobile, and the combined effects of oedema and fibrosis may eventually result in stricture formation and obstruction. The lesions may be localised to one segment of the gut, or multiple with apparently normal bowel intervening. The cobblestone appearance of the mucosa results from intercommunicating crevices or fissures surrounding islands of mucous membrane, which are raised up by the underlying inflammation and oedema and can be compared with the pseudopolypi of ulcerative colitis. The mesentery is thickened and oedematous and the regional lymph nodes are enlarged and often contain epithelioid granulomas. Anal lesions are common, whereas oral lesions are much less frequent. The four typical histological features of Crohn's disease are (1) sarcoid-like granuloma containing multinucleated giant cells and epithelioid cells, (2) focal aggregations of lymphocytes, (3) deep fissuring and ulceration, and (4) transmural inflammation. Not all cases show all of these features.

In a large series (615 cases) of mainly adult patients (Farmer, Hawk and Turnbull, 1975), the distribution of the lesions expressed as a percentage of the total number of patients was as follows: ileocolic (41), small gut (28.6), colon (27) and anorectal (3.4). The distribution of lesions in children with Crohn's disease seen at The Hospital for Sick Children is shown in Table 6.2. There is also evidence that minor abnormalities are frequently present in an apparently normal gut.

Clinical features

The physician must be constantly aware of the variety of ways in which Crohn's disease may present and of the insidious nature of the disease. The presenting symptoms are frequently vague and non-specific and can lead to

Table 6.2 Distribution of lesions in children with Crohn's Disease

Site of lesions	Percentage of children affected
Small bowel only	65
Ileum only	60
Large bowel only	20
Small and large bowel	15
Ileum involvement in all cases	80
Anal lesions	60

Table 6.3 Presenting clinical features in a combined series of 32 children with Crohn's Disease

Presenting features	Number of patients
Growth failure and/or weight loss	16
Abdominal pain	6
Fever	3
Perianal lesions	3
Diarrhoea	2
Nil	2

serious delays in diagnosis. For example in a series of 19 children (Dyer, 1975) the delay in diagnosis following the initial symptoms was over a year in 10 and over three years in seven of these patients. The difficulties are further demonstrated by the initial diagnosis which included anorexia nervosa, hypopituitarism and urinary tract infection. The presenting features and the symptoms and signs at diagnosis in a combined series of 32 children (Dyer, 1975; Nixon, 1976) are shown in Tables 6.3 and 6.4, respectively.

Crohn's disease has been reported in the neonatal period and in early infancy, but the relationship between this form of the disease and that seen in the older child is still uncertain. The clinical presentation is usually acute, often with intestinal obstruction. Jejunal Crohn's disease should be considered in children with failure to thrive, finger-clubbing, fever, anaemia and a raised erythrocyte sedimentation rate in whom there are no localising signs. Colonic disease presents with features which are often difficult to distinguish from ulcerative colitis; patchy lesions of the colon or right-sided colitis are suggestive. Earlier suggestions that this is a more benign form of the disease have now been shown to be incorrect.

Anaemia occurs in over 60 per cent of patients and is due to a combination of factors such as bone marrow depression, blood loss, anorexia, and defective

Table 6.4 Clinical features at time of diagnosis in a combined series of 32 children with Crohn's Disease

Clinical features	Percentage of total number of patients
Growth failure and/or weight loss	78
Anorexia	75
Diarrhoea	65
Abdominal pain	65
Fever	60
Lassitude	55
Perianal lesions	40
Abdominal mass	25
Finger-clubbing	25
Melaena	15

absorption of iron, folate and vitamin B_{12}. The erythrocyte sedimentation rate is usually raised in active disease. Increased protein loss into the gut is common and may lead to hypoproteinaemia.

Diagnosis

Radiology

Barium studies of the small and large bowel provide the best evidence of the presence, localisation, severity and extent of the disease. The main radiological features are the mucosal abnormalities and signs of obstruction. In addition to the mucosal changes, in early small bowel disease there is irritability of the terminal ileum, oedema of the ileocaecal valve and extrinsic pressure from enlarged regional lymph nodes. In advanced disease the classic 'string sign' is seen, in which oedema, spasm and fibrosis almost occlude the terminal ileum. In the large bowel the features distinguishing Crohn's disease from ulcerative colitis are the patchy distribution of the lesions, their varied nature, the presence of eccentric structures and the sparing of the rectum. In total colonic involvement many of these distinguishing features disappear and a separation from ulcerative colitis may not be possible.

Endoscopy

Sigmoidoscopy and biopsy, usually under general anaesthesia, will be diagnostic when the distal bowel is involved. Fibre optic endoscopy permits inspection and biopsy of the whole large bowel and is particularly useful in differentiating total colonic Crohn's disease from total ulcerative colitis when radiological examination has been equivocal. Any chronic perianal lesion should be biopsied even in the absence of any other symptoms or signs of Crohn's disease. A rectal suction biopsy should always be taken from the rectum as histological abnormalities may be present in macroscopically normal mucosa.

Management

The natural history of the disease, its capacity to involve extensive segments of gut and its notorious tendency to recur following surgery complicate the planning of management. General measures should be aimed at treating any anaemia and malnutrition and controlling troublesome diarrhoea. Dietary management includes a high protein-calorie diet, and substitution of medium-chain triglycerides for dietary long-chain triglycerides may improve fat absorption and reduce steatorrhea in some patients; a low residue diet may occasionally be helpful. Iron and vitamin supplements should be administered as indicated. The value of elemental-type diets has not yet been established.

Specific medical measures

There are no specific drugs which have been shown to be unequivocally effective in Crohn's disease. Nevertheless corticosteroids in doses similar to those used in ulcerative colitis are generally considered to be the drugs of choice for inducing a remission. Sulphasalazine has been recommended in children (British Medical Journal, 1975), and side effects from this drug have been claimed to be less frequent than in adults. Azathioprine by itself or in combination with corticosteroids has been reported to be effective in inducing and maintaining a remission (Harries and Lloyd, 1971; Willoughby *et al.*, 1971). Other authors have been less convinced of its benefits. The place of drugs such as metronidazole and dapsone in the treatment of Crohn's disease remains to be established.

Surgery
The high tendency to recurrence has inhibited physicians from recommending surgical treatment, particularly in children for whom the recurrence rate is highest. The recurrence rate is approximately 50 per cent after five years, and recurrences continue for up to 15 to 20 years (de Dombal *et al.*, 1971).

The limitations of medical treatment result in up to 90 per cent of patients coming to surgery (Fielding, 1972).

The indications for surgery may result from acute attacks of chronic disease. Emergency indications are relatively rare but include perforation, severe haemorrhage, acute obstruction and toxic megacolon. Chronic indications include growth retardation, delayed puberty, recurrent obstruction, disabling disease with loss of schooling, fistulae, intra-abdominal sepsis, severe perianal disease and remote complications such as arthritis, eye lesions and pyoderma gangrenosum.

The aim of surgery is to eradicate diseased bowel and to perform an end-to-end anastomosis. This is relatively simple when the disease is localised, as in terminal ileal lesions, but may be impossible when the disease is more extensive. Since the extent of the inflammatory process is often greater than is apparent to the naked eye, the level of resection should be confirmed by histological examination of frozen sections at operation. A simple bypass operation should be reserved for severely ill patients with small intestinal obstruction. Intravenous feeding may be necessary to improve the patient's general condition prior to major surgery. Ileorectal anastomosis is possible when the colon is extensively involved provided the rectum is healthy. When the rectum is also involved proctocolectomy with a permanent ileostomy is necessary. The immediate mortality rate following surgery is about 3 per cent and is almost confined to patients with severe disease. The majority of children show a dramatic improvement in general health following surgery, and for a few patients this improvement is permanent.

Complications

Toxic megacolon
Toxic megacolon, with or without perforation, is much rarer in Crohn's disease than in ulcerative colitis; the management is essentially the same.

Fistulae
Fistulae are common and may lead to abscess cavities, palpable abdominal masses, pain and persistent fever. Fistulae also develop between adjacent segments of intestine or to adjacent parts of the urinary and genital tracts.

Extraintestinal lesions unrelated to fistula formation

Arthritis, eye lesions and skin lesions such as erythema nodosum are much less common than in ulcerative colitis. Ankylosing spondylitis may precede bowel symptoms by several years. Abnormalities of liver function with or without histological evidence of pericholangitis may also complicate the disease. Carcinoma of the small or large bowel has been reported, and the incidence is greater than that seen in the general population (Weedon *et al.*, 1973) but the risk is much less than for ulcerative colitis. Hyperoxaluria and renal calculi may complicate terminal ileal disease or resection.

ACUTE TERMINAL ILEITIS AND ITS RELATION TO CROHN'S DISEASE

Among patients with signs and symptoms suggesting acute appendicitis, a small proportion (about one in 400) will be found at operation to have an acute inflammatory lesion of the terminal ileum. The distal 10 to 15 cm of the ileum is red and oedematous, the mesentery is thickened and the regional lymph nodes enlarged; the appendix and caecum are usually normal. The nature of this lesion and its relationship to Crohn's disease are uncertain. Crohn described it as an acute form of Crohn's disease, but other workers have disputed this (Thomasson and Havia, 1973). Kewenter, Hulten and Kock (1974) described 68 cases seen over a 20-year period and reported that 15 per cent were subsequently proven to have Crohn's disease. In Europe and the United States infections with *Yersinia enterocolitica* (Weber, Finlayson and Mark, 1970) and in Japan infestation with the fish nematode Anisalis (Hayasaka, Ishikura and Takayama, 1971) have been shown to be associated with the lesion. It seems probable that the acute terminal ileitis has several causes including Crohn's disease. It is controversial what the correct surgical procedure should be. Since the incidence of postoperative fistulae is no greater after appendicectomy than after a simple laparotomy, it is probably safest to remove the appendix provided the caecum is healthy. Histological examination of the appendix may also provide diagnostic information.

References

Aylett, S. O. (1971) Ileorectal anastomosis: review 1952–1968. *Proceedings of the Royal Society of Medicine,* **64,** 967.

Binder, S. C., Patterson, J. F. & Glotzer, D. J. (1974) Toxic megacolon in ulcerative colitis. *Gastroenterology,* **66,** 909.

British Medical Journal (1975) Sulphasalazine for Crohn's disease? *British Medical Journal,* **2,** 297.

Broberger, O. & Lagercrantz, (1966) Ulcerative colitis in childhood and adolescence. *Advances in Pediatrics,* **14,** 9.

Crohn, B. B. (1967) Granulomatous diseases of the small and large bowel. A historical survey. *Gastroenterology,* **52,** 767.

Crohn, B. B., Ginzburg, L. & Oppenheimer, G. D. (1932) Regional ileitis; pathological and clinical entity. *Journal of the American Medical Association,* **99,** 1323.

Davidson, M. (1967) Juvenile ulcerative colitis. *New England Journal of Medicine,* **277,** 1408.

Davidson, M., Bloom, A. A. & Kugler, M. M. (1965). Chronic ulcerative colitis of childhood. *Journal of Pediatrics,* **67,** 471.

de Dombal, F. T. (1971) Ulcerative colitis: epidemiology and aetiology, course and prognosis. *British Medical Journal,* **1,** 649.

de Dombal, F. T., Burton, I. & Goligher, J. C. (1971) Recurrence of Crohn's disease after primary excisional surgery. *Gut*, **12**, 519.

Devrode, G. J., Taylor, W. F., Sauer, W. G., Jackman, R. J. & Stickler, G. B. (1971) Cancer risk and life expectancy of children with ulcerative colitis. *New England Journal of Medicine*, **285**, 17

Dissanayake, A. S. & Truelove, S. C. (1973) A controlled therapeutic trial of long-term maintenance treatment of ulcerative colitis with sulphasalazine (Salazopyrin). *Gut*, **14**, 923.

Dyer, N. H. (1975) Chronic inflammatory disorders. Part I. Crohn's disease. In *Paediatric Gastroenterology*, Ch. 13, p. 411, ed. Anderson, C. & Burke, V. Oxford: Blackwell.

Edwards, F. C. & Truelove, S. C. (1963) The course and prognosis of ulcerative colitis. *Gut*, **4**, 299.

Eode, M. N. (1970) Liver disease in ulcerative colitis. I. Pathology, etiology and pathogenesis. *Annals of Internal Medicine*, **72**, 475.

Farmer, R. G. & Brown, C. H. (1966) Ulcerative proctitis: course and prognosis. *Gastroenterology*, **51**, 219.

Farmer, R. G., Hawk, W. A. & Turnbull, R. B. (1975) Clinical patterns in Crohn's disease: a statistical study of 615 cases. *Gastroenterology*, **68**, 627.

Fielding, J. F. (1972) Crohn's disease of the small intestine and stomach. *British Journal of Hospital Medicine*, **5**, 767.

Goligher, J. C. (1971) Surgical treatment of ulcerative colitis. *Proceedings of the Royal Society of Medicine*, **64**, 973.

Hammer, B., Ashurst, P. & Naish, J. (1968) Disease associated with ulcerative colitis and Crohn's disease. *Gut*, **9**, 17.

Harries, J. T. & Lloyd, J. K. (1971) Azathioprine in the treatment of Crohn's disease. *Acta Paediatrica Scandinavica*, **60**, 363.

Hayasaka, H., Ishikura, H. & Takayama, T. (1971) Acute regional ileitis due to Anisalis larvae. *International Surgery*, **55**, 8.

Jayson, M. I., Salmon, P. R. & Harrison, W. J. (1970) Inflammatory bowel disease in ankylosing spondylitis. *Gut*, **11**, 506.

Kaplan, H. P., Portnoy, B., Binder, H. J., Amatruda, T. & Spiro, H. (1975) A controlled evaluation of intravenous adrenocorticotropic hormone and hydrocortisone in the treatment of acute colitis. *Gastroenterology*, **69**, 91.

Kewenter, J., Hulten, L. & Kock, N. G. (1974) The relationship and epidemiology of acute terminal ileitis and Crohn's disease. *Gut*, **15**, 801.

Kirsner, J. B. (1975) Problems in the differentiation of ulcerative colitis and Crohn's disease of the colon: the need for repeated diagnostic evaluation. *Gastroenterology*, **68**, 187.

McEwen, C., Lingg, C. & Kirsner, J. B. (1962) Arthritis accompanying ulcerative colitis. *American Journal of Medicine*, **33**, 923.

Mitchell, D. N. & Rees, R. J. W. (1970) Agent transmissible from Crohn's disease tissue. *Lancet*, **2**, 168.

Morson, B. C. (1968) Histopathology of Crohn's disease. *Proceedings of the Royal Society of Medicine*, **61**, 79.

Nixon, H. H. (1976) Personal communication.

Perrett, A. D., Higgins, G., Johnston, H. H., Massarella, G. R., Truelove, S. C. & Wright, R. (1971) The liver in ulcerative colitis. *Quarterly Journal of Medicine*, **158**, 211.

Rosenberg, J. L., Wall, A. J., Levin, B., Binder, H. J. & Kirsner, J. B. (1975) A controlled trial of azathioprine in the management of chronic ulcerative colitis. *Gastroenterology*, **69**, 96.

Thomasson, B. & Havia, T. (1973) Is acute terminal ileitis a precursor of Crohn's disease. *Acta Chirwigica Scandinavica*, **139**, 192.

Truelove, S. C. & Witts, L. J. (1954) Cortisone in ulcerative colitis. Preliminary report on therapeutic trial. *British Medical Journal*, **2**, 375.

Truelove, S. C. & Witts, L. J. (1955) Cortisone in ulcerative colitis. Final report on therapeutic trial. *British Medical Journal*, **2**, 1041.

Turnbull, R. B., Weekley, F. L., Hawk, W. A. & Schofield, P. (1970) Choice of operation for the toxic megacolon phase of non-specific ulcerative colitis. *Surgical Clinics of North America*, **50**, 1151.

Weber, J., Finlayson, N. B. & Mark, J. B. D. (1970) Mesenteric lymphadenitis and terminal ileitis due to Yersinia pseudotuberculosis. *New England Journal of Medicine*, **283**, 172.

Weedon, D. D., Shorter, R. G., Duane, M., Ilstrup, M. S., Huizenga, K. A. & Taylor, W. F. (1973) Crohn's disease and cancer. *New England Journal of Medicine*, **289**, 1099.

Willoughby, J. M. T., Kumar, P. J., Beckett, J. & Dawson, A. M. (1971) Controlled trial of azathioprine in Crohn's disease. *Lancet*, **2**, 944.

Wright, R. (1970) Ulcerative colitis. *Gastroenterology*, **58**, 875.

Wright, R., Lumsden, K., Sevel, D. & Truelove, S. C. (1965) Abnormalities of the sacro-iliac joints and uveitis in ulcerative colitis. *Quarterly Journal of Medicine*, **34**, 229.

7. Long-term effects and management of intestinal resection

H. B. Valman

- Adaptation
- Absorption of bile salts and lipids
- Absorption of water-soluble vitamins and iron
- Absorption of water and electrolytes
- Hormonal changes
- Physical and intellectual development
- Stagnant loop syndrome
- Hyperoxaluria
- General aspects of management after small intestinal resections
- Resection of the large intestine

The long-term effects of an intestinal resection depend both on the site and length of intestine removed. Short resections of a few centimetres, as is often the case in intestinal atresia, present no problems, whereas removal of more than 30 cm of small intestine will result in long-term effects. This chapter will concentrate on the effects of small intestinal resections, and large intestinal resections will be discussed briefly.

The commonest cause for intestinal resection, and the usual ages for the resection to be performed, are listed in Table 7.1. Of these, the commonest

Table 7.1 Causes and usual ages for intestinal resection in childhood

Cause of intestinal resection	Usual age for resection
Small intestine	
Volvulus associated with malrotation or omphalocoele	Newborn
Stenosis or atresia of jejunum or ileum	Newborn
Necrotising enterocolitis	Newborn
Meconium ileus	Newborn
Re-duplication of intestine	Newborn
Crohn's disease	Childhood
Large intestine	
Hirschsprung's disease	Infancy following colostomy in newborn
Ulcerative colitis	Childhood

reason for an extensive resection in childhood is a volvulus secondary to a developmental anomaly of the intestine such as a malrotation, or an omphalocoele.

ADAPTATION

Structural

Several animal studies have provided evidence of structural adaptation after resection of the small intestine. Flint (1912) noted hypertrophy of villi in the remaining small intestine after resection in dogs, and Dowling and Booth (1967) showed that resection of either the jejunum or ileum was followed by an increase in the diameter of the small intestine, all layers of the gut wall and in the height of the villi; these changes were most marked following jejunal resections and were shown to be due to increased topical nutrition by transposition studies.

Resection of the colon is followed by an increased villous height in the ileum (Wright and Tilson, 1974), whereas Perry (1973) was unable to demonstrate any evidence of structural adaptation in the rat colon following jejunal resection. A considerable increase in the diameter of the large intestine has been observed in an 11-year-old boy following a massive resection of the small intestine and right colon in the neonatal period (unpublished observation). The severity of diarrhoea after small intestinal resection varies with the length of large intestine preserved, suggesting that the colon plays an important role in adaptation.

There is no good evidence that a compensatory increase in the length of the small intestine occurs after resection. It has been difficult to obtain evidence in man because of the wide variation in the normal length of the gut, but a large retrospective autopsy study showed the mean length of the small intestine in full-term infants to be 266 cm, and for preterm infants it was 190 cm (Reiquam, Allen and Akers, 1965); the infants with the shortest intestines had developmental abnormalities of their intestines. Damage to the intestinal vasculature during intrauterine development may result in atresia and a reduction in the length of the intestine. Infants with volvulus or atresia, the commonest reasons for resections, are likely to have a shorter small intestine than average, and there is no substitute for direct measurement of the remaining intestine at laparotomy. The mean length of the adult small intestine is 614 .cm with a range of 304 to 863 cm, and this is attained by about the age of 5 years.

Functional

Animal experiments have shown that there is an adaptive increase in passive diffusion of bile salts and electrolytes in the jejunum following ileal resection, and that after jejunal resection absorptive rates of vitamin B_{12} and bile salts are supranormal, probably due to an increase in the number of active transport sites following adaptive ileal hyperplasia (Perry, 1973). Using an intubation technique in man Dowling and Booth (1966) showed that following resection glucose absorption was increased in the residual jejunum compared with control subjects. An improvement in fat absorption can also occur within a few months of resection. Resection of the colon is followed by an increase in the rate of water and electrolyte absorption in the ileum (Wright and Tilson, 1974), whereas

Perry (1973) was unable to demonstrate any evidence of colonic adaptation after jejunal resection in the rat. Adaptive changes may involve a number of hormones which will be discussed later.

ABSORPTION OF BILE SALTS AND LIPIDS

For a more detailed account of the absorption of bile salts and lipids the reader is referred to a recent review (Clark and Harries, 1975). Normally about 97 per cent of the bile salts secreted by the liver are absorbed from the small intestine and pass via the portal vein back to the liver, so completing the enterohepatic circulation (Fig. 7.1). A highly efficient active transport system in the ileum is

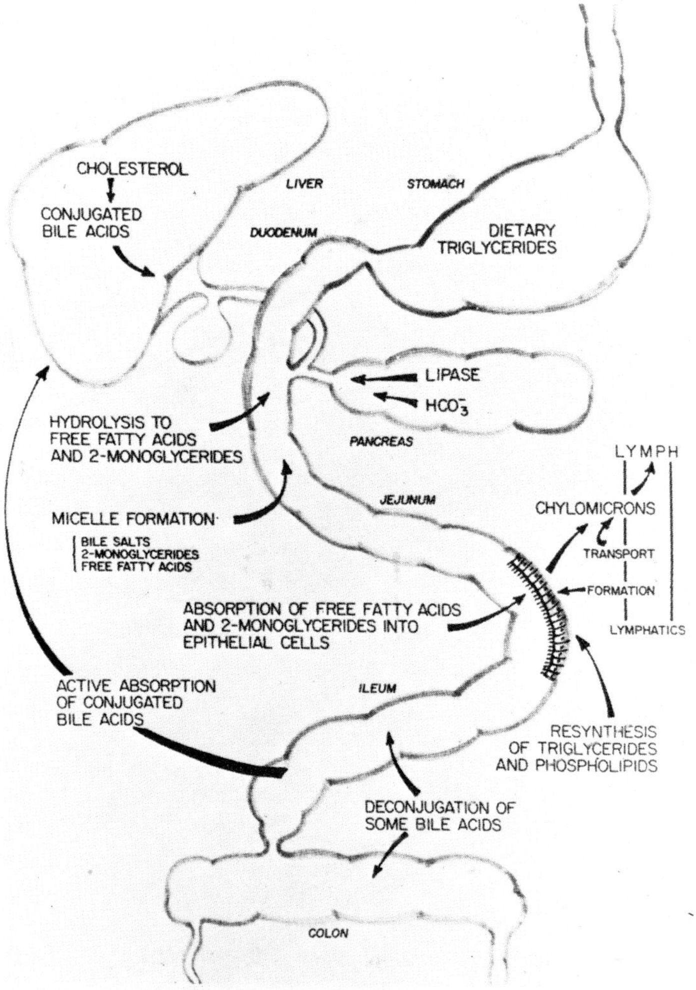

Fig. 7.1 The enterohepatic circulation of bile salts and their role in fat absorption. (By kind permission of Alan F. Hofmann, from Davenport)

Table 7.2 Clinical and laboratory details of 12 children with small intestinal resections

Case no.	Reason for resection and age[a]	Remaining small intestine (cm at laparotomy)	Remaining terminal ileum (cm at laparotomy)[b]	Age at assessment (years)	Period since supplementary vitamins given[c]
1	Multiple atresia (N)	—	30	16	4
2	Volvulus and malrotation (N)	—	15	15	14
3	Atresia (N)	—	0	14	12
4	Volvulus and malrotation (N)	65	12	9	7
5	Volvulus and duplication (N)	65	2	8	NG
6	Volvulus and atresia (N)	80	0	8	7
7	Septum (N)	78	10	8	NG
8	Volvulus and malrotation (N)	40	26	3	0·5
9	Long-segment Hirschsprung's disease (1·5 and 2·5)	—	0	8	NG
10	Volvulus and malrotation (3)	127	7	8	NG
11	Sickle-cell disease with infarction (5)	—	2	7	NG
12	Tuberculosis and stagnant loop (10)	155	0	14	NG
Normal values					

[a]N = newborn; numerals = years
[b]Measured from ileocaecal valve

responsible for most of the reabsorption, but some passive diffusion occurs from both the jejunum and colon. The extent of this passive diffusion depends on the concentration and the degree of ionisation of the bile salt, which varies with the dissociation constant of the bile acid and pH in the intestinal lumen. The total bile salt pool is normally 2·5–4 g and this circulates 6 to 12 times a day, twice or three times with each meal. The liver synthesises 0·5 g of bile salts from cholesterol each day to replace faecal losses, and synthesis is controlled by a negative feedback mechanism. Bile salts facilitate the absorption of fatty acids and monoglycerides released from dietary triglyceride by pancreatic lipase and are essential for the absorption of the fat-soluble vitamins. Above a critical micellar concentration (CMC) in aqueous solutions bile salts spontaneously form polymolecular aggregates called micelles. These micelles have the capacity to solubilise insoluble lipids such as fatty acids, monoglycerides, cholesterol and the fat-soluble vitamins within their central hydrocarbon cores; they are then called mixed micelles. Since the lumen of the small intestine presents a predominantly aqueous environment, bile salt micelles provide a mechanism for transporting insoluble lipids to the brush border of the mucosa where they can be absorbed.

After ileal resection the liver can compensate for the increased faecal losses of

Table 7.2 contd.

Vitamin B_{12} absorption with intrinsic factor (% of dose retained)	Faecal fat (g per day)	Plasma vitamin A (iu/100 ml)	Serum vitamin D[d] (ng/ml)	Serum vitamin E (mg/100 ml)	Prothrombin time(s)
77	21	273	4·7	0·6	14
72	—	—	—	—	—
4	26	260	12·0	0·5	14
28	9	—	20·0	0·9	14
—	—	—	—	—	—
12	—	—	6·2	0·7	—
18	—	—	—	—	—
82	—	—	16·0	0·9	15
39	—	—	3·3	0·9	—
0	24	125	12·2	0·6	14
18	4	197	—	0·8	16
4	—	184	6·6	0·9	18
>40	<4·5	70–200	3·8–32·8	0·4–1·2	14–18

[c]NG = never given; numerals = years
[d]25-hydroxycholecalciferol

bile salts by increasing its synthetic rate by a factor of up to eight. With extensive resections this compensatory capacity of the liver is inadequate, and the concentrations of bile salts within the lumen of the jejunum are markedly reduced. Removal of only 40 cm of terminal ileum in adult man is associated with a 30 per cent reduction in bile salt absorption.

The ratio of bile salts to cholesterol is decreased in the gall bladder bile of patients with ileal resections and is probably the reason for the high incidence of gallstones in patients with resection of the ileum.

In a recent study of 12 children with extensive resections of the ileum, none had diarrhoea which persisted for longer than a year after the resection (Valman, 1976). All the patients were able to tolerate a normal diet without diarrhoea, but steatorrhoea persisted in four of the five children tested (Table 7.2). Two fat balances were performed, one on a normal fat intake and the second on a high fat intake. The results showed that the percentage of the intake that was excreted was constant for a given patient, and similar observations have been made in adults following ileal resection (Booth, Alldis and Read, 1961). The absence of diarrhoea when the children were receiving normal diets contrasts with the observations of Booth, MacIntyre and Mollin (1964), who found that a low fat diet was necessary in their adult patients in order to prevent severe diarrhoea and electrolyte disturbances. Two of eight children had low fasting serum cholesterol levels and two factors are probably involved, depletion of the cholesterol pool by excessive bile salt synthesis and loss of ileal mucosa which is the most active part of the small intestine with regard to cholesterol synthesis. Despite long periods without vitamin supplements serum levels of the fat-soluble vitamins were normal in the majority (Table 7.2), and serum calcium, phosphorus, sodium, potassium and magnesium levels were normal in all 12 children. These findings are difficult to reconcile with current concepts on the physiology of lipid absorption.

ABSORPTION OF WATER-SOLUBLE VITAMINS AND IRON

Using the whole body counter technique, Valman and Roberts (1974) showed vitamin B_{12} malabsorption in eight of 11 children following resection of more than 45 cm of ileum, and in two patients with 15 cm or more of terminal ileum remaining absorption was normal. In the presence of malabsorption serum levels of vitamin B_{12} remained normal for several years, puberty being a particularly vulnerable time. Although information on the site and length of ileum removed was useful in predicting whether vitamin B_{12} deficiency was likely to develop, an absorption test was necessary for accurate prediction and the institution of rational treatment prior to the onset of complications. The whole body counter technique is particularly suitable for children, since it does not involve the collection of urine or faeces, injections or admission to hospital.

Apart from one child with sickle-cell disease, the other 11 children in the above series had normal haemoglobin, serum and red cell folate, and iron levels, whilst receiving no supplements except for vitamin B_{12} when indicated. Anderson (1965) noted that seven years after a resection preserving only 15 cm of jejunum, which was performed at the age of 14 years, there was no deficiency of iron or folic acid. Similarly, Booth *et al.* (1964) found no deficiency of these substances after distal resections in adults.

ABSORPTION OF WATER AND ELECTROLYTES

Hofmann (1972) has suggested that patients with ileal resections fall into two groups depending on the length resected, which determined whether the liver was able to compensate by an adequate increase in bile salt synthesis. Following short resections compensatory bile salt synthesis is adequate and malabsorption of fat is not a prominent feature; excessive quantities of conjugated bile salts enter the colon, are degraded by the resident colonic bacterial flora to toxic secondary bile acids, and these substances induce the colonic mucosa to secrete fluid and electrolytes which results in watery diarrhoea. In these patients the oral administration of cholestyramine, an anion exchange resin which sequestrates bile salts, improves the diarrhoea. Following larger resections the increased bile salt synthesis is unable to keep pace with the greater malabsorption of bile salts, and malabsorption of fat is predominant. In patients with severe steatorrhoea troublesome watery diarrhoea may also occur; this is probably due to the production of hydroxy fatty acids by colonic bacteria and the toxic effects of these acids on the colonic mucosa.

HORMONAL CHANGES

Alterations in the metabolism of hormones and their possible role in adaptation following intestinal resection have been recently reviewed by Dowling and Riecken (1974). Following massive small intestinal resection hypersecretion of gastric acid may occur. Strauss, Gerson and Yalow (1974) found high fasting plasma levels of a high molecular weight gastrin, 'big gastrin', in four patients after massive small intestinal resections and suggested that this resulted from the absence of a gastrin-inhibitory factor normally present in the distal small intestine.

The increased villous height in the ileum after resection of the colon and also during lactation may be due to hormonal factors. Glucagon secreted by the small intestine or pancreas may be a candidate, since raised circulating levels of enteroglucagon occur during lactation. In a patient with an enteroglucagon-secreting tumour of the kidney, high circulating levels of enteroglucagon were associated with small bowel enlargement and massive villus hyperplasia which disappeared when the tumour was removed (Gleeson *et al.*, 1971). It is not known whether the adaptation seen after increased topical nutrition following jejunal resection is related to the release of local or systemic hormones or possibly increased blood flow.

Experimentally induced diabetes in rats is associated with an increased villous height, enhanced absorption of glucose and amino acids in the jejunum and ileum, and of bile salts in the ileum. In man, however, diabetes mellitus is not associated with enhanced absorption of glucose, although an injection of glucagon is followed by a transient increase in absorption both in diabetics and healthy controls. Hypophysectomy in rats is followed by a marked decrease in the height of the villi and a reduction in glucose absorption, and both effects are reversed by hormonal replacement. Little is known of the effects of long-term corticosteroid treatment in man, but one study in rats showed atrophic changes in the small intestinal mucosa. Hyperthyroidism in animals is associated with a marked increase in villous height and the opposite changes are found in hypothyroidism.

PHYSICAL AND INTELLECTUAL DEVELOPMENT

Physical

The children with extensive resections described previously (Table 7.2) had weights which were appropriate for their heights, indicating that none of them had persistent malnutrition. They tended to be shorter than their siblings, but only two were below the third centile compared with the height expected from their parents. This suggests that the long period of malnutrition experienced by many of these children postoperatively was followed by a slight and permanent reduction in the eventual height which would have been expected from the parental size (Valman, 1976). Each patient reached his ultimate centile by the age of 3 years and remained on it even after puberty. Two children who had a low-fat, high-protein diet for about 10 years after neonatal resections grew particularly poorly compared with the rest of the group. The poor palatability of the diet may have been associated with a low total calorie intake.

Intellectual

Quantitative assessment of brain cells by DNA determination has suggested that temporary periods of malnutrition during critical phases of brain development may be followed by a permanent reduction in the total number of brain cells and mental retardation (Dobbing, 1972). Severe malnutrition in early infancy is believed to cause permanent mental retardation. In most studies it has been difficult to separate the effects of an episode of malnutrition from chronic food and social deprivation. A group of children who survived malnutrition after extensive resection of the small intestine in the neonatal period and who returned to normal homes provided an opportunity to separate these two effects (Valman, 1974). Assessment of intelligence by the 'draw a man' test, together with school reports, showed that the incidence of mental retardation was no higher in this group than in the normal population.

STAGNANT LOOP SYNDROME

Stagnation of small intestinal contents, usually due to an anatomical abnormality, is followed by colonisation with anaerobic bacteria and malabsorption of fat, vitamin B_{12} and nitrogen; patchy morphological abnormalities of the mucosa occur in some patients. The pathophysiological mechanisms responsible for the steatorrhoea are controversial. Bacterial deconjugation of bile salts results in reduced luminal concentrations of conjugated bile salts, and this may lead to impaired micellar solubilisation of lipids and steatorrhoea; alternatively free dihydroxy bile acids, such as deoxycholic acid, may have a direct effect on the mucosal phase of fat transport. Both mechanisms may operate simultaneously. In the experimental animal deoxycholic acid also inhibits the jejunal absorption of glucose, amino acids, water and electrolytes, inactivates the mucosal enzyme adenosine triphosphatase, and at high concentrations produces gross morphological damage (Sladen and Harries, 1972; Guiraldes *et al.*, 1975). In our series the stagnant loop syndrome commonly followed small intestinal resections when the anastomosis was by the end-to-side method. At present the proximal dilated part of the intestine is routinely resected and an end-to-end anastomosis carried out, and complications are less common. Following resections symptoms of a stagnant loop syndrome are usually insidious and not always recognised. The presenting features may be a recurrence of diarrhoea or poor growth, anaemia or rickets. Accurate diagnosis is important since treatment with antibiotics, with or without surgery, is often extremely effective. Barium meal and follow-through may show a localised dilated loop of intestine, though the diameter of the whole of the remaining small intestine is often increased for several months following a resection. Direct intubation of the small intestine is the most reliable method of diagnosis. Aspirated juice is examined for anaerobic and aerobic bacteria and for the presence of free bile acids.

HYPEROXALURIA

Hyperoxaluria and renal calculi following small intestinal resection in adults was first described by Smith *et al.* (1970), and this association has subsequently been confirmed by others. In children Valman, Oberholzer and Palmer (1974) documented hyperoxaluria in four of 10 children with ileal resections, and there was no relationship between the degree of hyperoxaluria and the length of ileum resected. McCollum *et al.* (1975) have shown that hyperoxaluria may occur in a wide variety of malabsorptive states as well as following small intestinal resection, and that treatment of the underlying condition (e.g. gluten-free diet in coeliac disease) corrects the hyperoxaluria.

The colon is responsible for a significant proportion of the normal intestinal absorption of oxalate, and hyperoxaluria does not occur following ileostomy or in patients who have had extensive ileal resection and colectomy. The mechanisms for the hyperoxaluria have not been clearly elucidated, but available evidence suggests that certain fatty acids and bile acids alter permeability of the colonic mucosa to oxalate leading to enhanced absorption of the dicarboxylic acid and hyperoxaluria (Saunders, Sillery and McDonald, 1975). An oxalate-free diet is effective in reducing urinary oxalate output but has been restricted to patients with recurrent renal stones since it is unpalatable and difficult to manage. Because of the risk of renal calculi urinary oxalate should be measured regularly in children following intestinal resections, and dietary treatment considered in those with hyperoxaluria.

GENERAL ASPECTS OF MANAGEMENT AFTER SMALL INTESTINAL RESECTIONS

A year after resection a normal diet can usually be tolerated, but a few patients may require a low-fat, high-protein diet to control diarrhoea. Frequent reassessment of calorie requirements is important in order to ensure that the infant's diet is adequate for his expected weight. Occasionally severe bouts of diarrhoea occur with rapid dehydration and hypoglycaemia, and patients with extensive resections should be readmitted to hospital at an early stage of severe diarrhoea. Following resections in the newborn, supplements of water and fat-soluble vitamins, folic acid and iron should be given until the age of 2 years but are usually unnecessary after that time.

The liver stores of vitamin B_{12} last for at least two years, and no supplements are required until that time. Vitamin B_{12} absorption should be formally assessed one to two years after ileal resections and, if absorption is severely impaired, intramuscular injections of hydroxycobalamin can be given once every three months for life. Alternatively, serum levels of vitamin B_{12} can be regularly determined and the vitamin administered if levels fall.

Cholestyramine may be useful in controlling watery diarrhoea following ileal resections. Its poor palatability and the increased steatorrhoea which it causes are immediate disadvantages, and there is a possibility of long-term effects such as vitamin A and folic acid deficiencies.

Urinary oxalate should be determined at regular intervals and investigation of the urinary tract should be considered in the presence of hyperoxaluria.

RESECTION OF THE LARGE INTESTINE

Resection of the large intestine is followed by watery diarrhoea which improves after a few months, and this is associated with an increased villous height in the ileum (Wright and Tilson, 1974). The commonest reason for resection of the large intestine in infants is Hirschsprung's disease and, in older children, chronic inflammatory bowel disease. No studies concerned with the long-term effects of large intestinal resections have been reported in children. Removal of the colon in piglets resulted in them not reaching their genetic potential for size (Wilkinson and McCance, 1973). If a child with an ileostomy has diarrhoea, urgent readmission to hospital for intravenous fluids may be necessary.

References

Anderson, C. M. (1965) Long term survival with six inches of small intestine. *British Medical Journal,* **1,** 419–422.

Booth, C. C., Alldis, D. & Read, A. E. (1961) Studies on the site of fat absorption. Fat balances after resection of varying amounts of small intestine in man. *Gut,* **2,** 168–174.

Booth, C. C., MacIntyre, I. & Mollin, D. L. (1964) Nutritional problems associated with extensive lesions of the distal small intestine in man. *Quarterly Journal of Medicine,* **33,** 401–420.

Clark, M. L. & Harries, J. T. (1975) Absorption of lipids. In *Intestinal Absorption in Man,* ed. McColl, I. & Sladen, G. E., p. 187. London: Academic Press.

Dobbing, J. (1972) *Lipids, Malnutrition and the Developing Brain. Ciba Foundation Symposium jointly with the Nestle Foundation,* ed. Elliott, K. & Knight, J. Amsterdam: Associated Scientific Publishers.

Dowling, R. H. & Booth, C. C. (1966) Functional compensation after small bowel resection in man. *Lancet,* **2,** 146.

Dowling, R. H. & Booth, C. C. (1967) Structural and functional changes following small intestinal resection in the rat. *Clinical Science,* **32,** 139.

Dowling, R. H. & Riecken, E. O. (1974) *Intestinal Adaptation.* Stuttgart: Schattauer Verlag.

Flint, J. M. (1912) The effect of extensive resections of small intestine. *Johns Hopkins Medical Journal,* **23,** 127–144.

Gleeson, M. H., Bloom, S. R., Polak, J. M., Henry, K. & Dowling, R. H. (1971) Endocrine tumour in kidney affecting small bowel structure, motility and absorptive function. *Gut,* **12,** 773–782.

Guiraldes, E., Lamabadusuriya, S. P., Oyesiku, J. E. J., Whitfield, A. E. & Harries, J. T. (1975) A comparative study on the effects of different bile salts on mucosal ATPase and transport in the rat jejunum in vivo. *Biochimica et Biophysica Acta,* **389,** 495–505.

Hofmann, A. F. (1972) Bile acid malabsorption caused by ileal resection. *Archives of Internal Medicine,* **130,** 597–605.

Hofmann, A. F. (1973) The chemistry of intraluminal digestion. *Mayo Clinic Proceedings,* **48,** 617.

McCollum, J. P. K., Ogilvie, D., Muller, D. P. R., Manning, J., Packer, S. & Harries, J. T. (1975) Hyperoxaluria in children with hepatic, pancreatic and intestinal dysfunction. *Archives of Disease in Childhood,* **50,** 824.

Perry, P. M. (1973) Bile salt absorption following small bowel resection. M. D. Thesis, University of London.

Reiquam, C. W., Allen, R. P. & Akers, D. R. (1965) Normal and abnormal small bowel lengths: an analysis of 389 autopsy cases in infants and children. *Americal Journal of Diseases of Children,* **109,** 447–451.

Saunders, D. R., Sillery, J. & McDonald, G. B. (1975) Regional differences in oxalate absorption by rat intestine: evidence for excessive absorption by the colon in steatorrhoea. *Gut,* **16,** 543–554.

Sladen, G. E. & Harries, J. T. (1972) Studies on the effects of unconjugated dihydroxy bile salts on rat small intestinal function in vivo. *Biochimica Biophysica Acta,* **288,** 443–456.

Smith, L. H., Hofmann, A. F., McCall, J. T. & Thomas, P. J. (1970) Secondary hyperoxaluria in patients with ileal resection and oxalate nephrolithiasis. *Clinical Research,* **18,** 541 (abstract).

Strauss, E., Gerson, C. D. & Yalow, R. S. (1974) Hypersecretion of gastrin associated with short bowel syndrome. *Gastroenterology,* **66,** 175–180.

Valman, H. B. (1974) Intelligence after malnutrition caused by neonatal resection of ileum. *Lancet,* **1,** 425–427.

Valman, H. B. (1976) Diet and growth after resection of ileum in childhood. *Journal of Pediatrics,* **88,** 41.

Valman, H. B. & Roberts, P. D. (1974) Vitamin B_{12} absorption after resection of ileum in childhood. *Archives of Disease in Childhood,* **49,** 932–935.
Valman, H. B., Oberholzer, V. G. & Palmer, T. (1974) Hyperoxaluria after resection of ileum in childhood. *Archives of Disease in Childhood,* **49,** 171–173.
Wilkinson, A. W. & McCance, R. A. (1973) Clinical and experimental results of removing the large intestine soon after birth. *Archives of Disease in Childhood,* **48,** 121–126.
Wright, K. & Tilson, M. D. (1974) Changes in structure and function of the small intestine after colectomy. In *Intestinal Adaptation,* ed. Dowling, R. H. & Riecken, E. O., pp. 99–107. Stuttgart: Schattauer Verlag.

8. The effects of malnutrition on structure and function

B. A. Wharton

Nutritional deficiencies
Abnormalities of individual organs
Bacteria and bile
Absorption of individual dietary constituents
Concluding remarks

In general those organs undergoing a high rate of cell turnover are the more susceptible to nutritional influences, and so organs such as the pancreas and the intestinal mucosa are particularly vulnerable. The thin atrophied small intestine was commented on in some of the earliest descriptions of starvation by morbid anatomists.

Following a brief introduction to nutritional deficiency this chapter describes the structural and biochemical changes occurring in the individual digestive and absorptive organs of malnourished children and then considers the digestion and absorption of individual nutrients. Much of the evidence is derived from developing countries where primary nutritional deficiency in childhood is common. The mechanisms have worldwide relevance, however, in the clinical management of any malnourished children whether the malnutrition is due to a primary dietary deficit or is secondary to some other disorder, such as chronic infection or malabsorption.

NUTRITIONAL DEFICIENCIES

In many countries a large proportion of the children do not get enough to eat. The diet is commonly insufficient in amount and lacks essential nutrients. Furthermore, infectious diseases are common so that appetite is depressed and utilisation of the small amount of food eaten is poor. Apart from these deficiencies of major nutrients, other more specific deficiencies may also result in gastrointestinal dysfunction.

Protein-energy deficiency

The FAO-WHO Expert Committee on Nutrition recommended the use of the term 'protein-calorie deficiency' rather than 'protein-calorie malnutrition' but this should now be revised to 'protein-energy deficiency'. The syndrome of protein-energy deficiency includes kwashiorkor, marasmus and intermediate or unspecified disorders. As a public health concept, marasmus and kwashiorkor and the apparently intermediate disorders can be grouped together as protein-

Table 8.1 The Wellcome classification of malnutrition

Designation	Weight as a percentage of the Boston median weight for age	Oedema
Kwashiorkor	60–80%[a]	Present
Marasmic kwashiorkor	Less than 60%	Present
Marasmus	Less than 60%	Absent
Underweight	60–80%[b]	Absent

[a]The occasional child who is very oedematous may be above 80 per cent.
[b]Eighty per cent of the Boston median is approximately the third centile; the Boston data were used as an international standard of reference, not necessarily as a standard of excellence to which all children should conform.

energy deficiency, but there is some debate whether this is justifiable on clinical or biochemical grounds. Biochemically some workers regard marasmus as successful adaptation to nutritional stress, and kwashiorkor as failure of that adaptation. The classification of protein-energy deficiency has received considerable attention in recent years (Waterlow, 1972) and the Wellcome classification has the merit of simplicity, as is shown in Table 8.1.

Diarrhoea of varying severity is a constant feature of kwashiorkor, whereas this is not necessarily so in marasmus. Weaning results in the consumption of food which is contaminated by various micro-organisms and is nutritionally inferior both in quality and often in quantity to breast milk, so that the gastrointestinal tract is stressed by both infection and malnutrition. The concept of 'weanling diarrhoea' as a major problem in the child health of developing countries is now firmly accepted.

Other deficiencies

The B vitamins are essential for normal intestinal function, and diarrhoea and/or malabsorption may be a feature of beriberi and pellagra. These dietary deficiencies occur in South-east Asia and South Africa, and may be associated with some degree of protein-energy deficiency. Folic acid and vitamin B_{12} deficiency may also result in gastrointestinal dysfunction but is rarely due to a dietary deficit alone. Iron deficiency has been implicated as a primary factor in the pathogenesis of an enteropathy, but the evidence for this is not firm. Dietary iron deficiency in preschool children is common throughout the world; chronic blood loss will aggravate any dietary deficiency, and on a worldwide basis hookworm infestation is the most common cause of chronic blood loss in childhood. The detailed aetiology and features of these deficiencies are available in standard works on nutrition (Jelliffe, 1968; Davidson, Passmore and Truswell, 1975).

ABNORMALITIES OF INDIVIDUAL ORGANS

Salivary glands

In kwashiorkor the salivary glands are atrophied, particularly the parotid gland. There is shrinking and degranulation of the enzyme-secreting cells but mucus cells are relatively unaffected (Trowell, Davies and Dean, 1954). Salivary amylase activity increases with age, and this is independent of dietary starch. Activity is reduced in infants with marasmus secondary to severe malabsorption, rising rapidly as the nutritional state improves. Children with cystic fibrosis, however, even though they may be malnourished, show normal or increased salivary amylase activity. Following malnutrition in adults, the parotid glands often become prominent; this occurs in children occasionally and is probably a true hypertrophy following atrophy.

Stomach

At post mortem the stomach of children with protein-energy deficiency is not so markedly thinned as the intestine (Trowell *et al.*, 1954); there is no detailed information available on gastric function or histology.

Jejunum

Mucosal morphology

In kwashiorkor the jejunal mucosa usually shows varying degrees of partial villous atrophy, but subtotal villous atrophy is unusual and occurs in only a minority of affected children who have been studied (Wharton, 1975). Electron microscopy has shown accumulation of lipid droplets in epithelial cells at the tips and sides of the villi, mainly in the apical cytoplasm, with very little fat in the Golgi apparatus as would be normally expected. These findings are similar to those in abetalipoproteinaemia (Theron, Wittmann and Prinsloo, 1971). The mucosa of marasmic children has been reported less frequently, but in general is nearer normal than in kwashiorkor.

There is a wide variation in the jejunal morphology of children from the developing parts of the world who are not overtly malnourished. At birth only finger-shaped villi are found, but during childhood ridges and convolutions predominate, particularly in the proximal small intestine (Chacko *et al.*, 1960; Cook, Kajubi and Lee, 1969). Is the partial villous atrophy observed in children with kwashiorkor attributable then to the malnutrition process, or are the changes no more than one would expect to find in children from a similar environment who were not overtly malnourished? There are three main pieces of evidence to suggest kwashiorkor itself causes a mucosal lesion: first, protein-deficient monkeys develop partial villous atrophy (Deo and Ramalingaswami, 1964); secondly, a gradual improvement, usually over many months, is observed in the jejunal appearances following an initial episode of kwashiorkor (James, 1971; Schneider and Viteri, 1972); and finally, the completely flat mucosa found in a number of Chilean children and the occasional Ugandan child with kwashiorkor are abnormal even by tropical standards. On balance, therefore, there is reasonable, but circumstantial, evidence that kwashiorkor results in abnormalities of the jejunal mucosa, but only occasionally does it cause subtotal villous atrophy.

Partial villous atrophy has been described in association with other nutritional deficiencies such as pernicious anaemia, folate deficiency, pellagra and iron deficiency.

Mucosal enzymes

A mixed deficiency of disaccharidases occurs in about two-thirds of patients with malnutrition and, as in other causes of jejunal atrophy, deficiency of lactase is most marked. In many countries where malnutrition occurs, however, genetically determined isolated lactase deficiency also occurs (see Ch. 11). Some children with isolated lactase deficiency may become malnourished, and the underlying disorder may play a role in the pathogenesis of the malnutrition and will certainly aggravate any intestinal abnormality induced by malnutrition (Cook, 1967). For these reasons it is sometimes difficult to be sure of the aetiology of sugar malabsorption in an individual malnourished child. As the child recovers the disaccharidase levels rise but may not reach normality for several months or years. In some African series low lactase levels persisted for some years even when other disaccharidases were normal, possibly because the lactase deficiency was genetically determined rather than secondary to the malnutrition. Disaccharidase levels in marasmic children in Jamaica were found to be less frequently and less severely depressed, but in only a few children were they completely normal (James, 1971).

In the few children studied, jejunal dipeptidases have been reduced, but absorption of amino acids using *in vitro* uptake techniques has been normal (Kumar, Ghai and Chase, 1971; Woodd-Walker, Hansen and Saunders, 1972). These biochemical abnormalities of the mucosa are at least partly secondary to the morphological changes described above. There may, however, be intrinsic changes in the metabolism of the enterocyte induced by the malnutrition or possibly by associated infection. Levin (1969) concluded that disaccharidase deficiency in malnutrition is secondary to associated infection, but this is based on animal work only.

Ileum

If malnutrition results in villous atrophy of the jejunum the same process might be expected to also cause an ileal lesion. Evidence on this in man is sparse, but a postmortem study in adults suggests the ileum is more severely affected than the jejunum (Passmore, 1947). In protein-deficient monkeys partial villous atrophy is more severe in the ileum than the jejunum, and B_{12} absorption is impaired (Deo and Ramalingaswami, 1964). The effects of malnutrition on vitamin B_{12} absorption and bile salt metabolism are considered later.

Large intestine

In kwashiorkor there is atrophy of the surface epithelium of the distal colon and rectum, cellular infiltration of the lamina propria and disorganisation of the vascular pattern; in contrast to the small intestine these abnormalities disappear within a few weeks of instituting treatment (Redmond *et al.*, 1971).

Pancreas

Exocrine function

The pancreas is atrophic in kwashiorkor (Trowell *et al.*, 1954); there is disruption of the acinar pattern with a loss or diminution of secretory granules, and on electron microscopy virtually all the organelles within the acinar cell are altered. Changes in the ducts, however, are minimal. These changes are associated with a reduced pancreatic enzyme activity in the duodenal juice, trypsin being less affected than other enzymes. Despite the reduced enzyme output, the volume and pH of the pancreatic secretions are normal. In most children exocrine pancreatic function returns to normal following treatment of an episode of kwashiorkor, but in a small proportion pancreatic insufficiency persists for several years. Danus *et al.* (1970) found that marasmic children in Chile had a reduced production of amylase and lipase, but the volume, pH and bicarbonate content of the secretions were normal.

Endocrine function

Blood glucose levels can be either high or low in kwashiorkor. The causes of this abnormal handling of glucose are probably many (see Wharton, 1975), but one factor is the reduced insulin production which occurs in response to a glucose load in the majority of patients. The intravenous glucose tolerance test is much nearer normal in children with marasmus than in kwashiorkor as are insulin/glucose ratios. No histological or ultrastructural studies of the beta cells or of glucagon production have been reported.

Long-term effects

The rate of disappearance of intravenously administered glucose and the rate of insulin secretion increase during the initial treatment of kwashiorkor but remain abnormal for several years. Eventually pancreatic function returns to normal in the majority, but it is possible that the effects of malnutrition in early life may play a role in the pathogenesis of chronic pancreatic disease, which is commonly seen in adults and older children in developing countries; also, malnutrition may account for the high proportion of patients with diabetes who have evidence of exocrine pancreatic disease.

Liver

The liver may be affected not only by the quantity or quality of the normal constituents of the diet but also by abnormal constituents, such as various toxins.

Protein-energy deficiency

Fatty infiltration of the liver (up to 50 per cent of its wet weight) is found in almost all children with kwashiorkor (Waterlow, 1948; Trowell *et al.*, 1954). The hepatic accumulation of fat may be secondary to the reduced plasma lipoprotein levels, so that triglyceride cannot be transported out of the hepatocytes; plasma β-lipoprotein levels, however, are not universally low in these children (Flores *et al.*, 1974). Synthesis of other plasma proteins, such as albumin and transferrin, is considerably reduced and many amino acids are handled abnormally. Grossly fatty livers are not found in marasmic children, possibly because plasma lipoprotein levels are normal, but excessive fat may be present microscopically. The hepatocytes are reduced in size, whereas the reverse is the case in kwashiorkor (Bhamarapravati, 1975). Biochemical evidence of liver cell necrosis (raised levels of serum bilirubin, transaminases and isocitrate dehydrogenase) occurs in only a few countries but, when present, carries a poor prognosis. The classical picture of hepatocellular failure is rarely seen, and fears of protein intoxication during the early stages of treatment are unfounded.

The reduced plasma proteins quickly regenerate during treatment of kwashiorkor. Even after three weeks, however, when the plasma albumin is usually normal and excessive fat has disappeared, the hepatocytes may continue to show ultrastructural appearances of repair. The liver eventually recovers, however, and some years after an overt episode of malnutrition there is no evidence of liver disease or damage (Cook and Hutt, 1967).

Dietary toxins

Three specific dietary toxins affect the liver, aflatoxin from peanut meal, hypoglycin in ackee fruit, and bush tea made from senecio.

Aflatoxin. Since the discovery that aflatoxin, produced by *Aspergillus flavus* growing in peanut meal, was responsible for the death of large numbers of turkeys in England this substance has been studied in considerable detail. It causes hepatoma in rats and trout, and fatty infiltration going on to cirrhosis in rhesus monkeys. A low-protein diet is known to increase the risk of liver damage. Aflatoxin is of clinical importance since it may be related to primary liver cancer (British Medical Journal, 1975), which is very common in Africa and South-east Asia and has its highest incidence in Mozambique, where it reaches an incidence of 15 per 1000 children, compared to 0·2 per 1000 in the United States (Higginson, 1963).

Hypoglycin. Ackee fruit (*Blighia sapida*) is often eaten in Jamaica. Unripe fruit may cause 'vomiting sickness', particularly in malnourished children, and is associated with hypoglycaemia, depletion of hepatic glycogen and fatty infiltration of the liver (Jelliffe and Stuart, 1954). Hypoglycin is believed to inhibit gluconeogenesis and to promote leucine build-up.

Bush tea. Veno-occlusive disease occurs most commonly in children of the Caribbean islands, particularly Jamaica, but has also been observed in South Africa, Egypt and India. It occurs mainly in preschool children but older children and adults may also be affected (Stuart and Bras, 1957). About half show a complete clinical, biochemical and histological recovery. Death in the acute stage is usually due to hepatocellular failure, whereas in the chronic stage haematemesis and liver failure are equally responsible. The hepatic vein occlusion seems to be due to the consumption of toxins from *Crotalaria* and *Senecio* plants which are used to make 'bush tea' in Jamaica. These plants are now known to be associated with similar lesions in man and in animals in many others parts of the world (Stuart and Bras, 1957).

BACTERIA AND BILE

Bacterial contamination of the upper gastrointestinal tract occurs in malnourished children but the interpretation of such findings meets the same difficulties as encountered in the interpretation of jejunal morphology; control data from adequately nourished children living in the same environment is either lacking or if it is available shows a similar degree of bacterial contamination. At present the available evidence suggests that bacterial colonisation of the small intestine is more likely to be related to the microbiological environment than to the patient's nutritional state (Mata *et al.*, 1972); the relationship between the integrity of the immunological status of the gut and bacterial colonisation, however, has not been defined in malnourished children.

High concentrations of free bile acids in the duodenum have been reported in children with kwashiorkor, but similar abnormalities were found in adequately nourished children and there was little change following treatment. However, while conjugated bile acids were present in normal concentrations in the controls, they were reduced in the patients with kwashiorkor and increased during treatment (Schneider and Viteri, 1974). The high concentrations of free bile acids in these patients was presumably related to bacterial colonisation, and the reduction in conjugated acids may have been related to the nutritional state per se; whether this reflects altered function of the liver or ileum is not known. At present it is not clear to what degree disturbances of bile acid metabolism contribute to the pathogenesis of the intestinal abnormalities in children with malnutrition.

ABSORPTION OF INDIVIDUAL DIETARY CONSTITUENTS

Having considered the various lesions and associated biochemical abnormalities which can be induced by malnutrition in different digestive organs, their effects on the absorption of individual dietary constituents will now be considered.

Protein

Nitrogen balances in children with kwashiorkor suggest that nitrogen absorption from milk protein is almost normal (70 to 90 per cent), and retention is very high (20 to 50 per cent), falling to normal after treatment. In most investigations vegetable proteins have been reasonably absorbed (60 to 80 per cent), but retention (12 to 30 per cent) has been well below that of milk protein (see Wharton, 1975). Whole milk protein is absorbed as well as prehydrolysed casein and lactalbumin. Balances are rarely performed in ill children, however, so these figures may be misleading when considering the acutely ill child. When malnutrition is associated with diarrhoea nitrogen absorption is markedly reduced.

Fat

Steatorrhoea occurs in children with kwashiorkor but its pathogenesis is not clear. Viteri *et al.* (1964) and Schneider and Viteri (1974) studied children with kwashiorkor, and their observations suggest that defective micellar solubilisation of the products of lipolysis is more important than defective pancreatic lipolysis of dietary triglyceride in the production of steatorrhea. As previously discussed chylomicron formation may be also defective (Theron *et al.*, 1971) and may contribute to the fat malabsorption. Following treatment, fat absorption returns to normal within a month or more, which is relatively slower than recovery in xylose and nitrogen absorption (Viteri *et al.*, 1973).

Carbohydrates

The reduced levels of salivary and pancreatic amylase presumably limit digestion of starch, and a poor rise in blood glucose following an oral load of starch may be found many years after an overt episode of kwashiorkor; there is little evidence, however, concerning the digestion of starch during the early stages of treatment.

The reduced levels of jejunal disaccharidases previously described are associated with varying degrees of sugar malabsorption. The different techniques of assessing sugar malabsorption result in varying degrees of emphasis on its importance. A poor rise in blood glucose following a lactose load does not necessarily imply a clinically important intolerance, and similarly some children who are intolerant of a sugar load will often progress satisfactorily without any dietary manipulation. The reduced insulin levels and slow disappearance of intravenously administered glucose make oral sugar load tests particularly difficult to interpret. Whatever the differences of emphasis, however, sugars are not absorbed normally by children with kwashiorkor. Disaccharide malabsorption can be demonstrated by techniques such as faecal lactic acid and sugar chromatography, and jejunal perfusion. Monosaccharide malabsorption may also occur, particularly in children who are not only malnourished but also have intestinal infections. Dietary restriction of carbohydrate, however, is only occasionally necessary for successful treatment. Clinical sugar intolerance in kwashiorkor resolves within three weeks of hospital admission, but biochemical indicators of malabsorption, particularly of lactose, may persist much longer. Xylose absorption returns to normal very rapidly during the first few days of treatment in children with kwashiorkor (Viteri *et al.*, 1973).

Water and minerals

Jejunal perfusion studies in malnourished children have shown that children admitted with acute diarrhoea secreted fluid into the jejunum, while those patients without diarrhoea absorbed fluid. After treatment secretion reversed to absorption (James, 1970; James, Drasar and Miller, 1972). These findings are similar to those found in cholera where profuse jejunal secretion persists for several days.

Balance studies have shown that sodium and potassium absorption in children without diarrhoea is relatively normal with little change during treatment, whereas the absorption of calcium, phosphorus and magnesium is depressed, improving during treatment. Magnesium and potassium absorption are inversely related to stool weight, being higher when the stool weight is small, presumably indicating losses of these minerals due to diarrhoea. Similarly the reduced absorption of calcium and phosphorus that occurs probably reflects some degree of steatorrhoea (see Wharton, 1975). Zinc and copper deficiency may also occur in kwashiorkor.

Changes in the plasma, whole body or tissue levels of many minerals, however, cannot be explained solely by malabsorption. Rather, they may reflect the dietary intake of the mineral concerned and/or the abnormal intermediary metabolism of malnutrition.

Vitamins

Deficiencies of all the fat-soluble vitamins are known to occur in kwashiorkor, but the geographical variations in prevalence suggest that the vitamin content of the diet itself rather than malabsorption is more important, particularly for vitamin A.

Megaloblastic anaemia occurs in about 10 per cent of children with kwashiorkor and is usually attributed to folic acid deficiency. Although malabsorption of the vitamin can be demonstrated, the vitamin content of the diet is an important factor in the pathogenesis of the deficiency.

Malabsorption of vitamin B_{12} can be demonstrated by the Schilling test and is not corrected by intrinsic factor (Alvarado *et al.*, 1973). Concentrations of the circulating B_{12} transport protein, transcobalamin II, are increased in kwashiorkor (Grassman and Retief, 1969). The defect in absorption must therefore be due to other mechanisms such as pancreatic insufficiency, and/or bacterial colonisation of the small bowel and/or an ileal lesion.

CONCLUDING REMARKS

A number of nutrients are handled abnormally by the malnourished child, sometimes due to a defect in absorption and sometimes due to an abnormality of intermediary metabolism. Abnormalities of absorption may be related to the changes which occur in small intestinal morphology, the pancreas, intestinal flora and bile salt metabolism, but it is often difficult to ascribe the malfunction to one particular cause. Indeed, the pathogenesis of the malabsorption of a particular nutrient might well be multifactorial, e.g. the possible causes of steatorrhoea or of vitamin B_{12} malabsorption in a child with kwashiorkor. The dietary content of a particular nutrient may often be more important than malabsorption in the pathogenesis of its deficiency in a malnourished child.

The intestine, liver and pancreas of the marasmic child have been studied less intensively and less frequently than in kwashiorkor, but intestinal function is probably less embarrassed in such children so long as they do not have diarrhoea. This may make many of the observations made in developing countries on children with kwashiorkor less applicable to the problems seen in temperate areas, where malnutrition is usually of the marasmic variety and secondary to some other cause. However, the clinical problems presented by a child with advanced kwashiorkor in Africa and one with a severe postenteritis malabsorption in Britain have many similarities, such as hypothermia, hypoglycaemia, drowsiness, diarrhoea, dangers of fluid overload and infection. In each case the tight circle of malnutrition, diarrhoea and malabsorption has to be broken (Wharton, 1970).

References

Alvarado, J., Vargas, W., Diaz, N. & Viteri, F. E. (1973) Vitamin B_{12} absorption in protein calorie malnourished children during recovery: influence of protein depletion and of diarrhoea. *American Journal of Clinical Nutrition*, **26**, 595.

Bhamarapravati, N. (1975) The liver in protein-calorie malnutrition: an ultrastructural study. In *Protein-Calorie Malnutrition*. Ed. Olson, R. E. p. 299, New York: Academic Press.

British Medical Journal (1975) More on the aflatoxin-hepatoma story. *British Medical Journal*, **2**, 647.

Chacko, C. J. G., Paulson, K. A., Mathan, V. I. & Baker, S. J. (1960) The villous architecture of the small intestine in the tropics: a necropsy study. *Journal of Pathology*, **98**, 146.

Cook, G. C. (1967) The practical significance of lactase deficiency in childhood. *Journal of Tropical Pediatrics*, **13**, 85.

Cook, G. C., Kajubi, S. K. & Lee, F. D. (1969) Jejunal morphology of the African in Uganda. *Journal of Pathology*, **98**, 157.

Cook, G. C. & Hutt, M. S. R. (1967) The liver after kwashiorkor. *British Medical Journal*, **3**, 454.

Danus, O., Urbina, A. M., Valenzuela, I. & Solimano, G. (1970) The effect of refeeding on pancreatic exocrine function in marasmic children. *Journal of Pediatrics*, **77**, 334.

Davidson, S., Passmore, R. & Truswell, A. S. (1975) *Human Nutrition and Dietetics*. 6th edition. Edinburgh: Churchill Livingstone.

Deo, M. G. & Ramalingaswami, V. (1964) Absorption of Co^{58} labelled cyancobalamin in protein deficiency. An experimental study in the rhesus monkey. *Gastroenterology*, **46**, 167.

Flores, H., Seakins, A., Brooke, O. G. & Waterlow, J. C. (1974) Serum and liver triglycerides in malnourished Jamaican children with fatty liver. *American Journal of Clinical Nutrition*, **27**, 610.

Grassman, R., & Retief, F. P. (1969) Serum vitamin B_{12} binding proteins in kwashiorkor. *British Journal of Haematology*, **17**, 237.

Higginson, J. (1963) The geographical pathology of primary liver cancer. *Cancer Research*, **23**, 1624.

James, W. P. T. (1970) Sugar absorption and intestinal motility in children when malnourished and after treatment. *Clinical Science*, **39**, 305.

James, W. P. T. (1971) Effects of protein-calorie malnutrition on intestinal absorption. *Annals of New York Academy of Science*, **176**, 244.

James, W. P. T., Drasar, B. S. & Miller, C. (1972) Physiological mechanism and pathogenesis of weanling diarrhoea. *American Journal of Clinical Nutrition*, **25**, 564.

Jelliffe, D. B. (1968) *Infant Nutrition in the Subtropics and Tropics. Passim*. Geneva: WHO.

Jelliffe, D. B. & Stuart, K. L. (1954) Acute toxic hypoglycaemia in the vomiting sickness of Jamaica. *British Medical Journal*, **1**, 75.

Kumar, V., Ghai, O. P. & Chase, H. P. (1971) Intestinal dipeptide hydrolase activities in undernourished children. *Archives of Disease in Childhood*, **46**, 801.

Levin, B. (1969) Disorders of carbohydrate digestion and absorption. *Journal of Clinical Pathology*, **22**, Suppl. 2, 24.

Mata, L. J., Jimenez, F., Cordon, M., Rosales, R., Priera, E., Schneider, R. E. & Viteri, F. (1972) Gastrointestinal flora of children with protein-calorie malnutrition. *American Journal of Clinical Nutrition*, **25**, 1118.

Passmore, R. (1947) Mixed deficiency diseases in India. A clinical description. *Transactions of the Royal Society of Tropical Medicine and Hygiene*, **41**, 189.

Redmond, A. B. D., Kaschula, R. O. C., Freeseman, C. & Hansen, J. D. L. (1971) The colon in kwashiorkor. *Archives of Disease in Childhood*, **46**, 470.

Schneider, R. E. & Viteri, F. E. (1972) Morphological aspects of the duodenojejunal mucosa in protein-calorie malnourished children and during recovery. *American Journal of Clinical Nutrition*, **25**, 1092.

Schneider, R. E. & Viteri, F. E. (1974) Luminal events of lipid absorption in protein-calorie malnourished children: relationship with nutritional recovery and diarrhoea. 1. Capacity of the duodenal content to achieve micellar solubilisation of lipids. *American Journal of Clinical Nutrition*, **27**, 777.

Stuart, K. L. & Bras, G. (1957) Veno-occlusive disease of the liver. *Quarterly Journal of Medicine*, **26**, 291.

Theron, J. J., Witmann, W. & Prinsloo, J. G. (1971) The fine structure of the jejunum in kwashiorkor. *Experimental and Molecular Pathology*, **14**, 184.

Trowell, H. C., Davies, J. N. P. & Dean, R. F. A. (1954) *Kwashiorkor. passim*. London: Arnold.

Viteri, F. E., Behar, M., Arroyave, G. & Scrimshaw, N. S. (1964) Clinical aspects of protein malnutrition. In *Mammalian Protein Metabolism*, ed. Munro, H. M. & Allison, J. B., Vol. 2, p. 523. London: Academic Press.

Viteri, F. E., Flores, J. M., Alvarado, J. & Behar, M. (1973) Intestinal malabsorption in malnourished children before and during recovery. *American Journal of Digestive Diseases*, **18**, 201.

Waterlow, J. C. (1948) Fatty liver disease in infants in the British West Indies. *Medical Research Council Special Report*, Series No. 263. London, H.M.S.O.

Waterlow, J. C. (1972) Classification and definition of protein-calorie malnutrition. *British Medical Journal*, **3**, 566.

Wharton, B. A. (1970) The child with kwashiorkor—30 years on. In *Alimentary and Haematological Aspects of Tropical Disease*, p. 420, ed. Woodruff, A. W. London; Arnold.

Wharton, B. A. (1975) Gastrointestinal problems in children of developing countries. In *Paediatric Gastroenterology*, p. 569, ed. Anderson, C. M. & Burke, V. Oxford: Blackwell.
Woodd-Walker, R. B., Hansen, J. D. L. & Saunders, S. J. (1972) The *in vitro* uptake of lysine and alanine by human jejunal mucosa in protein-calorie malnutrition, in gastroenteritis and after neomycin. *Acta Paediatrics Scandinavica*, **61**, 140.

9. Small intestinal enteropathies

J. A. Walker-Smith and Anne Kilby

Coeliac disease
Transient intolerance to dietary proteins
Bacterial and viral enteritis
Giardiasis
Tropical sprue
Acrodermatitis enteropathica
Eosinophilic gastroenteropathy
Histiocytosis X
Other enteropathies

The term small intestinal enteropathy describes the presence of a morphological abnormality of the small intestinal mucosa which may occur in a variety of disorders. In children routine small intestinal biopsies are taken from the fourth part of the duodenum or just distal to the D-J flexure, and so provide information concerning the mucosa of the proximal small intestine. From a diagnostic point of view it is fortunate that most enteropathies chiefly affect the proximal mucosa, though the enteropathy associated with infective enteritis in infancy may be variable in distribution and affect the ileal mucosa predominantly. The enteropathy may be of uniform severity, as in coeliac disease (Creamer and Leppard, 1965), or patchy, as in dermatitis herpetiformis and infective enteritis (Walker Smith, 1972; Schreiber, Blacklow and Trier, 1973).

The presence of a small intestinal enteropathy may be a primary feature of the disease process, as in coeliac disease, or a secondary feature, as in protein-energy malnutrition. Table 9.1 lists the disorders in childhood where a small intestinal enteropathy has been described, based on biopsy and autopsy studies and on observations of specimens obtained at laparotomy.

COELIAC DISEASE

This condition was first described in the second century A.D. by a Greek physician, Aretaeus the Cappodocian, who wrote of the 'coeliac affection' in adults (Dowd and Walker Smith, 1974). Nearly 800 years later Dr Samuel Gee (1888) described a similar disorder in children, giving a vivid and accurate clinical account of the condition as we now recognise it. In 1950 Dicke made his great discovery that dietary gluten was the toxic factor and that withdrawal of gluten leads to a complete clinical remission. Seven years later Sakula and

Table 9.1 Causes of small intestinal enteropathies in childhood

Coeliac disease	
Transient dietary protein intolerance	cows' milk protein
	soy protein
	gluten
Bacterial and viral enteritis	
Giardiasis	
Tropical sprue	
Protein-energy malnutrition	
Intestinal lymphangiectasia	
Acrodermatitis enteropathica	
Eosinophilic gastroenteropathy	
Histiocytosis X	
Non-specific enterocolitis	
Drugs, e.g. methotrexate	
Radiation enteritis	
Lymphoma	
Crohn's disease	
Iron deficiency	

Shiner (1957) reported the first small intestinal biopsy in a child with coeliac disease, describing the typical flat appearance of the mucosa now recognised to be characteristic of this disorder. Despite these major advances the basic pathophysiology operating in coeliac disease remains uncertain.

Definition

Coeliac disease results from a gluten-induced enteropathy which predominantly affects the proximal small intestinal mucosa and which usually leads to malabsorption and biochemical and clinical abnormalities; withdrawal of dietary gluten results in complete remission, but the intolerance to gluten is permanent. The condition may present in childhood or in adult life.

Aetiology

Gluten is the germ protein of wheat and also of several other cereals and, whilst it is clear that gluten is toxic to all patients with coeliac disease, the mechanism by which it exerts its toxic effects is far from clear. Gluten is a large complex molecule and consists of a mixture of four heterogeneous classes of proteins: gliadins, glutenins, albumins and globulins. Techniques such as starch-gel electrophoresis have shown the gliadin fraction to contain about 40 different components, and most interest has centred around the α-gliadin fraction which has been shown to be the most toxic component (Kendall *et al.*, 1972). Enzymatic degradation of gluten or gliadin suggests that the toxic portion of the α-gliadin molecule is a polypeptide with a molecular weight of less than 15 000 (Kowlessar, 1967; Dissanayake *et al.*, 1974). As α-gliadin is present in variable amounts in different wheats, it is possible that some wheats are more toxic than others.

Controversy exists regarding the basic mechanism by which gluten induces mucosal abnormalities, and there are two schools of thought.

Primary mucosal peptidase deficiency

This theory was first put forward by Frazer (1956), who proposed that a primary deficiency of an intracellular peptidase resulted in accumulation of a toxic peptide which caused cell damage and villous atrophy. Several workers have shown mucosal dipeptidase deficiency in untreated coeliac disease, but levels return to normal with treatment (Douglas and Peters, 1970). Douglas and Booth (1970) found no evidence to support this theory in studies of the rate of liberation of amino acids from gluten-peptides using normal mucosa and mucosa from patients with treated coeliac disease. Cornell and Townley (1973) have shown that a toxic fraction of gliadin (fraction 9) is defectively hydrolysed by mucosa from treated children; in this study, however, it was not made clear for how long the patients had been treated or whether other markers of mucosal function had returned to normal. At present there is no good evidence to support a primary peptidase deficiency.

Immunological abnormality

In recent years a great deal of evidence has accumulated indicating that a variety of immunological abnormalities are present in patients with coeliac disease, but whether the toxic effects of gluten are mediated by a primary immune process remains controversial. There is both direct and indirect evidence of immunological abnormalities in untreated patients.

Most notable amongst the direct evidence is the demonstration of disturbances in humoral reactivity, such as elevated titres of circulating antibodies to various dietary proteins and reticulin, and abnormalities of serum immunoglobulin concentrations and plasma-containing immunoglobulin cell concentrations in the lamina propria, and evidence of complement activation. Serum IgG and IgM concentrations are usually reduced, whereas IgA levels are raised (Kenrick and Walker Smith, 1970; Asquith, Thompson and Cooke, 1969), but there is considerable variation in the frequency of these abnormalities. Both the elevated levels of dietary protein antibodies and the abnormalities of serum immunoglobulins return to normal following treatment. Data on the quantification of immunoglobulin-containing plasma cells in lamina propria are variable according to the age of the patient. In untreated children both IgA- and IgM-containing cells are increased (Savilahti, 1972) and our findings are similar (see Figs. 9.5 and 9.6); in some children IgE cells may be raised (Kilby, Walker Smith and Wood, 1975). In untreated adults IgA cells are normal or reduced and IgM cells are raised; following a gluten challenge both IgA and IgM cells increase, and the magnitude of the rise in IgA cells is directly related to the duration of treatment prior to challenge (Lancaster-Smith, Kumar and Clark, 1974). Thus local IgA production is probably stimulated initially in both children and adults, only later to become exhausted. Shiner and Ballard (1972) found antibody, mainly IgA, in the basement membrane of the small intestinal epithelial cells after gluten challenge in children; in addition they observed deposition of complement and immune complexes in the lamina propria. Within one to six hours of gluten challenge in adults, there is evidence of serum complement consumption, and complement-binding immune complexes appear in the serum (Doe, Henry and Booth, 1974). The first morphological changes following gluten challenge occur in the lamina propria, not the surface epithelial cells, and involve the basement membrane of the epithelial cells, the endothelial cells of small blood vessels, and connective tissue fibrils and inflammatory cells (Shmerling and Shiner, 1970). Using *in vitro* culture techniques Falchuk, Gebhard and Strober (1974) have studied the pathogenesis of gluten toxicity in biopsy specimens from patients with coeliac disease. Their results suggest that gluten peptides are not directly toxic but that activation of an endogenous effector mechanism is first required; they propose this to be a local immune system, which elaborates a humoral material, which in turn reacts with the gluten peptides, the complex mediating the toxic effects of gluten; they suggest that the humoral material is a locally produced gluten antibody. Finally, Ezoke *et al.* (1974) have described lymphocyte-dependent serum antibodies which can co-opt lymphocytes known as K or Killer cells to attack gluten-labelled targets.

Direct evidence of abnormalities in cellular reactivity include increased numbers of interepithelial lymphocytes in the small intestinal mucosa of untreated patients (Ferguson and Murray, 1971), and gluten stimulation of lymphocytes (Holmes, Asquith and Cooke, 1972).

The indirect evidence for an immune abnormality includes the occasional report of gluten shock and the improvement in the mucosal abnormality following steroid therapy (Wall *et al.*, 1970).

This review clearly indicates that a number of immunological abnormalities occur in patients with coeliac disease, but how fundamental or primary these are in the pathogenesis of the disease remains unknown. On the evidence available it seems possible that an allergic reaction of the Gell and Coombs classification, Types I, III or IV, may occur; such a reaction could be a primary phenomenon or be secondary to a high concentration of a toxic fragment of gluten which has been incompletely digested due to a peptidase deficiency. Thus the two theories of enzyme deficiency and immunological abnormality are not mutually exclusive (Asquith, 1974a).

Genetic and environmental factors

Coeliac disease only occurs in those parts of the world where gluten is ingested, such as Britain, Europe, North America, Australia and the Punjab region of the Indian subcontinent; it has not yet been documented in China, Japan or Africa, nor in West Indians or American Negroes. A partial explanation for this geographical distribution may be related to the predisposition of people possessing the histocompatibility antigen HL-A8 to develop coeliac disease, since nearly all countries from which coeliac disease has been reported have a high frequency of this antigen (NcNeish *et al.*, 1974). The reported incidence of coeliac disease within the British Isles shows considerable variation, ranging from between one in 2000 and one in 6000 in England (Carter, Sheldon and Walker, 1959) to one in 300 in West Ireland (Mylotte *et al.*, 1973); part of the reason for this wide variation may be related to the applied diagnostic criteria. The familial occurrence of coeliac disease is well known, and it has been suggested that the condition is inherited as a dominant gene with incomplete penetrance. The discordance for the condition in monozygotic twins, however, argues strongly

Table 9.2 Discordance for coeliac disease in monozygotic twins

Authors	Mucosal biopsy	Response to diet	Diagnosis confirmed by gluten challenge	Assessment of Monozygosity
Hoffman *et al.*, 1966	Flat	Clinical	No	Blood groups and dermatoglyphics
Carter *et al.*, 1959	Not done	Clinical	No	Blood groups
Walker Smith, 1973	Flat	Clinical and histological	Yes	Blood groups, dermatoglyphics and placental examination
McNeish and Nelson, 1974	Flat	Clinical and histological	Yes	Blood groups

against such a mode of inheritance (see Table 9.2). The most probable explanation for the familial occurrence of coeliac disease is that susceptibility to a number of environmental factors is inherited by polygenic variation (McCrae, 1969).

Pathology

The proximal small intestinal mucosa is abnormal whereas the distal mucosa is usually normal; however, direct instillation of gluten into the ileum induces mucosal abnormalities in patients with coeliac disease but not in normal individuals (Rubin *et al.*, 1960), indicating that the whole length of the small intestinal mucosa is sensitive to gluten. The proximal distribution of the mucosal abnormality accords with the concept of a noxious agent in the diet becoming completely hydrolysed in the gut lumen, so that by the time it reaches the ileum it is no longer toxic.

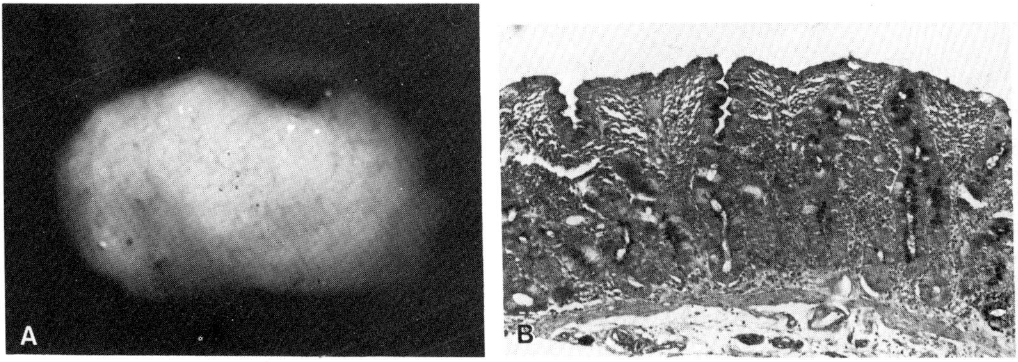

Fig. 9.1 A Dissecting microscopic appearances of proximal jejunal mucosa in untreated coeliac disease showing flat cobbled mucosal surface.

Fig. 9.1 B Light microscopic appearances of proximal jejunal mucosa in untreated coeliac disease (PAS stain, magnified × 104). The normal villous architecture is lost and the mucosa is flat; the surface epithelial cells are abnormal and the lamina propria is infiltrated with plasma cells.

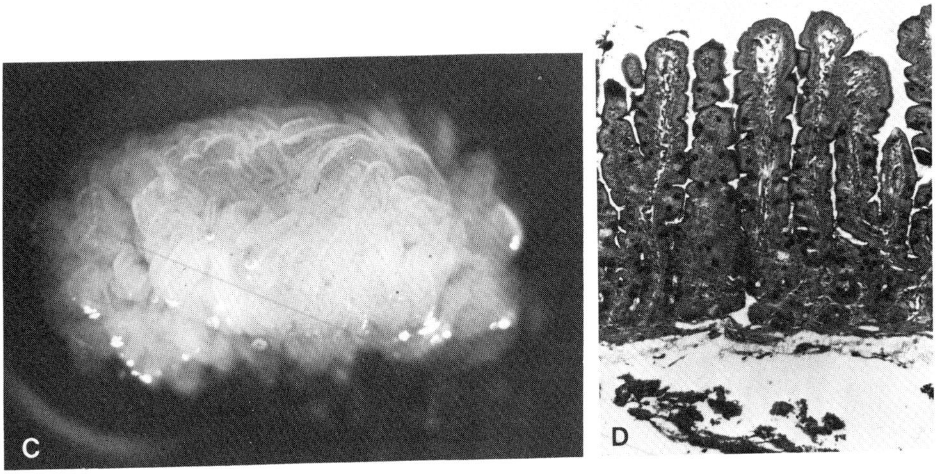

Fig. 9.1 C Dissecting microscopic appearances of proximal jejunal mucosa in treated coeliac disease showing normal leaf and finger shaped villi.

Fig. 9.1 D Normal light microscopic appearances of proximal jejunal mucosa in treated coeliac disease (PAS stain, magnified × 104).

The characteristic dissecting and light microscopic appearances of the proximal small intestinal mucosa in untreated coeliac disease are shown in Figure 9.1A and B; with treatment the mucosal lesion reverts completely to normal (Fig. 9.1C and D). Kinetic studies have shown that the turnover rate of the surface epithelial cells is increased in untreated coeliac disease (Wright *et al.*, 1973); the increased loss of epithelial cells from the villous tips into the lumen is accompanied by a compensatory increase in crypt cell replication, which ultimately results in villous atrophy and elongated hyperplastic crypts, i.e. hyperplastic villous atrophy. The normally columnar epithelial cells with their basally located oval nuclei may become pseudostratified or cuboidal with the nuclei spherical and pyknotic. These changes are accompanied by a quantitative increase in lamina propria plasma cells with a concomitant decrease of lymphocytes, and an increase in interepithelial cell lymphocytes. An analogy has been drawn between the gluten-induced increase in cell turnover rate and the increased turnover of erythrocytes in haemolytic anaemia, and the word 'enterocyte' has been coined and widely used to refer to the surface epithelial cells of the mucosa (Booth, 1968). When examined under the dissecting or stereomicroscope the mucosa of children with coeliac disease is completely flat or featureless, or it may have a flat mosaic appearance with irregular areas divided by grooves (Fig. 9.1A). When examined histologically under the light microscope the mucosa has an appearance described as subtotal or total villous atrophy, or simply a flat mucosa. The severity of the proximal mucosal lesion has generally been regarded to be uniform, but recent studies in adults suggest

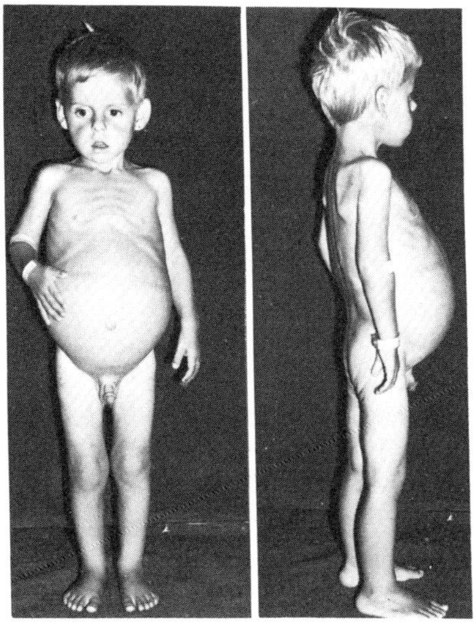

Fig. 9.2 Classical features of coeliac disease showing muscle wasting and abdominal distention.

that the lesion may be 'patchy' with areas of flat mucosa adjacent to less abnormal mucosa. At present the finding of anything but a flat biopsy in a child who presents with suspected coeliac disease should alert the physician to the possibility of an alternative diagnosis. Further studies using multiple biopsy techniques and rigid diagnostic criteria are required to determine whether the mucosal lesion in childhood coeliac disease is patchy. There is no natural recovery of the mucosal lesion. The time required for the mucosa to return to normal following the institution of a gluten-free diet in an individual child may sometimes be surprisingly long, for example up to a year and perhaps longer.

Clinical features

The majority of children present before the age of 2 years. The interval between the introduction of gluten-containing foods and the development of symptoms, however, is variable and although most children become symptomatic within six months of starting cereals, others may present in late childhood. In young infants acute symptoms such as diarrhoea and vomiting may occur after the first ingestion of gluten and mimick the clinical picture of acute infective enteritis. It is now a common but unnecessary practice to introduce cereals to babies aged only 2 to 3 weeks. As a result coeliac disease is presenting at an earlier age (Anderson, Gracey and Burke, 1972), and it is in this very young age group that an acute onset is more likely to occur.

The classical features of abnormal stools, anorexia, vomiting, abdominal distention and muscle wasting (Fig. 9.2) occur in approximately half the children presenting before the age of two years (unpublished observations); frequently there is a history of irritability, apathy and delay or regression of motor development, and hypotonia may be present. Tables 9.3 and 9.4 show the age at the onset

Table 9.3 Age of children with coeliac disease at onset of symptoms

Series	Years studied	Number of patients	0–6 months	7–12 months	13–24 months	2–5 years	6 years and over
Young and Pringle, 1971	1950–1969	63	25	29	9	0	0
Hamilton *et al.*, 1969	1964–1968	42	10	11	12	8	1
Walker Smith and Kilby (unpublished)	1972–1975	42	26	9	3	2	2

Table 9.4 Age of children with coeliac disease at time of diagnosis

Series	Years studied	Number of patients	0–6 months	7–12 months	13–24 months	2–5 years	6 years and over
Young and Pringle, 1971	1950–1969	91	–	33	37	18	3
Hamilton *et al.*, 1969	1964–1968	42	0	6	16	15	5
Walker Smith and Kilby (unpublished)	1972–1975	42	8	14	10	4	6

of symptoms and the age at diagnosis, respectively, of children with coeliac disease in three independent series.

A diagnosis of coeliac disease should never be dismissed because of the absence of classical features since the condition has a wide spectrum of presentation. The bowel pattern may vary from bouts of explosive watery diarrhoea in the young infant to bulky offensive stools in the older child; episodes of diarrhoea may alternate with constipation, and occasionally constipation may be a presenting feature. The typical irritability and fretfulness may be absent. Older children may present with symptoms of more insidious onset, such as persistent iron deficiency anaemia, small stature or delayed puberty, and they may or may not have a history of gastrointestinal symptoms; there may be little to find on physical examination apart from short stature.

Investigations

Peroral intestinal biopsy, prior to starting a gluten-free diet, is mandatory for the diagnosis of coeliac disease and should probably only be performed in centres with experience in the preparation and interpretation of mucosal specimens; the only rare exception is when diagnostic biopsy should be deferred in the acutely ill child with a dilated small bowel (i.e. 'coeliac crisis'), when biopsy is more likely to be complicated by bleeding and/or perforation. These two complications are exceptionally uncommon in experienced centres. A number of screening tests such as quantification of faecal fat, serum iron and folate, red cell folate, serum reticulin antibodies and urinary xylose following an oral load have been recommended but are far from ideal. Rolles *et al.* (1973) have applied the one-hour blood xylose test as a screening test and reported a high degree of discrimination between children with and without coeliac disease. Lamabadusuriya, Packer and Harries (1975), using a somewhat different oral loading dose

Table 9.5 Established causes of a flat small intestinal mucosa

Coeliac disease
Cows' milk protein intolerance
Soy protein intolerance
Acute viral and bacterial enteritis
Protein-energy malnutrition
Tropical sprue
Giardiasis

of xylose, did not find the test as reliable and reported three children with flat mucosae due to coeliac disease who had normal one-hour blood xylose concentrations.

A clinical suspicion of coeliac disease is the single most important indication for biopsy. The early performance of this investigation avoids time-consuming and equally discomforting investigations, and reduces the duration of hospitalisation to a minimum by providing a rapid diagnosis.

Diagnostic criteria

The demonstration of a flat, small intestinal mucosa followed by a clinical response to the dietary withdrawal of gluten used to be considered an adequate basis for a definitive diagnosis of coeliac disease. The recognition of other causes of a flat mucosa (see Table 9.5) and the probable existence of a syndrome of transient gluten intolerance have necessitated stricter diagnostic criteria. A

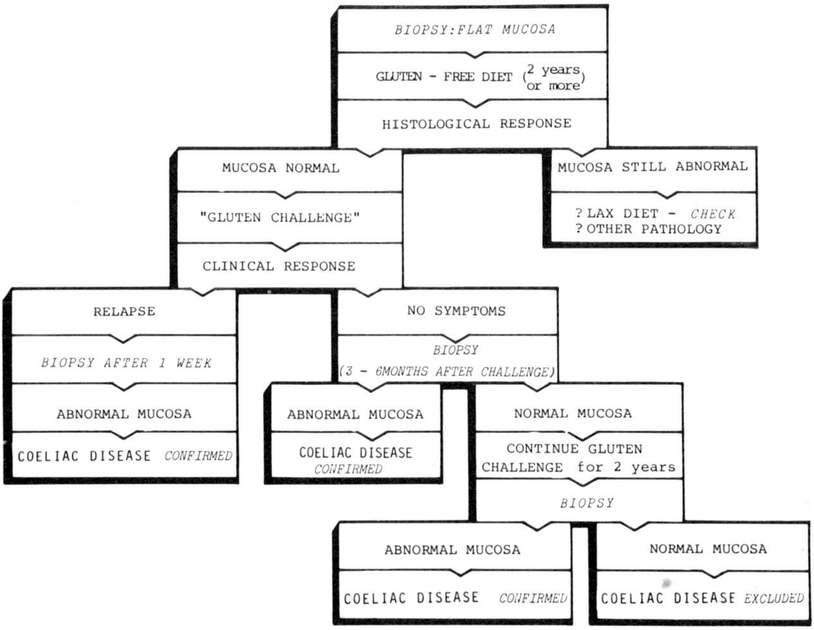

Fig. 9.3 Diagnostic criteria and investigatory regime for coeliac disease

definitive diagnosis of coeliac disease (i.e. permanent gluten intolerance) can be made only when gluten-induced mucosal abnormalities have been demonstrated following initial diagnosis and treatment. A scheme for such a diagnostic programme is illustrated in Figure 9.3, and we have applied this to 32 children with a past diagnosis of coeliac disease (unpublished observations). In 23 of the patients the diagnosis was based on a flat mucosal biopsy and the clinical response to a gluten-free diet; in the remaining nine children biopsy was not performed. After two years of returning to a normal diet, four of the children who had an initial flat biopsy had normal biopsies, and two of the nine patients who did not have initial biopsies also had normal biopsies. After returning to a normal diet vague symptoms were common and unreliable in predicting which children developed mucosal abnormalities; such symptoms are probably related to the anxiety associated with returning to the 'toxic' gluten-containing diet. This study emphasises the necessity of applying strict diagnostic criteria, and similar findings have been reported by others (Packer, Rowlatt and Harries, 1975).

Complications

Retarded growth and development

Severe growth retardation and delayed puberty are less common complications than formerly but may still occur as a mode of presentation. Vanderschueren-Lodeweyckx *et al.* (1973) found evidence of growth hormone deficiency in nine out of 13 children with coeliac disease. Thus coeliac disease should be considered as a diagnostic possibility in children of short stature who have growth hormone deficiency.

Skeletal abnormalities

Rickets and osteoporosis are uncommon complications of coeliac disease nowadays.

Hypoproteinaemia

Hypoalbuminaemia, hypogammaglobulinaemia and hypoprothrombinaemia may all occur. Hypoalbuminaemia occurs in about a third of cases and is mainly due to intestinal loss of protein. Hypoprothrombinaemia is secondary to malabsorption of vitamin K and can be rapidly corrected with intramuscular vitamin K_1 (1 mg); this should be done prior to diagnostic biopsies.

Anaemia

Iron deficiency anaemia is quite common. Although serum and/or red cell folate levels are often reduced, megaloblastic anaemia is most unusual. The combination of iron and folate deficiency should suggest the possibility of coeliac disease.

Milk intolerance

Intolerance to the lactose or protein moieties of cows' milk may occasionally be present at the time of diagnosis in infants (Young and Pringle, 1971; Visakorpi and Immonen, 1967). Withdrawal of dietary disaccharides and/or cows' milk protein should only be considered if gastrointestinal symptoms persist following the institution of a gluten-free diet. Reduced activity of mucosal disaccharidases is an almost invariable finding in untreated coeliac disease and is not by itself an indication for a disaccharide-free diet; clinical intolerance is the only indication for such diets.

Neoplastic disease

Untreated adult coeliac disease may be complicated by lymphoma and carcinoma (Harris *et al.*, 1967), and a gluten-free diet may protect against the development of carcinoma and reduce the incidence of lymphoma (Asquith, 1974b). The risk of children developing neoplastic disease is not known.

Associated diseases

Diabetes mellitus

This association is now well documented and in one patient hyperthyroidism was also present (Chambers, 1975). Autoimmune thyroiditis has also been reported in coeliac disease (MacLaurin, Mathews and Kilpatrick, 1972). It is noteworthy that Cudworth and Woodrow (1974) found that 54 per cent of patients with juvenile onset diabetes had the HL-A8 antigen. In the light of the predisposition to coeliac disease that possession of this antigen endows, perhaps this is a common factor between coeliac disease and diabetes mellitus.

Isolated IgA deficiency

An association between IgA deficiency and coeliac disease has been described by a number of observers. Unlike the other abnormalities of serum immunoglobulins described in children with coeliac disease, this is not influenced by a gluten-free diet (Savilahti, Pelkonen and Visakorpi, 1971). Thus IgA deficiency appears to be a disorder that predisposes to coeliac disease but, in fact, only a small proportion of children with this deficiency develop the disorder. Savilahti (1974) reported four out of 29 children with IgA deficiency who also had coeliac disease, the rest having normal small intestinal morphology.

Dermatitis herpetiformis

Although there is an association between dermatitis herpetiformis and coeliac disease, it is uncommonly seen in childhood. The severity of the enteropathy in dermatitis herpetiformis varies from patient to patient and may be patchy in any one individual patient (Brow *et al.*, 1971). Both the enteropathy and the skin lesions may respond to withdrawal of dietary gluten (Kumar *et al.*, 1973).

Other associations

Both cystic fibrosis and alpha-1-antitrypsin deficiency have been reported in children with coeliac disease, but the significance of these associations is uncertain.

Management

The specific treatment for coeliac disease is a gluten-free diet, and such a diet is generally regarded as one which is free of wheat, rye, oats and barley; maize (corn) and rice are harmless. The evidence that wheat and rye are toxic in childhood coeliac disease is well established, but the effect of oats and barley is controversial. Dissanayake, Truelove and Whitehead (1974) have provided some evidence that oats are not toxic in adults, but their period of observation following challenge with oats was far too short to draw firm conclusions. A survey of coeliac children in Britain showed that 12 per cent were upset by oats (Segall, 1974). The evidence that oats and/or barley are toxic in coeliac disease remains controversial, and further studies are required to clarify the situation.

Elimination of dietary gluten often leads to rapid clinical response within a few days, although in some children obvious improvement may be delayed. The first sign of improvement is a change of mood, the child becoming less irritable, clinging and withdrawn. There follows a gain in weight with further symptomatic relief such as improvement in diarrhoea. Anxiety, depression and preoccupation with the child and his illness are common in the mother and usually rapidly disappear as the child begins to recover (Gardiner, Porteous and Walker Smith, 1972). In the majority of patients a gluten-free diet is all that is required, and only in a minority is it necessary to temporarily exclude disaccharides and/or cows' milk protein. Ideally treated patients should be followed up by a centre experienced in coeliac disease and their progress and diet checked at regular intervals. The necessity for a life-long diet depends on the diagnostic criteria previously discussed.

TRANSIENT INTOLERANCE TO DIETARY PROTEINS

This group of clinical syndromes results from the sensitisation of an individual to one or more dietary proteins which have been absorbed through a permeable intestine and are temporary syndromes of variable duration in children. Abnormalities of the small intestinal mucosa have been reported in cows' milk protein, soy protein and gluten intolerances; the evidence for the existence of the first two disorders as entities is unequivocal, whereas the existence of transient gluten intolerance is controversial. The enteropathy is not always as severe as in coeliac disease, although a flat mucosa may be seen. Other clinically and immunologically recognised syndromes of dietary protein intolerance do exist, for example egg protein intolerance, but biopsy studies have not yet been reported in these disorders.

The mucosal abnormalities which occur in transient protein intolerance are generally considered to result from an allergic reaction, but the precise mechanisms involved in the pathogenesis of the enteropathy have not been defined. Schloss in 1911 was the first to relate gastrointestinal symptoms to an allergy to a particular food and he diagnosed egg allergy on the basis of positive skin tests using a protein fraction of ovomucoid. Skin tests have subsequently been recognised to be of limited value in the diagnosis of food allergy, but Schloss's concept of food allergy has become widely accepted in relation to several food proteins.

Cows' milk protein intolerance

This condition may manifest itself with a number of extraintestinal features such as eczema and asthma, but this account will be confined to the gastrointestinal effects of cows' milk allergy. The composition of cows' milk protein differs in a number of important ways to that of human milk. For example, the bovine protein contains beta-lactoglobulin and is low in immunoglobulins, whereas its human counterpart contains no beta-lactoglobulin and is rich in IgA, particularly colostrum (Ste-Marie, Lee and Brown, 1974). These differences have important implications, since beta-lactoglobulin is the protein moiety most often responsible for cows' milk protein intolerance (Visakorpi and Immonen, 1967).

Pathogenesis

It seems probable that excessive entry of dietary antigens across the intestinal mucosa occurs in infants with this disorder. This may be related to a transient immunodeficiency state such as transient IgA deficiency (Taylor *et al.*, 1973), or to non-specific mucosal damage from any cause. It is indeed possible that there may be two syndromes, a so-called primary disorder of immunological origin or a secondary disorder, a sequel of mucosal damage which in turn produces an immunological abnormality. Harrison, Wood and Walker Smith (1975) provided some evidence that acute enteritis (assumed to be infective in origin) may be followed by not only lactose intolerance but by more persistent and longer lasting cows' milk protein intolerance. Unlike coeliac disease HLA status is normal in this disorder, perhaps suggesting that environmental factors are more important than genetic ones (Kuitunen *et al.*, 1975). As in coeliac disease IgA- and IgM-containing plasma cells are quantitatively increased in the lamina propria (Savilahti, 1974), but IgE-containing cells are relatively increased compared with coeliac disease (Kilby, Walker Smith and Wood, 1975); in the latter study IgE cells decreased following a milk-free diet, only to reappear with milk challenge. The involvement of IgE in pathogenesis is also suggested by the finding of positive skin tests in some patients. Thus a Gell and Coombs (1968) type I reaction may be present. Evidence of complement activation (Mathews and Soothill, 1970) and of abnormalities in serum immunoglobulins and cell-mediated immunity suggests that more than one reaction may participate in the pathogenesis of this disorder.

Pathology

In the vast majority of patients the architecture of the proximal small intestinal mucosa is abnormal but the severity of the enteropathy is variable; in some the mucosa is flat and indistinguishable from that seen in coeliac disease (Kuitunen *et al.*, 1975). The lamina propria may be infiltrated by eosinophils (Silverberg and Davidson, 1974). The mucosa rapidly returns to normal on withdrawal of milk, only to relapse following challenge with milk (Walker Smith, 1975).

Clinical features

Presentation may be acute with vomiting and diarrhoea, or as a chronic syndrome characterised by less severe vomiting and diarrhoea with failure to thrive. The majority present with acute symptoms under the age of 6 months and have features indistinguishable from acute infective enteritis; lactose intolerance may accompany the protein intolerance, but is relatively short-lived compared with the intolerance to protein. There is usually a latent interval between the introduction of cows' milk and the onset of symptoms, but occasionally violent reactions, such as anaphylactoid shock, may immediately follow the infant's first contact with cows' milk. The chronic syndrome may present in a very similar fashion to coeliac disease with loose stools and failure to thrive. The syndrome may be accompanied by an iron deficiency anaemia due to intestinal blood loss with the sigmoidoscopic appearances of acute colitis (Gryboski, 1967).

Diagnostic criteria

Because of its transient nature rigid diagnostic criteria are not so necessary in cows' milk protein intolerance compared with coeliac disease; nevertheless accurate diagnosis is important. As with all dietary protein intolerances, diagnosis is based on the response to withdrawal and reintroduction of the offending protein and there is no specific laboratory test. Most clinicians base their diagnosis on the clinical response to the withdrawal of cows' milk and its reintroduction; a more definitive diagnosis is possible using sequential small intestinal biopsies.

Management

Treatment involves substituting cows' milk feeds with the commercially available cows' milk, protein-free formula feeds (see Francis, 1975). Goats' milk is sometimes used as a substitute, but cross-reactivity with cows' milk may be associated with intolerance to both milks. It is important to ensure that both liquid and solid feeds are free of cows' milk proteins. Disaccharide intolerance may accompany the protein intolerance, and in these circumstances disaccharides should also be withdrawn from the diet. The necessity for dietary treatment is always temporary, and reintroduction of a normal diet is usually possible by the age of 1 to 2 years; this is usually possible in the home, but a history of severe reactions, such as urticaria or anaphylactoid shock, is an absolute indication for reintroduction of a normal diet under very close medical supervision.

Soy protein intolerance

There have been a number of clinical reports of intolerance to soy protein, but it was not until recently that Ament and Rubin (1972a) established that the protein induced an enteropathy which resolved with dietary treatment and which reappeared when soy protein was reintroduced into the diet; they described a flat mucosal lesion indistinguishable to that found in coeliac disease. The frequency of soy protein intolerance may well increase with the more widespread use of soy-protein based infant feeds.

Gluten intolerance

Unequivocable evidence for a syndrome of transient gluten intolerance has not yet been documented. However, a number of children have been reinvestigated following a diagnosis of coeliac disease (based on the finding of a flat mucosa and a clinical response to a gluten-free diet), who have remained clinically well with a normal small intestinal mucosa for more than two years after the reintroduction of a gluten-containing diet (Lindberg and Meeuwisse, 1973; McNicholl, Egan-Mitchell and Fottrell, 1974; Packer, Rowlatt and Harries, 1975). A clinical response to the initial withdrawal of dietary gluten cannot be regarded as proof of temporary gluten toxicity; this can only be established by early reinvestigation and demonstration of gluten toxicity and the demonstration that such toxicity disappears after a time interval. Hence there is still controversy regarding the existence of this entity. If such an entity exists, it is most likely to occur in infancy and be secondary to conditions such as acute infective enteritis. This emphasises the necessity to reinvestigate, by means of gluten challenge and intestinal biopsy, infants diagnosed as coeliac disease before recommending a life-long diet.

BACTERIAL AND VIRAL ENTERITIS

Infective enteritis is a major problem in childhood throughout the world and is covered in detail elsewhere (see Ch. 10). This discussion will therefore be limited to the morphological appearances of the small intestinal mucosa in acute enteritis and in the 'postenteritis syndrome' (i.e. persistently loose stools and/or failure to thrive for longer than two weeks following an acute episode of diarrhoea with or without vomiting). Proof of an infecting agent being the primary pathophysiological factor is often not possible, and in many cases it can only be assumed that this is the case.

Acute disease

The evidence that a small intestinal enteropathy may accompany acute enteritis is derived from autopsy studies and from peroral biopsies performed during the acute phase of the disease.

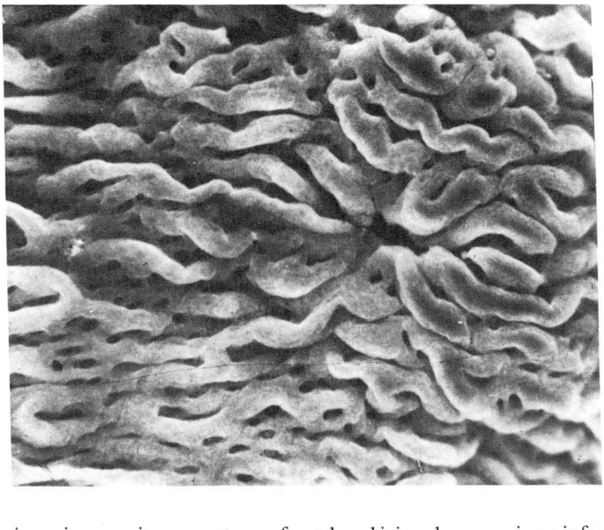

Fig. 9.4 Dissecting microscopic appearances of autolysed jejunal mucosa in an infant dying of acute enteritis, showing short thick ridges.

Using a modification of the technique described by Creamer and Leppard (1965), autopsy studies in children dying during the acute phase were first reported by Walker Smith (1972); the small intestine was placed in running water for 24 hours to allow the surface epithelium to slough off leaving the connective tissue 'cores' of the villi exposed, and the exposed basement membrane was then stained with ordinary ink. The three-dimensional morphology of the whole length of the small intestine could then be scanned with the dissecting microscope. Morphological abnormalities were found in seven of the 10 patients studied (see Fig. 9.4), and the severity and extent of the abnormalities were variable. In the majority the distribution of the enteropathy

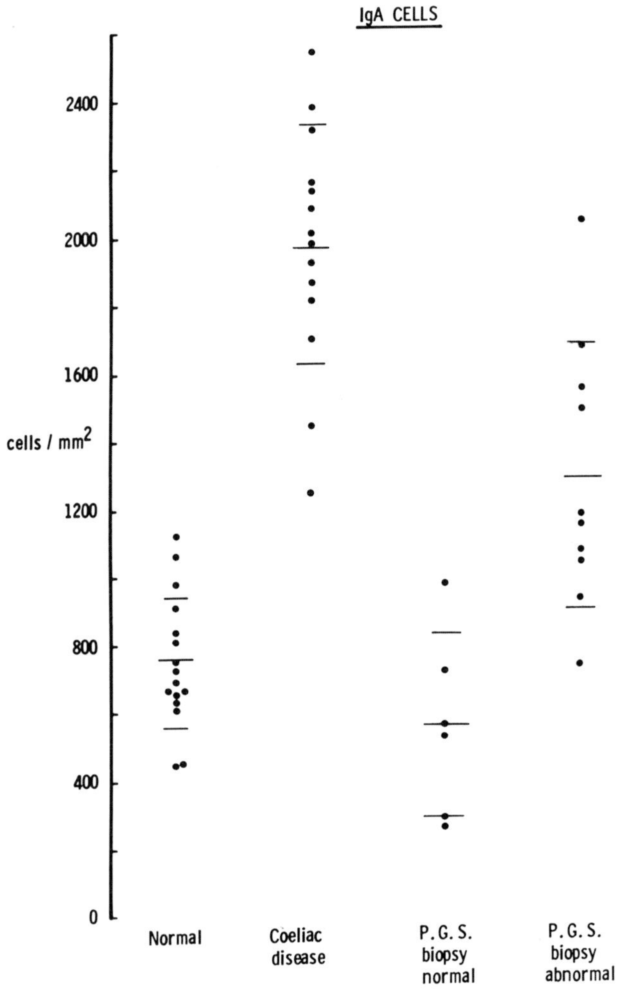

Fig. 9.5 IgA-containing cells in lamina propria of jejunal mucosa of children with coeliac disease, 'postgastroenteritis syndrome' (PGS), with normal and abnormal biopsies. Horizontal bars indicate mean values ± 1 s.d.

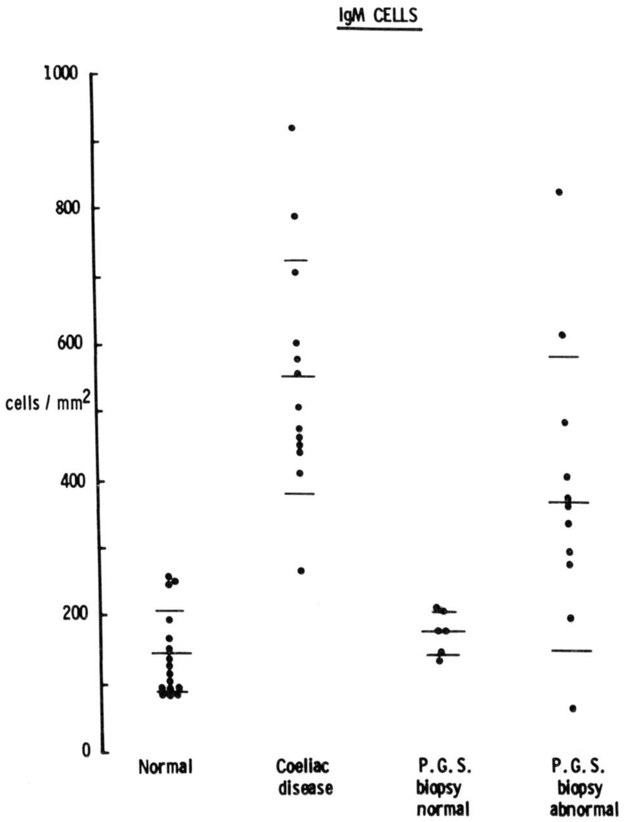

Fig. 9.6 IgM-containing cells in lamina propria of jejunal mucosa of children with coeliac disease, 'postgastroenteritis syndrome' (PGS), with normal and abnormal biopsies. Horizontal bars indicate mean values ± 1 s.d.

was proximal, but in one patient the whole of the small intestine was affected, whereas in another the ileum was chiefly involved. The mucosal lesions tended to be patchy in individual patients.

Barnes and Townley (1973) performed biopsies in 31 infants with acute enteritis; the mucosa was flat in five and 20 infants had less severe abnormalities. In three patients serial biopsies after three days, eight days and seven weeks showed significant improvement, but the interpretation of single biopsies as a guide to the overall state of the proximal small intestinal mucosa must be cautious in the light of the studies discussed above (Walker Smith, 1972). Moreover, patchy mucosal lesions have been reported in normal adults following administration of the Norwalk agent (Schreiber, Blacklow and Trier, 1973).

Chronic disease

Mucosal abnormalities have been well documented in a proportion of children who developed protracted diarrhoea following an acute episode of enteritis (Burke, Kerry and Anderson, 1965; Boyce, France and Walker Smith, 1974), the degree of abnormality ranging from a completely flat mucosa to varying degrees of villous shortening and surface cell changes. We have recently investigated 28 infants with protracted diarrhoea, of whom 22 had mucosal abnormalities of varying severity (unpublished observations); immunofluorescent studies showed increased numbers of IgA- and IgM-containing cells in the lamina propria of the patients with mucosal lesions, but numbers were normal in the absence of mucosal abnormalities (see Figs. 9.5 and 9.6). These changes in immunoglobulin-containing cells are similar but not usually so marked as in untreated coeliac disease and return to normal as the mucosa heals.

The pathogenesis of the enteropathy in both acute and protracted diarrhoea in infancy is not known; infective agents and various dietary proteins may play an individual and/or collective pathophysiological role, and further studies are required to define the mechanism(s) involved.

GIARDIASIS

Infestation with this flagellate protozoon is dealt with more fully elsewhere (see Ch. 12), and this discussion will be confined to the morphology of the small intestinal mucosa.

Giardiasis may be accompanied by gastrointestinal symptoms in both adults and children in the absence of recognisable immunodeficiency. In adult patients with hypogammaglobulinaemia Ament and Rubin (1972b), using a multiple biopsy technique, have shown patchy mucosal abnormalities and nodular lymphoid hyperplasia; the mucosal lesions varied in severity from flat to mild. Treatment with metronidazole was accompanied by a concomitant improvement in the mucosal abnormalities and the malabsorption and eradication of the giardia; the mucosal lesions, however, did not disappear completely in any of their patients. Improvement in mucosal abnormalities associated with giardiasis following eradication of the protozoon in the absence of an immunodeficiency state has only recently been convincingly demonstrated (D. Ogilvie and J. T. Harries, personal communication). They investigated a 7-year-old boy with Down's syndrome who had a six-month history of failure to gain weight and loose, bulky, offensive stools. Proximal small intestinal biopsy showed partial villous atrophy (Fig. 9.7 A), and giardia were identified in both duodenal juice and mucosa; tests of humoral and cell-mediated immunity were normal. Treatment with quinacrine (50 mg t.d.s. for three weeks) was associated with symptomatic improvement, and a repeat biopsy six weeks after completing quinacrine was normal (Fig. 9.7 B). These observations suggest that the protozoon can induce mucosal abnormalities in the absence of a recognisable immune deficiency state.

TROPICAL SPRUE (see Lindenbaum, 1973)

This poorly understood disorder is relatively uncommon in children compared with adults and is characterised by diarrhoea, megablastic anaemia, and malabsorption of vitamin B_{12}, folic acid and fat. The pathogenesis of this disorder is not known, but infection with bacterial overgrowth of the small intestine is of probable importance in the development of the condition. There

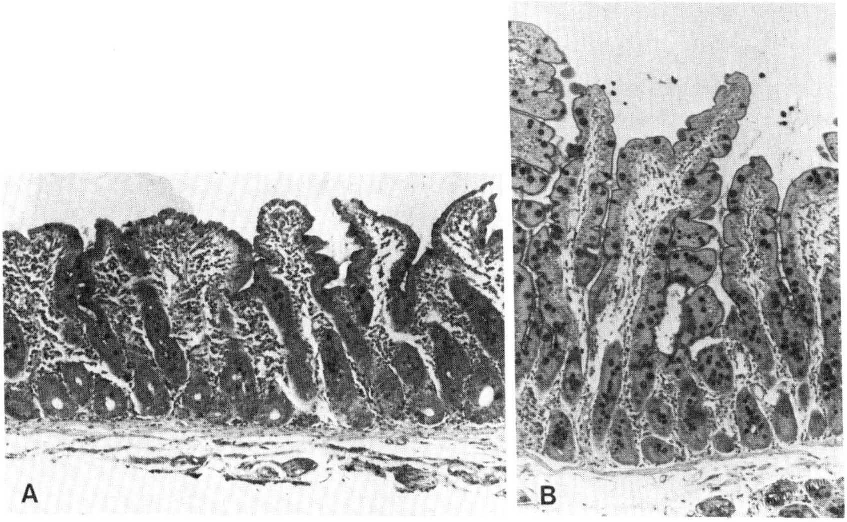

Fig. 9.7 A Light microscopic appearances of proximal jejunal mucosa in untreated giardiasis (PAS stain, magnified × 104). The normal villous architecture is lost, there is partial villous atrophy, the surface epithelial cells are abnormal and the lamina propria is infiltrated with chronic inflammatory cells.

Fig. 9.7 B Normal light microscopic appearances of proximal jejunal mucosa in treated giardiasis (PAS stain, magnified × 104)

is a non-specific enteropathy which affects the whole length of the small intestine; occasionally the mucosa is flat but usually the lesion is less severe. The condition responds to folic acid and/or antibiotic therapy. The diagnosis should be considered in children in non-tropical countries who have recently lived in an endemic area.

ACRODERMATITIS ENTEROPATHICA

This rare condition, an autosomal recessive inherited disorder, typically presents in infancy and is characterised by severe diarrhoea, failure to thrive, a rash at the mucocutaneous junctions and pressure areas, alopecia and dystrophy of the nails with or without paronychia (Neldner *et al.*, 1974). It does not occur in breast-fed babies, and characteristically presents at the time of weaning; untreated it is usually fatal. There have been conflicting reports of both abnormal and normal small intestinal mucosa in this condition; ultrastructural studies have indicated an abnormality of the Paneth cells (Lombeck *et al.*, 1974). There is good evidence that the clinical features of acrodermatitis enteropathica result from zinc deficiency (Moynahan, 1974) and that this deficiency state is due to a defect in zinc absorption. Treatment with oral zinc supplements results in a dramatic and sustained improvement (Moynahan, 1974).

EOSINOPHILIC GASTROENTEROPATHY (see Greenberger and Gryboski, 1973)

This syndrome is a disorder involving the stomach and/or small intestine and is characterised by eosinophilic infiltration of the gastrointestinal tract wall, eosinophilia and the development of gastrointestinal symptoms following the ingestion of certain specific dietary foods; improvement follows withdrawal of the offending dietary constituent(s) and/or corticosteroid therapy. The pathogenesis is not clearly understood but an allergic or immunological basis seems likely. Cows' milk protein intolerance may present as an eosinophilic gastroenteropathy. The disorder can be classified according to the extent of the eosinophilic infiltration: (1) primary mucosal involvement with malabsorption and protein loss, (2) muscle layer disease with obstructive features or (3) subserosal disease with eosinophilic ascites. The eosinophilic gastroenteropathy seen in childhood is almost invariably a primary mucosal disease. The jejunal mucosal enteropathy varies in severity. There may be mild eosinophilic infiltration of the lamina propria with preservation of villous pattern, or at the other extreme a severe infiltrative lesion with a flat mucosa; the mucosal lesion is patchy and, using multiple biopsy techniques, varying degrees of severity may be found in an individual patient.

HISTIOCYTOSIS X

Histiocytic infiltration of the small intestine may be present in infants with disseminated histiocytosis X (Letterer-Siwe syndrome). In an autopsy review of 12 cases (Keeling and Harries, 1973) the small intestine was found to be involved in six cases, four of whom had developed diarrhoea during the course of their illness; the ileum was most commonly affected but changes in the duodenum and jejunum were also found. The abnormalities included infiltration of the lamina propria with abnormal histiocytes and multinucleate giant cells; the villous architecture and epithelium were normal in all but one case, in which there was loss of the normal villous pattern. The cellular infiltration may impair intestinal function resulting in malabsorption.

OTHER ENTEROPATHIES

Small intestinal lymphomas, radiation enteritis, acute necrotising enterocolitis, chronic inflammatory disease, iron-deficiency anaemia and the administration of certain drugs may be associated with a small intestinal enteropathy and gastrointestinal symptoms. Although gastrointestinal symptoms commonly follow the administration of a variety of drugs, in only a few instances have small intestinal mucosal abnormalities been demonstrated. Methotrexate and high doses of neomycin may induce mucosal lesions (Dobbins, 1968); however, there is no evidence that therapeutic doses of neomycin produce mucosal damage. Mild mucosal changes have been reported to accompany iron-deficiency anaemia, but whether the iron deficiency is primary in the pathogenesis of the mucosal lesions has not been established.

References

Ament, M. E. & Rubin, C. E. (1972a) Soy protein—another cause of the flat intestinal lesion. *Gastroenterology*, **62,** 227.

Ament, M. E. & Rubin, C. E. (1972b) Relation of giardiasis to abnormal intestinal structure and function in gastrointestinal immunodeficiency syndromes. *Gastroenterology*, **62,** 216.

Anderson, C. M., Gracey, M. & Burke, V. (1972) Coeliac disease. Some still controversial aspects. *Archives of Disease in Childhood*, **47,** 292.

Asquith, P. (1974a) Immunology. *Clinics in Gastroenterology*, **3,** 213.

Asquith, P. (1974b) Discussion. In *Coeliac Disease*, p. 321, ed. Booth, C. C. & Dowling, R. H. Edinburgh: Churchill Livingstone.

Asquith, P., Thompson, R. A. & Cooke, W. T. (1969) Serum immunoglobulins in adult coeliac disease. *Lancet*, **2,** 129.

Barnes, G. L. & Townley, R. R. W. (1973) Duodenal mucosal damage in 31 infants with gastroenteritis. *Archives of Disease in Childhood*, **48,** 343.

Booth, C. C. (1968) Enteropoiesis: structural and functional relationships of the enterocyte. *Postgraduate Medical Journal*, **44,** 12.

Boyce, M. J., France, N. E. & Walker Smith, J. A. (1974) Small intestinal morphology in a group of infants and young children with delayed recovery after acute diarrhoea and vomiting. *Gut*, **15,** 827.

Brow, J. R., Parker, F., Weinstein, W. M. & Rubin, C. E. (1971) The small intestinal mucosa in dermatitis herpetiformis. I. Severity and distribution of the small intestinal lesion and associated malabsorption. *Gastroenterology*, **60,** 355.

Burke, V., Kerry, K. R. & Anderson, C. M. (1965) The relationship of dietary lactose in refractory diarrhoea in infancy. *Australian Paediatric Journal*, **1,** 147.

Carter, C., Sheldon, W. & Walker, C. (1959) The inheritance of coeliac disease. *Annals of Human Genetics*, **23,** 266.

Chambers, T. L. (1975) Coeliac disease, diabetes mellitus and hyperthyroidism. *Archives of Disease in Childhood*, **50,** 162.

Cornell, H. J., & Townley, R. R. W. (1973) Investigations of possible intestinal peptidase deficiency in coeliac disease. *Clinica Chimica Acta*, **43,** 113.

Creamer, B. & Leppard, P. (1965) Post mortem examination of a small intestine in the coeliac syndrome. *Gut*, **6,** 466.

Cudworth, A. G. & Woodrow, J. C. (1974) HLA antigens and diabetes mellitus. *Lancet*, **2,** 1153.

Dicke, W. K. (1950) Coeliakie. M.D. Thesis, University of Utrecht.

Dissanayake, A. S., Jerrome, D. W., Offord, R. E., Truelove, S. C. & Whitehead, R. (1974) Identifying toxic fractions of wheat gluten and their effect on the jejunal mucosa in coeliac disease. *Gut*, **15,** 931.

Dissanayake, A. S., Truelove, S. C. & Whitehead, R. (1974) Lack of harmful effect of oats on small-intestinal mucosa in coeliac disease. *British Medical Journal*, **4,** 189.

Dobbins, W. O. (1968) Drug-induced steatorrhoea. *Gastroenterology*, **54,** 1193.

Doe, W. F., Henry, K. & Booth, C. C. (1974) Complement in coeliac disease. In *Coeliac Disease*, ed. Hekkens, W. & Pena, A. Proceedings of the 2nd International Coeliac Symposium, p. 189. Leiden: Stenfert Kroese.

Douglas, A. P. & Booth, C. C. (1970) Digestion of gliadin peptides by normal human jejunal mucosa and by mucosa from patients with adult coeliac disease. *Clinical Science*, **38,** 11.

Douglas, A. P. & Peters, T. J. (1970) Peptide hydrolase activity of human intestinal mucosa in adult coeliac disease. *Gut*, **11,** 15.

Dowd, B. & Walker Smith, J. A. (1974) Samuel Gee, Aretaeus and the coeliac affection. *British Medical Journal*, **2,** 45.

Ezoke, W., Ferguson, N., Fakhri, O., Hekkens, W. Th. J. M. & Hobbs, J. R. (1974) Antibodies in the sera of coeliac patients which can co-opt K cells to attack gluten-labelled targets. In *Coeliac Disease*, ed. Hekkens, W. & Pena, A. Proceedings of the 2nd International Coeliac Symposium, p. 176. Leiden: Stenfert Kroese.

Falchuk, Z. M., Gebhard, R. L. & Strober, W. (1974) The pathogenesis of gluten sensitive enteropathy (coeliac sprue): organ culture studies. In *Coeliac Disease*, ed. Hekkens, W. & Pena, A. Proceedings of the 2nd International Coeliac Symposium, p. 107. Leiden: Stenfert Kroese.

Ferguson, A. & Murray, D. (1971) Quantitation of intra-epithelial lymphocytes in human jejunum. *Gut*, **12,** 988.

Francis, D. E. M. (1975) *Diets for Sick Children*. 3rd edition. Oxford: Blackwell.

Frazer, A. C. (1956) Growth defect in coeliac disease. *Proceedings of the Royal Society of Medicine*, **49,** 1009.

Gardiner, A., Porteous, N. & Walker Smith, J. A. (1972) The effect of coeliac disease on the mother child relationship. *Australian Paediatric Journal,* **8,** 39.

Gee, S. J. (1888) On the coeliac affection. *St. Bartholomew's Hospital Reports,* **24,** 17.

Gell, P. G. H. & Coombs, R. R. A. (1968) Classification of allergic reactions responsible for hypersensitivity and disease. In *Clinical Aspects of Immunology,* ed. Gell, P. G. H. & Coombs, R. R. A., p. 575. Oxford: Blackwell.

Greenberger, N. & Gryboski, J. D. (1973) Allergic disorders of the intestine and eosinophilic gastroenteritis. In *Gastrointestinal Disease,* ed. Sleisenger & Fordtran, Chap. 81, p. 1066. Philadelphia: Saunders.

Gryboski, J. D. (1967) Gastrointestinal milk allergy in infants. *Pediatrics,* **40,** 354.

Hamilton, J. R., Lynch, M. J. & Reilly, B. J. (1969) Active coeliac disease in childhood. *Quarterly Journal of Medicine,* **38,** 135.

Harris, O. D., Cooke, W. T., Thompson, H. & Waterhouse, J. A. H. (1967) Malignancy in adult coeliac disease and idiopathic steatorrhoea. *American Journal qf Medicine,* **42,** 899.

Harrison, M., Wood, C. B. S. & Walker Smith, J. A. (1975) Sugar malabsorption in cows milk protein intolerance. *Archives of Disease in Childhood,* **50,** 746.

Hoffman, H. N., Wollaeger, E. E. & Greenberg, E. (1966) Discordance for non tropical sprue in a monozygotic twin pair. *Gastroenterology,* **51,** 36.

Holmes, G. K. T., Asquith, P. & Cooke, W. T. (1972) Cell mediated mechanisms in adult coeliac disease. *Gut,* **13,** 324.

Keeling, J. W. & Harries, J. T. (1973) Intestinal malabsorption in infants with Histiocytosis X. *Archives of Disease in Childhood,* **48,** 350.

Kendall, M. J., Schneider, R., Cox, P. S. & Hawkins, C. E. (1972) Gluten subfractions in coeliac disease. *Lancet,* **2,** 1065.

Kenrick, K. G. & Walker Smith, J. A. (1970) Immunoglobulins and dietary protein antibodies in childhood coeliac disease. *Gut,* **11,** 635.

Kilby, A., Walker Smith, J. A. & Wood, C. B. S. (1975) Small intestinal mucosa in cows' milk allergy. *Lancet,* **1,** 53.

Kowlessar, O. D. (1967) Effect of wheat proteins in coeliac disease. *Gastroenterology,* **52,** 893.

Kuitunen, P., Visakorpi, J. K., Savilahti, E. & Pelkonen, P. (1975) Malabsorption syndrome with cows' milk intolerance: clinical findings and course in 54 cases. *Archives of Disease in Childhood,* **50,** 351.

Kumar, P. J., Silk, D. B. A., Marks, R., Clark, M. L. & Dawson, A. M. (1973) Treatment of dermatitis herpetiformis with corticosteroids and a gluten free diet: a study of jejunal morphology and function. *Gut,* **14,** 280.

Lamabadusuriya, S. P., Packer, S. & Harries, J. T. (1975) Limitations of xylose tolerance test as a screening procedure in childhood coeliac disease. *Archives of Disease in Childhood,* **50,** 34.

Lancaster-Smith, M., Kumar, P. & Clark, M. L. (1974) Immunological phenomena following gluten challenge in the jejunum of patients with adult coeliac disease and dermatitis herpetiformis. In *Coeliac Disease,* ed. Hekkens, W. & Pena, A. Proceedings of the 2nd International Coeliac Symposium, p. 173. Leiden: Stenfert Kroese.

Lindberg, T. & Meeuwisse, G. (1973) Transient coeliac disease—does it exist? *Acta Paediatrica Scandinavica,* Supplement 236, 56.

Lindenbaum, J. (1973) Tropical enteropathy. *Gastroenterology,* **64,** 637.

Lombeck, I., von Bassewitz, D. B., Becker, K., Tinschmann, P. & Kastner, H. (1974) Ultrastructural findings in acrodermatitis enteropathica. *Pediatric Research,* **8,** 82.

MacLaurin, B. P., Mathews, N. & Kilpatrick, J. A. (1972) Coeliac disease associated with autoimmune thyroiditis, Sjögern's syndrome and a lymphocytotoxic serum factor. *Australian & New Zealand Journal of Medicine,* **4,** 401.

Mathews, T. S. & Soothill, J. F. (1970) Complement activation after milk feeding in children with cows' milk allergy. *Lancet,* **2,** 893.

McCrae, W. N. (1969) Inheritance of coeliac disease. *Journal of Medical Genetics,* **6,** 129.

McNeish, A. S. & Nelson, R. (1974) Coeliac disease in one of monozygotic twins. *Clinics in Gastroenterology,* **3,** 143.

McNeish, A. S., Rolles, C. J., Nelson, R., Kyaw Myint, T. O., Mackintosh, P. & Williams, A. F. (1974) Factors affecting the differing racial incidence of coeliac disease. In *Coeliac Disease,* ed. Hekkens, W. & Pena, A. Proceedings of the 2nd International Coeliac Symposium, p. 330. Leiden: Stenfert Kroese.

McNicholl, B., Egan-Mitchell, B. & Fottrell, P. F. (1974) Varying susceptibility in coeliac disease. In *Coeliac Disease,* ed. Hekkens, W. & Pena, A. Proceedings of the 2nd International Coeliac Symposium, p. 413. Leiden: Stenfert Kroese.

Moynahan, E. J. (1974) Acrodermatitis enteropathica: a lethal inherited human zinc deficiency disorder. *Lancet,* **2,** 399.

Mylotte, M. J., Egan-Mitchell, B., Fottrell, P. F., McNicholl, B. & McCarthy, C. F. (1973) Incidence of coeliac disease in the West of Ireland. *British Medical Journal,* **60,** 703.

Neldner, K. H., Hagler, L., Wise, W. R. *et al.* (1974) Acrodermatitis enteropathica: a clinical and biochemical survey. *Archives of Dermatology,* **110,** 711.

Packer, S., Rowlatt, R. J. & Harries, J. T. (1975) Reappraisal of a past diagnosis of 'coeliac disease'. *Acta Paediatrica Scandinavica,* **64,** 144.

Rolles, C. J., Kendall, M. J., Nutter, S. & Anderson, C. M. (1973) One hour blood xylose screening test for coeliac disease. *Lancet,* **2,** 1043.

Rubin, C. E., Brandborg, L. L., Phelps, P. A. & Taylor, H. C. (1960) Studies of coeliac sprue. *Gastroenterology,* **38,** 28.

Sakula, J. & Shiner, M. (1957) Coeliac disease with atrophy of the small intestine mucosa. *Lancet,* **2,** 876.

Savilahti, E. (1972) Intestinal immunoglobulins in children with coeliac disease. *Gut,* **13,** 958.

Savilahti, E. (1974) Immunofluorescence in coeliac disease. In *Coeliac Disease,* ed. Hekkens, W. & Pena, A. Proceedings of the 2nd International Coeliac Symposium, p. 163. Leiden: Stenfert Kroese.

Savilahti, E., Pelkonen, P. & Visakorpi, J. K. (1971) IgA deficiency in children. A clinical study with special reference to intestinal findings. *Archives of Disease in Childhood,* **46,** 665.

Schloss, O. M. A. (1911) A case of allergy to common foods. *American Journal of Disease of Children,* **3,** 41.

Schreiber, D. S., Blacklow, N. R. & Trier, J. S. (1973) The mucosal lesion of the proximal small intestine in acute infectious nonbacterial gastroenteritis. *New England Journal of Medicine,* **288,** 1318.

Segall, E. (1974) Oats and coeliac disease. *British Medical Journal,* **4,** 589.

Shiner, M. & Ballard, J. (1972) Antigen-antibody reactions in the jejunal mucosa in childhood coeliac disease after gluten challenge. *Lancet,* **1,** 1202.

Shmerling, D. H. & Shiner, M. (1970) The response of the intestinal mucosa to the intraduodenal instillation of gluten in patients with coeliac disease. In *Coeliac Disease,* ed. Booth, C. C. & Dowling, R. H. Edinburgh: Churchill Livingstone.

Silverberg, M. & Davidson, M. (1974) Milk (bovine) protein gastrointestinal hypersensitivity associated with eosinophilic gastroenteropathy in children. *Acta Paediatrica Scandinavica,* **63,** 651.

Ste Marie, M. T., Lee, E. M. & Brown, W. R. (1974) Radioimmunological measurements of naturally occurring antibodies. Antibodies reactive with Escherichia Coli or bacteroides fragilis in breast fluids and sera of mothers and newborn infants. *Pediatric Research,* **8,** 815.

Taylor, B., Norman, A. P., Orgel, H. A., Stokes, C. R., Turner, M. W. & Soothill, J. F. (1973) Transient IgA deficiency and pathogenesis of infantile atopy. *Lancet,* **2,** 111.

Vanderschueren-Lodeweyckx, M., Wolter, M., Molla, A., Eggermont, E. & Eeckels, R. (1973) Plasma growth hormone in coeliac disease. *Helvetica Paediatrica Acta,* **28,** 349.

Visakorpi, J. K. & Immonen, P. (1967) Intolerance to cows' milk and wheat gluten in the primary malabsorption syndrome in infancy. *Acta Paediatrica Scandinavica,* **56,** 49.

Walker Smith, J. A. (1972) Uniformity of dissecting microscope appearances in proximal small intestine. *Gut,* **13,** 17.

Walker Smith, J. A. (1973) Discordance for childhood coeliac disease in monozygotic twins. *Gut,* **14,** 374.

Walker Smith, J. A. (1975) Cows' milk protein intolerance; transient food intolerance of infancy. *Archives of Disease in Childhood,* **50,** 347.

Wall, A. J., Douglas, A. P., Booth, C. C. & Pearse, A. G. E. (1970) Response of the jejunal mucosa in adult coeliac disease to oral prednisolone. *Gut,* **11,** 7.

Wright, N., Watson, A., Morley, A., Appleton, D., Marks, J. & Douglas, A. (1973) The cell cycle time in the flat (avillous) mucosa of the human small intestine. *Gut,* **14,** 603.

Young, W. & Pringle, E. M. (1971) 110 children with coeliac disease. *Archives of Disease in Childhood,* **46,** 421.

Acknowledgements. We should like to thank the Department of Medical Illustration, St Bartholomew's Hospital, for the production of the figures. We should also like to express our thanks to our colleagues, in particular Dr N. E. France, Professor C. B. S. Wood, Dr A. M. Dawson, Dr M. Lancaster-Smith and Dr Mary Harrison, for their helpful advice, and Dr O. D. Fisher and Dr M. Stoneman for referring patients with coeliac disease.

10. Infective diarrhoea and vomiting

J. H. Tripp and J. T. Harries

Predisposing factors
Infecting agents and pathophysiology
Clinical features
Differential diagnosis of acute diarrhoea and/or vomiting
Management
Early complications
Protracted diarrhoea
Prognosis

Infective diarrhoea, with or without vomiting, is one of the major health problems in the world today and carries an appreciable mortality and morbidity. This is particularly the case during infancy and in those developing parts of the world where malnutrition is common. In an inter-American investigation of mortality in childhood, diarrhoeal disease constituted the major underlying cause of death in children under the age of 5 years (Puffer and Serrano, 1973). In India 1·4 million children die each year from diarrhoeal disease, and these figures do not take into account cholera (Registrar General and Census Commissioner, 1972). In developing countries the highest incidence of diarrhoeal disease is during the second year of life, when the attack rate may be as high as three per child per annum and the mortality 36 per 1000 (Gordon, 1971). The peak incidence of diarrhoeal disease and malnutrition occurs together and is related to the age of weaning, so that in a community where weaning is early the peak incidence of diarrhoea is correspondingly early. Seasonal variations are common with a peak incidence in the summer in tropical countries. Massive epidemics may follow natural disasters such as floods or droughts when endemic disease may become epidemic. Of the recorded bacterial pathogens Shigellae are the commonest although, for reasons discussed later, enteropathogenic strains of *E. coli* may more frequently cause diarrhoea than is established by serological testing.

In the developed world the incidence of diarrhoeal disease has greatly decreased over the last 25 years mainly due to improved social, hygienic and medical standards. Nevertheless, diarrhoea is the fifth commonest cause of death in children under the age of 1 year in England and Wales (Registrar General, 1972).

In contrast to developing countries the peak incidence in developed countries is during the first year of life, when about 10 per cent of infants will have an episode of acute diarrhoeal disease with a mortality rate of 40 per 100 000 live births (Registrar General, 1958–1972). The commonest recognisable pathogenic agents have been *E. coli* (particularly in severe newborn nursery outbreaks) and Salmonellae. *E. coli* and Shigellae infections are transmitted by human to human contact, whereas Salmonellae infections (apart from *S. typhi*) result from the ingestion of contaminated food (e.g. poultry). As discussed later, recent work suggests that certain viruses and enteropathogenic strains of *E. coli* may be far more important aetiological agents than hitherto supposed.

Little information is available on the long-term sequelae of affected children, but permanent intellectual and/or neurological deficits may result from disease in early infancy, particularly if the diarrhoea is complicated by hypernatraemia or is protracted and leads to impaired nutrition.

The term 'gastroenteritis' is somewhat unsatisfactory since it implies that an inflammatory process is present in the stomach and intestine. There is no good evidence, however, that the gastric mucosa is affected, and the intestinal mucosa is structurally normal in patients with cholera as well as in those with diarrhoea due to toxin-producing strains of *E. coli.* Nevertheless this nomenclature is widely applied as a diagnostic term to patients who develop acute diarrhoea and/or vomiting, and for convenience sake it is used in parts of this chapter.

Parasitic infections are dealt with elsewhere (see Chs. 12 and 17) and this chapter considers bacterial and viral diarrhoea. It should be remembered, however, that 'enteropathogenic' parasites, bacteria and viruses, may all coexist in the intestinal lumen of a patient with diarrhoea when identification of the causative pathogen may not be possible.

PREDISPOSING FACTORS

Colonisation of the bowel by sufficient numbers of bacteria or viruses will result in disease in susceptible individuals. Colonisation will depend on a complex series of interactions between the external environment, the infecting agent, the host and its endogenous bowel flora. Knowledge on many aspects of these interactions is fragmentary.

The external environment

In the developing parts of the world the most important predisposing factors lie in the external environment. An excellent plan of action to combat infective diarrhoea and malnutrition in children under the age of 2 years was formulated at the Fifth Caribbean Health Ministers Conference in 1973 and should serve as a model to other developing countries. The plan includes improvement of environmental health services (e.g. adequate and safe water supplies, sewage disposal, solid waste disposal), development of infant welfare clinics, campaigns to encourage breast feeding, family planning advice, improved management and follow-up of diarrhoeal disease and malnutrition, health and nutrition education of the public and economic and agricultural measures. Improved nutrition in infancy is probably one of the most important factors which will reduce morbidity and mortality.

Interactions between the host and the infecting agent

The ecology of the gut flora reflects intricate relationships between the host and its micro-organisms and is of great importance in determining whether a particular organism will produce disease. Little is known of the numbers and types of viruses normally present in the alimentary tract compared with the available information on the bacterial flora. There is no information on the bacterial flora along the whole gastrointestinal tract of the normal child as there is for adults (Williams and Drasar, 1972). In the adult small gut aerobic bacteria predominate, total counts varying from 10^3–10^4/ml in the jejunum to 10^5–10^7/ml in the distal ileum. In contrast, 99 per cent of the bacteria in the colon and faeces are anaerobes, predominantly bacteroides and bifidobacteria in counts of 10^{10}–10^{11}/g.

The stools of breast-fed babies contain a relative and absolute preponderance of bifidobacteria compared to *E. coli*/coliform species, whereas the reverse is the case in bottle-fed babies. During weaning the faecal flora becomes similar to that of adults (Mata, Mejicanos and Jimenez, 1972).

Interactions between bacteria

Many favourable interactions occur between the resident bacterial flora of the alimentary tract which are important in maintaining the normal ecology (Bryant, 1972). For example, certain bacteria such as *Bacteroides ruminicola* produce branched-chain organic acids which are essential for growth of other bacteria; lactose-fermenting bacteria derive substrate from other bacteria, and hydrogen and carbon dioxide produced by some bacteria are necessary for the growth of others.

The resident bacterial flora possess a number of mechanisms which protect the host from pathogens and maintain the normal ecosystem (Grady and Keusch, 1971a; Bryant, 1972), e.g. (1) substrate competition, (2) maintenance of hydrogen ion concentration and redox potential, (3) production of short chain organic acids which have bactericidal properties when in a protonated state and (4) synthesis of colicines which are bactericidal to certain strains of *E. coli*.

Gastric juice

One of the functions of gastric acid secretion is to prevent the passage of viable ingested micro-organisms to more distal regions of the alimentary tract (Drasar, Shiner and McLeod, 1969). The protective role of the intact stomach in bacterial diarrhoea is supported by abundant evidence of the sensitivity of pathogens to acid. Salmonellosis is commoner in patients following gastrectomy (Waddell and Kunz, 1956) and individuals with hypochlorhydria and/or gastrectomy are more susceptible to cholera (Hurst, 1934; British Medical Journal, 1975). An unidentified inhibitory substance may also contribute to the stomach's protective influence (Smith, 1966).

Small intestinal motility

The motility of the small intestine is probably the most important mechanism in the maintenance of its relative sterility. Inhibitory studies using opiates, ganglion blockers, antiperistaltic pouches and ligation provide good evidence on how reduced motility favours conditions for pathogens to colonise the small bowel (Grady and Keusch, 1971b). This may contribute to the susceptibility of opium addicts to severe attacks of cholera (Gorbach, 1975). Impaired motility may also result in overgrowth of the small bowel by bacteria not normally considered pathogenic and, as a result of substrate metabolism, e.g. bile salt degradation (Guiraldes *et al.,* 1975), result in diarrhoea.

Mucosal binding of bacteria

Mucosal binding of bacterial pathogens is a prerequisite to colonisation and the production of disease. Studies on toxigenic strains of *E. coli* in newborn pigs have shown that a surface antigen (K88 antigen) is an essential virulence determinant and, because of its adhesive properties, enables the bacteria to attach to the mucosa and proliferate (Smith and Linggood, 1971; Jones and Rutter, 1972). Attachment to the mucosa is also dependent, however, on the adhesive properties of the mucosa, and this may be genetically determined (Rutter *et al.,* 1975); these latter studies suggest that the susceptibility of young infants to bacterial diarrhoea may partly be genetically determined.

Immune systems

Endogenous. Concentrations of immunoglobulin A (IgA) are high in intestinal secretions, suggesting that secretory IgA may be an important defence mechanism against infection; this is not supported, however, by the observation that the bacterial flora of individuals with selective IgA deficiency is no different to controls (Brown *et al.,* 1972). In contrast, patients with hypogammaglobulinaemia have moderate to excessive numbers of anaerobic bacteria in the small gut (Brown *et al.,* 1972). The role of immunodeficiency, whether primary or acquired, as a predisposing factor to infectious diarrhoea is not at present clear.

Exogenous. Breast-fed babies are much less likely to develop infectious diarrhoea compared with their bottle-fed counterparts (Gerrard, 1974), and the present decline of breast feeding throughout the world is particularly disturbing. The mechanism of the protective effect of breast feeding is multifactorial and includes a reduced risk of contamination, the presence in milk of immunoglobulins, particularly IgA (Gerrard, 1974; Stoliar *et al.*, 1975), and the presence of an iron binding protein (lactoferrin), which in association with immunoglubulins is bacteriostatic (Bullen *et al.*, 1972). Bifidobacteria predominate in the faeces of breast-fed babies and may contribute to the low frequency of Shigella and other enteropathogens during breast feeding (Mata *et al.*, 1972). The relatively low pH of the faeces of breast-fed babies may also play a protective role (Bullen and Willis, 1971). Finally, both breast and cows' milk contain non-specific antiviral factors (T. H. J. Mathews and D. A. J. Tyrrell, personal communication).

Other interactions

Bacteria may regulate the turnover of epithelial cells and influence brush border enzyme activity (Savage, 1972). Lysozyme in *Succus entericus* is

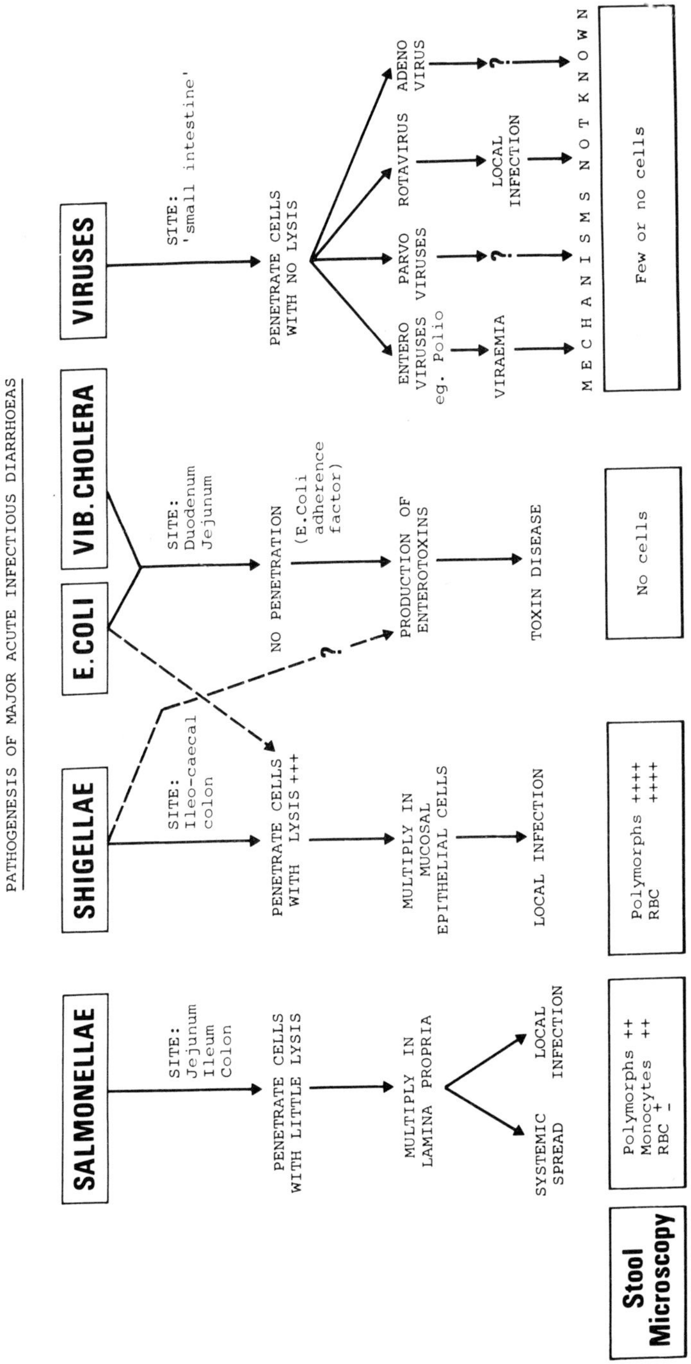

Fig. 10.1 Pathogenesis of the major acute infectious diarrhoeas (by kind permission of W. C. Marshall)

bactericidal and is, at least in part, synthesised by the Paneth cells of the crypts (Peeters and Vantrappen, 1975). Plasmids are extrachromosomal genetic components of certain bacteria which can be transferred from one bacterial strain to another by conjugation. They regulate the biosynthesis of a variety of bacterial products that play a role in survival of bacteria and in their interactions with the host and other bacteria. Of particular importance is the fact that synthesis of both heat-stable and heat-labile *E. coli* enterotoxins is plasmid-controlled, raising the possibility that toxin pathogenicity may be transferable from one bacteria to another (Gyles, 1972); the K88 antigen of enteropathogenic strains of *E. coli* in young piglets is also under plasmid control.

INFECTING AGENTS AND PATHOPHYSIOLOGY

Figure 10.1 shows a simplified scheme of the pathogenesis of the major acute infectious diarrhoeas in childhood.

Bacteria

Over the last 20 years the reported incidence of pathogenic bacteria cultured from the stools of children under the age of 2 years with acute diarrhoea has varied from 4 to 33 per cent (Cramblett *et al.*, 1971), the commonest organisms being 'enteropathogenic' strains of *E. coli*, Salmonellae and Shigellae. Recently it has become clear that enterotoxin-producing strains of *E. coli* can result in diarrhoea in both adults and children, and also that the somatic serotypes of these strains are often not the recognised enteropathogenic ones (Gorbach *et al.*, 1975; Sack *et al.*, 1975). Thus the term 'enteropathogenic' as applied to serotypes of *E. coli* needs to be redefined. The detection of enterotoxin-producing strains of *E. coli* with techniques such as ligated rabbit loops and tissue culture may well show that the aetiological importance of bacteria in childhood diarrhoea is considerably greater than previous reports have indicated.

Table 10.1 lists the established bacterial pathogens in man together with other bacterial species which have been implicated, but not proven, in producing sporadic diarrhoeal disease. Curiously cholera is rare in infants under the age of 1 (Mosley, Bevenson and Barui 1968). Some types of staphylococci produce toxins in food; disease results from ingestion of preformed toxins, and the

Table 10.1 Bacterial pathogens in diarrhoeal disease

Established pathogens	Possible pathogens
Escherichia Coli	*Pseudomonas aeruginosa*
Salmonellae	*Aeromonas hydrophila*
Shigellae	*Edwardsiella tarda*
Vibrio cholerae	
Vibrio parahaemolyticus	*Bacillus cereus*
Clostridium perfringens	*Bacillus subtilis*
Staphylococci	*Vibrio fetus*
Yersinia enterocolitica	

majority of outbreaks of food poisoning caused by staphylococci are due to coagulase-positive species. *Vibrio parahaemolyticus* is a marine organism and is mainly found in Japan; it has been a major cause of outbreaks of food poisoning and this is probably due to the Japanese custom of eating raw fish (Zen-Yoji, 1968). *Clostridium perfringens* is one of the commonest causes of food-borne diarrhoea (Center for Disease Control, 1970) and can cause a fatal enteritis known as 'Darmbrand' in Germany and 'pig-bel' in the highlands of New Guinea. Infections with *Yersinia enterocolitica* have been responsible for both sporadic and epidemic outbreaks of acute gastroenteritis (Toivanen *et al.*, 1973). Other bacteria have been implicated as occasionally causing diarrhoea (Table 10.1).

Classification

Enteropathogenic bacteria may be broadly classified as invasive or non-invasive. Invasive organisms (e.g. Salmonellae, Shigellae and some strains of *E. coli*) penetrate the mucosa of the distal small intestine and colon to produce morphological abnormalities and dysentery (i.e. passage of blood, mucus and pus in the stools). Studies on Salmonella and Shigella diarrhoea in monkeys have shown that the jejunum is morphologically normal but in a secretory state with respect to fluid and electrolytes (Rout *et al.*, 1974; Rout *et al.*, 1975). Thus dysentery results from mucosal disruption, and diarrhoea from jejunal secretion overwhelming the reabsorptive capacity of the injured colon. *Shigella dysenteriae* can also produce an enterotoxin which induces small intestinal secretion of fluid and electrolytes (Donowitz, Keusch and Binder, 1975), and it is possible that other invasive pathogens may also have this capacity.

The non-invasive enteropathogens (e.g. *V. cholera* and *E. coli*) elaborate enterotoxins in the small intestine and induce secretion without affecting mucosal structure. The absorptive defect is confined to the small bowel and colonic function is normal. Diarrhoea results from the small intestinal secretions overwhelming the normal reabsorptive capacity of the colon. *V. cholera* and *E. coli* produce heat-labile (LT) enterotoxins which are antigenically similar and which act in a similar fashion, as will be discussed later. *E. coli* also produces a non-antigenic heat-stable (ST) toxin which appears to act in a different way to the LT toxins; its role in human disease is not yet as well established as that for the LT toxins. As previously discussed synthesis of both *E. coli* LT and ST toxins are under plasmid control.

Pathophysiology

Since the successful purification of cholera toxin major advances have been made in our understanding of the precise mechanisms which mediate the secretory effects of bacterial toxins, and the reader is referred to the following excellent detailed reviews: Banwell and Sherr, 1973; Field, 1974; Kimberg, 1974. Both cholera and *E. coli* LT toxins are thought to act in an identical fashion. The toxins bind to the brush border of the surface epithelial cells and activate the enzyme adenyl cyclase, which is located in the basolateral membranes of the cell. Adenyl cyclase catalyses the conversion of adenosine triphosphate to cyclic adenosine 3′,5′-monophosphate (cyclic-AMP). The resulting high intracellular concentrations of cyclic-AMP induce secretion of fluid and electrolytes across the brush border into the small intestinal lumen to produce profuse diarrhoea. Although the precise mechanisms by which cyclic-AMP affects the brush border ion transport systems have not been clearly defined, a model has been proposed (Schultz, Frizzell and Nellans, 1974). Certain strains of *S. typhimurium*, traditionally considered not to elaborate enterotoxin, have also been shown to activate mucosal adenyl cyclase and produce small intestinal secretion of fluid and electrolytes (Giannella *et al.*, 1975).

Current evidence suggests that the secretory effects of *S. dysenteriae* and *E. coli* ST toxins are mediated by some other process than the adenyl cyclase system (Donowitz *et al.*, 1975).

The invasive pathogens penetrate the mucosa of the colon and distal small gut to produce enteritis or dysentery, but the factors which control the invasive process are poorly understood. A number of Salmonellae strains invade the bloodstream, but this is extremely uncommon with Shigellae infections.

Viruses

Certain viral infections may be associated with diarrhoea (e.g. measles, hepatitis, poliomyelitis and influenza), and mild morphological abnormalities of the small intestinal mucosa have been reported in patients with acute viral hepatitis (Sheehy, Artenstein and Green, 1964). Other viruses such as ECHO viruses, Coxsackie viruses, reoviruses and adenoviruses, have been incriminated as aetiological agents in diarrhoeal disease. Acute infectious non-bacterial gastroenteritis is second only to acute respiratory tract disease as the most common illness in the United States (Dingle *et al.*, 1953), and the reader is referred to an excellent review on the aetiology and pathogenesis of acute infectious non-bacterial gastroenteritis as seen in the United States by Blacklow *et al.* (1972). In recent years important advances have been made in identifying certain specific viruses which are probably of major aetiological importance in acute infantile diarrhoea and/or vomiting, and are considered below.

Prenatal infection

Certain intrauterine infections such as those caused by cytomegalovirus and rubella virus may be accompanied by diarrhoea dating from birth (unpublished observations). The association may be fortuitous and not necessarily indicate a causal relationship between the virus and the diarrhoea. Nevertheless, in the absence of an identifiable cause, intrauterine infection should be excluded in infants with diarrhoea dating from birth.

Postnatal infection

Evidence has accumulated in recent years from several parts of the world that a variety of viruses may be aetiological agents in acute diarrhoea and/or vomiting, both in adults and children (Lancet, 1975a). These include the Norwalk agent, Vellore virus-like particles and RNA viruses of approximately 70 to 80 nm in diameter ('reo-like virus', 'orbivirus', 'rotavirus' or 'duovirus').

Norwalk/Hawaii agents. An outbreak of acute vomiting and diarrhoea affected 50 per cent of the pupils of an elementary school in Norwalk, Ohio, in 1968 (Adler and Zickl, 1969). The incubation period was 48 hours, the disease lasted 24 hours and remitted spontaneously. The disease has been transmitted to healthy volunteers by administration of bacterial-free stool filtrates from affected individuals; the agent is a small (27 nm) ether-, acid- and heat-stable virus (Blacklow *et al.*, 1972). The spread of the disease is characteristically epidemic but it may also persist in an endemic form causing sporadic cases or localised outbreaks. The disease affects mainly older children and adults and has a peak incidence in the winter. Infection is associated with structural abnormalities of the small intestinal mucosa (Schreiber, Blacklow and Trier, 1973), whilst the gastric mucosa is unaffected (Widerlite *et al.*, 1975). The Hawaii particle is very similar if not identical to the Norwalk agent.

Rotavirus (synonyms: 'reo-like virus', 'orbivirus', 'duovirus'). This RNA virus was first incriminated as an aetiological agent in acute non-bacterial gastroenteritis by Bishop and her colleagues in 1973. Electron microscopy of the duodenal mucosa obtained from nine children aged 4 to 31 months with acute gastroenteritis demonstrated virus particles within the epithelial cells of six of the patients; no virus particles were observed in duodenal mucosa obtained from three of these children after clinical recovery. The mucosa showed patchy morphological abnormalities during the acute phase of the disease which reverted to normal following clinical recovery. Subsequently, electron-microscopic studies of faeces have suggested that the virus may be responsible

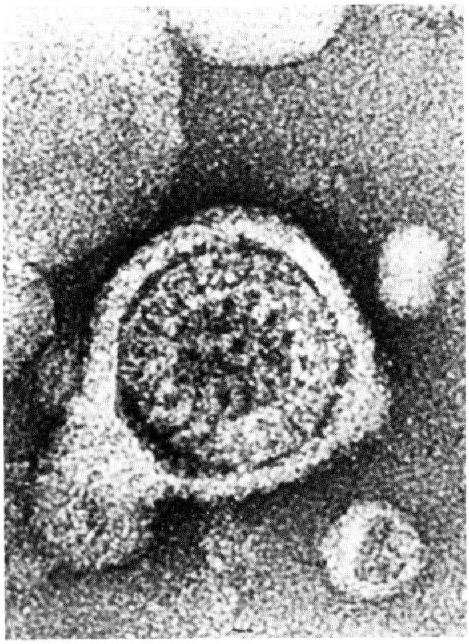

Fig. 10.2 Electronmicroscopic appearances of a rotavirus particle obtained from the stool of an infant with acute diarrhoea

for up to 50 to 60 per cent of acute gastroenteritis in children under the age of 5 years and that it may have a worldwide distribution (Davidson *et al.*, 1975; Flewett, Bryden and Davies, 1975; Lancet, 1975a.) Seroepidemiological studies will further clarify the importance of these agents in acute diarrhoeal disease. The virus consists of a core about 38 nm in diameter surrounded by an inner layer of capsomeres, which radiate outwards like the spokes of a wheel; an outer layer of capsomeres seems to be attached to the tops of the inner ones giving the characteristic appearance of a sharply defined rim surrounding the particle; the diameter of the virus particle is about 60 to 65 nm (Fig. 10.2).

The further characterisation of viral agents associated with gastrointestinal disease will depend on the development of appropriate tissue culture techniques; this development will, in turn, be a step towards the preparation of vaccines. The pathophysiological mechanisms by which viruses produce watery diarrhoea have not been defined.

CLINICAL FEATURES

Spread of both epidemic and sporadic infection in the community results from (1) contamination of food during its production (e.g. Salmonellae in poultry), (2) contamination of water supplies (e.g. cholera), (3) contamination of food or water prior to consumption (e.g. *E. coli*, Shigellae, and *S. typhi*) or (4) by unknown routes (e.g. rotavirus). Aggregation of affected cases within families or communities is common and may sometimes be helpful in incriminating a particular aetiological agent. Table 10.2 shows some of the salient features of the bacterial and viral enteric infections which are known to occur in children. In most instances the infecting agent cannot be accurately incriminated from the clinical features, and the symptoms and signs may be similar in disease caused by many of the listed agents.

The illness frequently begins with vomiting, which may be profuse and even projectile and may be the only symptom until the onset of diarrhoea six to 24 hours later. The stools are watery and in the severest cases, particularly those due to toxin-secreting strains of *E. coli*, may be of the 'rice water' type seen in cholera; parents may notice a distinct change in the smell of the stools. Because there is only a small amount of solid material in the stool it may be largely absorbed by the napkin leaving a misleadingly small stool. Blood staining is unusual and rarely gross except in dysenteric infections, but it is more frequent in very young infants. The illness is sometimes accompanied by colicky abdominal pain, more apparent in older children, and considerable abdominal distention may occur. A fever is frequently present particularly when the infecting agent is a bacterial pathogen, although this is not a useful diagnostic feature in individual cases. A mild pharyngitis, otitis or respiratory infection may be associated with the gastrointestinal symptoms.

Dehydration

As a result of vomiting and diarrhoea the child becomes dehydrated despite continuing to take oral fluids avidly. Skin elasticity becomes decreased, and this can be easily assessed in areas of loose attachment such as the back of the hand

Table 10.2 Features of bacterial and viral enteric infections

Agents	Disease types	Incubation periods	Comments
1. Bacteria			
E. Coli	(i) Enteritis	2–14 days	Epidemics; nurseries
	(ii) Toxin	12–48 hours	'Cholera infantum'; severe fluid losses; poor correlation with recognised serotypes
V. cholera	Toxin	12–48 hours	Human source; clear fluid stools ± mucus; very severe fluid losses
Shigellae	(i) Dysentery	1–5 days	Human source; fever
	(ii) Toxin	1–5 days	*S. dysenteriae*
Salmonellae	Enteritis	12–48 hours	Animal or human source; ± watery diarrhoea; occasionally leads to typhoid fever
Yersinia	Enteritis	7–10 days	Abdominal pain may mimick appendicitis; fever, rashes and arthritis
Staphylococci	(i) Enterocolitis	?	Superinfection after or during antibiotic therapy
	(ii) Toxin	2–6 hours	Preformed toxin in food
2. Viruses			
Norwalk/Hawaii	Not known	1–3 days	Mucosal damage; often mild disease
Rota/Duo	Not known	48 hours–?	Winter incidence; ?commonest single agent

Toxin: profuse watery diarrhoea without mucosal invasion; no pus cells in stools; lack of systemic symptoms such as fever.

Enteritis: mucosal invasion with diarrhoea and pus cells in stools; occasionally bloody diarrhoea; fever ±.

Dysentery: marked mucosal invasion with bloody diarrhoea and pus cells in stools; fever.

or the neck. The mouth and tongue are dry, thirst is apparent, urine is passed infrequently and ocular tension is diminished. Metabolic acidosis, if present, is apparent clinically as an increased respiratory rate. As the dehydration progresses the fontanelle becomes sunken, the eyes and face appear hollow and eventually a state of shock supervenes with cold extremities, cyanosis, mottling of the skin, irregular respirations and eventual circulatory collapse and death. In fulminant cases this clinical sequence is lost, and infants may present with severe or even terminal degrees of dehydration due to pooling of fluid in the distended bowel before the passage of the first diarrhoeal stool. Gastroenteritis is now recognised as one of the causes of sudden death in early infancy (McWeeney and Emery, 1975). The primary aim of the clinical examination is to determine as accurately as possible the degree and type of dehydration (see Table 10.3), with particular emphasis on the identification and immediate

Table 10.3 Clinical assessment of the degree and type of dehydration

Symptoms or signs	Normonatraemic 3–5[a]	6–9	>10	Hypernatraemic 3–5	6–9	>10	Hyponatraemic 3–5	6–9	>10
Thirst	+	++	±	+	++	+++	+	±	±
Dry mouth	+	++	+++		±	+			
Oliguria	+	++	+++	+	++		+	+	++
Skin elasticity	↓	↓↓	↓↓↓			↓	↓	↓↓	↓↓↓
Sunken eyes and ocular tension		↓	↓↓			↓		↓	↓↓
Fontanelle tension		↓	↓↓		N/↑	↑/↓		↓	↓↓
Apathy			+						+
Hyper-reflexia					+	++			
Convulsions			+		+	++			+
Tachycardia and hypotension		+	++			+		+	++
Cold extremities/cyanosis			+						+
Acidosis			±		++	+++		+	++

[a] Numerals indicate per cent dehydration; N denotes normal

treatment of the severely dehydrated child, who is at risk of sudden death. Information on recent weight loss is particularly helpful in rapidly assessing the degree of dehydration. In obese infants the usual clinical methods of assessing dehydration may grossly underestimate the actual degree of dehydration, probably because of the small amount of water present in adipose tissue. In such infants particular emphasis should be placed on signs not affected by obesity such as fontanelle and eyeball tension, dryness of the mouth, thirst, oliguria, tachycardia and hypotension.

Hypernatraemic (hypertonic) dehydration

The classical features of dehydration described above are those of normonatraemic (normotonic) dehydration which accounts for the dehydration seen in about 70 per cent of cases seen in Western industrialised nations (Finberg, 1970; unpublished observations). Although only accounting for about 20 per cent of infants admitted to hospital with gastroenteritis, hypernatraemic dehydration carries a mortality which is five to 10 times higher than the overall mortality in gastroenteritis. The incidence of hypernatraemia is highest in the winter (Finberg, 1973). Young infants are particularly likely to develop this complication, particularly if high osmolar milk feeds are continued during the illness. The clinical recognition of hypernatraemic dehydration may be difficult since, as shown in Table 10.3, many of the classical signs of dehydration can be absent. For example the skin feels 'doughy' and firm rather than inelastic, and fontanelle tension may be increased or decreased. Other biochemical disturbances are almost invariably present. These include a metabolic acidosis with tachypnoea, hyperglycaemia and hypocalcaemia; tetanic symptoms are very uncommon, and convulsions are only very rarely due to hypocalcaemia.

Signs of a central nervous disturbance appear much earlier than in other types of dehydration. The initial irritability and sometimes meningism may progress to generalised hyper-reflexia, spasticity and coma, and be accompanied by convulsions. Subdural effusions or haemorrhages or dural sinus thromboses may further complicate the picture.

Hypernatraemia should be suspected in any infant with gastroenteritis, particularly if he is under 6 months, who has an unexpectedly severe clinical disturbance (for the degree of clinical dehydration), severe acidosis or central nervous symptoms. It can be assumed that the infant is more than 7 per cent dehydrated if hypernatraemia (sodium >155 mmol/l) is confirmed.

Hyponatraemic (hypotonic) dehydration

Hyponatraemic dehydration is unusual in the United States of America and Europe, accounting for only 10 per cent of all cases, but is frequent and often severe in tropical countries, with plasma sodium levels as low as 80 mmol/l being recorded (Kingston, 1973). Whether this different incidence reflects climatic or other factors such as the type and usage of artificial feeds, underlying malnutrition, or different aetiological agents is not known. The symptoms and signs are in general similar to those seen in normonatraemic dehydration although they tend to be more apparent with the same degree of dehydration. Dryness of the mouth and mucous membranes is not a feature (see Table 10.3), and in severely affected patients excessive salivation and even lacrimation may occur.

DIFFERENTIAL DIAGNOSIS OF ACUTE DIARRHOEA AND/OR VOMITING

In addition to gastrointestinal infections, acute diarrhoea with or without vomiting may be the presenting features of other unrelated diseases (see Table 10.4) so that a careful general clinical assessment is essential in all cases. For example, vomiting and diarrhoea may occur in otitis media, upper respiratory tract infections, pneumonia, urinary tract infections, septicaemia and meningitis, and all these must be carefully excluded and promptly treated; the importance of excluding meningitis and the urgency of instituting appropriate therapy cannot be overemphasised. Surgical abdominal emergencies may masquerade as gastroenteritis and careful examination of the abdomen is mandatory; acute 'toxic' dilatation of the small gut may accompany acute infective enteritis and its associated metabolic disturbances, and such 'functional' obstruction may be extremely difficult to differentiate from anatomical causes of obstruction. In these circumstances a combined medical and surgical approach is essential, as in all infants presenting with acute gastrointestinal symptoms in whom there is any suspicion of an underlying obstructive lesion. A slow or atypical onset, severe pain, vomiting greatly in excess of diarrhoea, or blood in the stools are clues which should alert one to the possibility of a surgical condition. A history of previous constipation with or without abdominal distension may be the presenting features of Hirschsprung's disease with acute diarrhoea due to an enterocolitis. An unusual degree of abdominal distension, redness or oedema of the abdominal wall, the absence of

Table 10.4 Differential diagnosis of acute diarrhoea and/or vomiting in infancy

Gastroenteritis
Food poisoning
Systemic infections
Septicaemia
Meningitis
Urinary tract infections
Respiratory tract infections
Surgical conditions
Appendicitis
Intussusception
Hirschsprung's disease
Pyloric stenosis
Metabolic conditions
Diabetic precoma
Congenital adrenal insufficiency
Haemolytic-uraemic syndrome
Miscellaneous
Coeliac disease
Chronic inflammatory bowel disease
Immune deficiency states
Selective inborn errors of absorption
Cows' milk protein intolerance
Enterocolitis
Poisoning

hyperactive bowel sounds or the presence of abdominal tenderness are all indications for a surgical opinion. Rectal examination (specifically in relation to intussusception, acute appendicitis or Hirschsprung's disease) and erect and supine films of the abdomen are necessary when there is any clinical doubt as to the diagnosis. Marked abdominal distension with fluid levels is, however, quite consistent with uncomplicated acute gastroenteritis, as discussed above.

MANAGEMENT

Hospital admission is undesirable for the majority of patients with less severe forms of the disease, so that positive reasons should be clearly given when asking parents to continue coping with a vomiting and messy infant in their home if this is at all practicable. The parents, who are not unnaturally anxious, often stress that vomiting is severe, and a clear fluid test meal is often useful in assessing whether admission is necessary for this reason alone. Severe cases with profuse watery diarrhoea probably merit immediate admission before the onset of dehydration, which is likely to ensue.

Investigations

Two simple investigations are necessary in all cases of gastroenteritis, but both are frequently omitted. The patient must be accurately weighed to provide an estimate of dehydration if a recent previous weight is known, as well as to provide a base line for accurate assessment of day-to-day progress. Culture of a stool or rectal swab for bacterial pathogens may provide early warning of an impending epidemic or identify an asymptomatic excretor of a pathogen such as Salmonella. The presence of blood or pus cells in the stools may provide useful information as to the infecting agent, and microscopic examination of stools may be diagnostic of amoebic infection. The determination of plasma electrolytes and urea in severe disease is discussed later.

Use of antibiotics
A variety of antibiotics have been traditionally used in the routine management of gastroenteritis but there is no good evidence that they reduce morbidity or mortality and in some instances they may be positively harmful. Antibiotics prolong the duration of uncomplicated Salmonella enteritis, and the likelihood of a carrier state developing is increased (Dixon, 1965). In infections which have resulted in bacteraemia or septicaemia (e.g. typhoid fever), however, the use of appropriate antibiotics is unquestioned and essential for the control of the disease.

The routine use of antibiotics in hospitalised patients has been the subject of considerable controversy (British Medical Journal, 1972). Protagonists argue that non-absorbable antibiotics not only reduce the excretion of viable bacteria from infected patients but also protect uninfected patients and thereby reduce the risk of cross-infection. As yet no satisfactory controlled trial has been reported, and the question remains unresolved.

Use of antidiarrhoeal agents
As previously discussed the motility of the small gut is probably the single most important mechanism in maintaining its relative sterility compared with more distal parts of the intestine. For this reason antidiarrhoeal agents such as kaolin, opium derivatives, codeine and diphenoxylate hydrochloride (Lomotil) should be avoided since, by slowing intestinal transit, they may encourage the proliferation of pathogens and exacerbate disease, as well as prolong faecal excretion of the pathogen (DuPont and Hornick, 1973).

Mild dehydration
Although the vast majority of infants with gastroenteritis can be managed in the home, clinical vigilance is essential if tragedies are to be avoided. The successful management of mild dehydration depends on clear instructions to the parents and their willingness to comply with the suggested dietary modifications. When treating well-nourished infants we have adopted a regime of clear fluids, which is inappropriate in the management of malnourished children, as discussed later. Clear fluids should be administered over the first 24 hours followed by a gradual increase in the strength of the patient's normal diet over a period of three to four days. The composition of the clear fluids is a matter of some debate, and a variety of solutions have been recommended (see Table 10.5). In our view glucose should be included in such solutions, not only for provision of calories but also because of its physiological effect in stimulating fluid and electrolyte absorption and therefore in reducing the faecal losses of fluid. Low concentrations of sodium chloride should be used in those parts of the world where hyper-

Table 10.5 Recommended oral solutions in the management of gastroenteritis in infancy

	Composition (mmol/l)				
Solutions	Sodium	Chloride	Potassium	Bicarbonate	Glucose
WHO solution for cholera	120	97	25	48	110
Half-strength Darrow's	60	52	18	25 (as lactate)	—
Electrosol solution[a]	46	44	17	19	—
MRC (U.K.) solution	24	24	28	31	280
A[b]	80	70	18	28	100

[a] Electrosol tablets are flavoured with orange and prescribable; 8 tablets dissolved in 1 litre give the ionic concentrations shown above.
[b] See *Lancet* (1975b), **1**, 79.

natraemic dehydration is relatively common. The dangers of such solutions being made up in the home, particularly with regard to the addition of sodium chloride, should not be underestimated (Whitelaw, Dillon and Tripp, 1975), and the availability of preformed clear solutions to parents for the management of their children with gastroenteritis should be encouraged.

Regular, initially daily, reassessment by clinical examination and weighing is important in the recognition of insidious deterioration and to control the rate at which the infant is regraded on to a normal diet. Follow-up after the acute illness is desirable but often impractical and is probably unnecessary in a well-nourished child in whom there is rapid resolution of symptoms.

For social reasons it is sometimes necessary to admit patients with mild disease to hospital, and in these circumstances it is probably wise to delay their discharge until they have been returned to a normal diet.

Moderate dehydration

In industrialised countries infants with moderate degrees of dehydration (5 to 10 per cent) tend to be admitted to hospital for intravenous rehydration. In developing countries hospital staff and beds are at a premium, and oral rehydration is the rule. Using suitable oral glucose-electrolyte solutions such regimes have been highly successful in managing all but the most severely dehydrated patients (Lancet, 1975b).

Severe dehydration

A severely dehydrated infant presents a medical emergency that demands immediate and careful attention. Emergency therapy is directed towards restoring the plasma volume by the intravenous infusion of plasma (20 ml/kg) or normal saline (30 ml/kg). Severe acidosis (standard bicarbonate < 12 mmol/l) is treated by providing about half of the calculated deficit of bicarbonate; in the presence of severe clinical manifestations of acidosis 1 mmol/kg of sodium bicarbonate should be administered. The bicarbonate deficit is calculated as follows: Deficit = weight in kilogrammes × 0·6 × (24—observed standard bicarbonate in mmol/l), and half of this is given. Total correction or the correction of mild acidosis is not necessary (Heese *et al.*, 1966), and increases the risk of hypernatraemia.

Planned rehydration will depend on the electrolyte and acid-base status of the patient, so that blood for electrolytes, urea and standard bicarbonate should be taken at the earliest opportunity, preferably before starting treatment. During the first four hours, when the results of the plasma electrolyte determinations are often not available, the following empirical regime is recommended: 40 to 80 ml/kg of intravenous half normal saline; half strength Hartman's solution or half strength Darrow's solution are suitable for any of the three types of dehydration. Darrow's and Hartman's solutions, however, contain potassium (36 and 5 mmol/l, respectively) and are probably best avoided until urine flow is established.

Hyponatraemic (hypotonic) dehydration

Hyponatraemia may result from body losses of electrolytes exceeding those of water or from attempts at rehydration without appropriate electrolyte replacement. The body deficits of sodium and water are predominantly extracellular, and result in circulatory collapse due to contraction of the plasma volume with relatively minor disturbances of the intracellular compartment.

The requirements for the first 24 hours are estimated by addition of the calculated fluid deficit to the maintenance requirements (see Table 10.10 in Appendix A) for the estimated rehydrated weight of the infant (see Appendix A). The sodium deficit is calculated from the plasma sodium concentration and again added to the maintenance requirement (see Appendix A). Since the potassium concentration in diarrhoeal stools is usually slightly less than half the sodium concentration, the potassium deficit may be taken as half that of sodium in addition to the maintenance requirements. The administration of intravenous potassium is dangerous and a maximum safe dose in infants of 4 mmol/hour, and a maximum concentration of 40 mmol/l in the infused fluid, is recommended. This means that intravenous replacement is often necessarily incomplete and must be made up by the oral route over the subsequent few days.

Examples of the calculations necessary to arrive at an appropriate regime for the management of infants with any of the three types of dehydration are provided in Appendix A.

Normonatraemic (normotonic) dehydration

Calculation of the fluid deficit is identical to that for hyponatraemic dehydration but, since by definition the plasma sodium is normal, no precise calculation of the sodium deficit can be made. However, the sodium deficit can be approximately estimated by assuming that the fluid lost has a concentration of sodium half that of normal saline. In very mild hyponatraemia the formal calculation may give a sodium deficit less than that calculated for normonatraemia; the greater value for the deficit should therefore be used in such a situation.

Hypernatraemic (hypertonic) dehydration

In hypernatraemic dehydration the hypertonicity of the extracellular fluid results in osmotic gradients and a loss of intracellular water, potassium and other electrolytes. The physiological response to hypernatraemia is an increased excretion of sodium by the kidney (via the aldosterone system) resulting in further losses of water and further dehydration of both extracellular and intracellular compartments. The emergency use of plasma or normal saline to increase the plasma volume and the administration of half normal saline over the first four hours is, as already discussed, appropriate for this type of dehydration; this treatment provides an amount of free water which does not decrease the sodium concentration in the extracellular fluid too rapidly. Rapid dilution of the increased extracellular sodium concentration will result in major osmotic gradients between the extra- and intracellular spaces and may cause convulsions (Hogan *et al.*, 1969). Convulsions, however, may not be of themselves a bad prognostic factor when occurring during rehydration of hypernatraemic patients (Morris-Jones, Houston and Evans, 1967). Since hypernatraemia *per se* may result in subdural effusions and haemorrhages (Finberg, 1973) reasonably rapid correction of the hypernatraemic state is desirable. There are therefore arguments to support both rapid rehydration with solutions containing relatively high sodium concentrations (e.g. 75 mmol/l) and slower rehydration with solutions of lower sodium content (e.g. 30 mmol/l). There is general agreement that electrolyte-free solutions should be avoided. Satisfactory results have been obtained using two-fifths normal saline (with other inorganic ions) administered at a rate of about 200 ml/kg/24 hours of the estimated rehydrated weight of the patient as well as with one-fifth normal saline given at a rate of 100 ml/kg/day of the estimated rehydrated weight (Bannister, 1975). In the latter study, however, the neurological condition of the patients tended to deteriorate during treatment, and calculation indicates that plasma osmolality would not have returned to normal for as long as three days in some of the patients. Our view is that the appropriate regime is a compromise between the relatively rapid correction of dehydration with solutions of high sodium content and the very slow correction with more dilute solutions. We would recommend a regime which provides a total fluid intake of 150 ml/kg/24 hours, fluid being administered as one-fifth normal saline in 4 per cent dextrose after the initial four hour period. To this is added potassium chloride at a concentration of 40 mmol/l.

Further management

In all three types of dehydration it is our policy to reintroduce oral feeds on the second day providing the diarrhoea is reduced, aiming to provide half the total fluid intake as an oral glucose electrolyte feed (see Table 10.5), and the rest intravenously. On the third day the baby's usual feeds are reintroduced in a dilute form (one-quarter or one-fifth strength), and increased to full strength in a step-wise fashion over the next few days.

Malnourished infants and children

The energy deprivation which would ensue if malnourished children were treated with a prolonged regime of clear fluids may be far more dangerous to the child than the continuing diarrhoea. For this reason it is recommended that a full calorie intake should be established by 24 hours, or at the most 48 hours, after starting treatment (D. C. Morley, personal communication).

Rehydration of infants with protein-energy deficiency (see Ch. 8) is complicated by (1) the fact that such patients may have chronic water and electrolyte disturbances prior to any acute diarrhoeal illness, (2) the impaired function of renal and other homeostatic mechanisms which are normal in well-nourished children, (3) the increased risk of hypoglycaemia during regrading of the patients on to a normal diet, and (4) the high incidence of food intolerances, particularly to lactose. It should also be remembered that pulmonary losses of water may be considerable in hot climates.

EARLY COMPLICATIONS

Anuria

Anuria is a common feature of severe dehydration, but urine flow is usually re-established within four to eight hours of instituting a rehydration regime. If no urine has been passed in the first eight hours intravenous frusemide (1–2 mg/kg) may induce a diuresis. The urine urea and osmolality can then be determined and a conclusion reached as to whether the anuria was secondary to dehydration or indicative of acute renal failure. If renal failure has occurred the fluid intake is reduced to allow sufficient fluid for rehydration but providing only 50 ml/kg/24 hours for maintenance requirements, and potassium is omitted from the regime. Even when the blood urea has reached very high levels such as 50 to 67 mmol/l (300–400 mg/100 ml), full recovery of renal function often occurs without resort to dialysis. Occasionally prolonged anuria or oliguria may be the result of renal vein thrombosis or medullary necrosis. In the former case the presence of blood in the urine, persistent oliguria or anuria, a raised blood urea and a palpable renal mass are useful diagnostic clues; the diagnosis is confirmed by intravenous pyelography which shows a non-functioning kidney in unilateral cases. Medullary necrosis may complicate gastroenteritis when, after an apparently normal polyuric phase during recovery from acute renal failure, there is a persistence of the polyuria with increased losses of cations, particularly sodium, and a raised blood urea (Chrispin, 1972); diagnosis is confirmed by intravenous pyelography. In many intances infants with renal vein thrombosis or medullary necrosis appear to make a complete clinical recovery, but it is not known whether they develop late complications such as hypertension.

Convulsions

Convulsions may occur in gastroenteritis in association with fever, dehydration, metabolic disturbances or during the treatment of hypertonic states. Anticonvulsants such as phenobarbitone may be helpful in the control of fits; it should be remembered that absorption of intramuscularly administered drugs may be impaired in dehydrated infants. Hypocalcaemia is probably not related to convulsions, and the administration of calcium has no place in management.

Hypokalaemia

A reduction in total body potassium is probably very common in gastroenteritis. Despite a total body deficit, plasma levels may remain normal in the dehydrated infant due to leakage of intracellular potassium into the extracellular compartments. Hypotension or bradycardia occurring during rehydration should alert the clinician to the possibility of hypokalaemia, and an electrocardiogram will show the characteristic changes of flattened T waves and later widening of the QRS complex. If renal function is adequate intravenous potassium can be safely administered.

Pulmonary oedema

Pulmonary oedema with or without peripheral oedema occurs most frequently in infants who are hypernatraemic, particularly if large amounts of fluid are given while they are severely acidotic (Finberg, 1970). The clinician should always be aware of the possibility of volume overload, and regular auscultation of the chest is necessary in very sick infants.

Hyperglycaemia

Hyperglycaemia often accompanies hypertonic dehydration and acidosis (Finberg, 1973), and blood glucose concentrations of over 28 mmol/l (500 mg/100 ml) may sometimes be found. Treatment with insulin is usually not necessary since blood glucose levels return to normal after correction of the acidosis and other biochemical disturbances. If insulin is used it must be given in very small quantities and with great caution if hypoglycaemia is to be avoided.

Hypoglycaemia

Hypoglycaemia may occur during a period of calorie deprivation, e.g. during intravenous therapy or during the early part of regrading the infant on to a normal diet. Malnourished infants are particularly at risk of developing hypoglycaemia.

Extraintestinal infections

Because of their ability to invade mucosa, Salmonellae, Shigellae and certain strains of *E. coli* may result in extraintestinal infection in children, particularly in neonates or if immunity is impaired. Extraintestinal infection is most commonly associated with Salmonella enteritis which can result in bacteraemia, septicaemia, meningitis and osteomyelitis, patients with sickle-cell disease being particularly susceptible to osteomyelitis. In patients with intestinal infection due to any of the invasive pathogens, careful monitoring of temperature and regular white blood counts and blood cultures are necessary so that early diagnosis and treatment of bacteraemia can be achieved.

PROTRACTED DIARRHOEA

Protracted diarrhoea is defined as four or more watery stools per day persisting for longer than two weeks in a child whose body weight either remains static or declines. The condition most commonly complicates acute gastroenteritis in infants under the age of 6 months. The acute illness can only be assumed to be infective since a pathogen can be identified in the stools of only a small

Table 10.6 Pathophysiology of protracted diarrhoea following acute enteric infections

Disaccharide intolerance	
Monosaccharide intolerance	
Cows' milk protein intolerance	
Gluten intolerance	
Bacterial overgrowth of the small intestine	
Intraluminal metabolism of substrates	Bile acids Hydroxy fatty acids Short-chain organic acids

proportion of patients. The condition can present major problems in management and may carry an appreciable mortality. Unless the disease process is arrested at an early stage severe malnutrition may ensue, the infant presenting the clinical features of protein-energy deficiency as seen in developing parts of the world (see Ch. 8).

Pathophysiology

A variety of pathophysiological mechanisms acting singly or in concert may result in protracted diarrhoea following acute enteric infections, and these are listed in Table 10.6. The morphology of the small intestinal mucosa is usually abnormal (see Ch. 9) but may be entirely normal.

Disaccharide intolerance

Since the disaccharidase enzymes are located at the brush border luminal poles of the absorptive cells, reduced activity can be anticipated to accompany any factor which induces mucosal damage. Lactase is the last enzyme to reach maturity during fetal development, and for this reason premature babies who develop enteric infection are particularly at risk of becoming lactose-intolerant. Of the three disaccharides lactose, sucrose and maltose, clinical intolerance to lactose is by far the most important entity. Following mucosal damage lactase is the last enzyme to recover; this may take several months and be preceded by complete recovery of mucosal morphology. For example, in a group of adults with tropical sprue who had been treated for three months to four years with folic acid or antibacterial agents, the morphology of small intestinal mucosa was found to be normal; sucrase and maltase activities were normal, but 63 per cent remained lactase-deficient (Gray, Walter and Colver, 1968). The development of clinical symptoms of disaccharide intolerance will depend not only on the magnitude of the decreased enzyme activity, but also on its extent along the small intestine. For example, proximal small intestinal lesions are usually not accompanied by intolerance simply because the unabsorbed disaccharides can be hydrolysed and absorbed by the remaining normal mucosa.

Symptoms include vomiting, abdominal distention and pain, and watery acid stools which are often frothy and result in perianal excoriation. The stools have a low pH and contain excessive amounts of reducing substances and short-chain organic acids such as acetic, propionic and lactic acids; these acids are derived from the fermentative actions of colonic bacteria on the unabsorbed

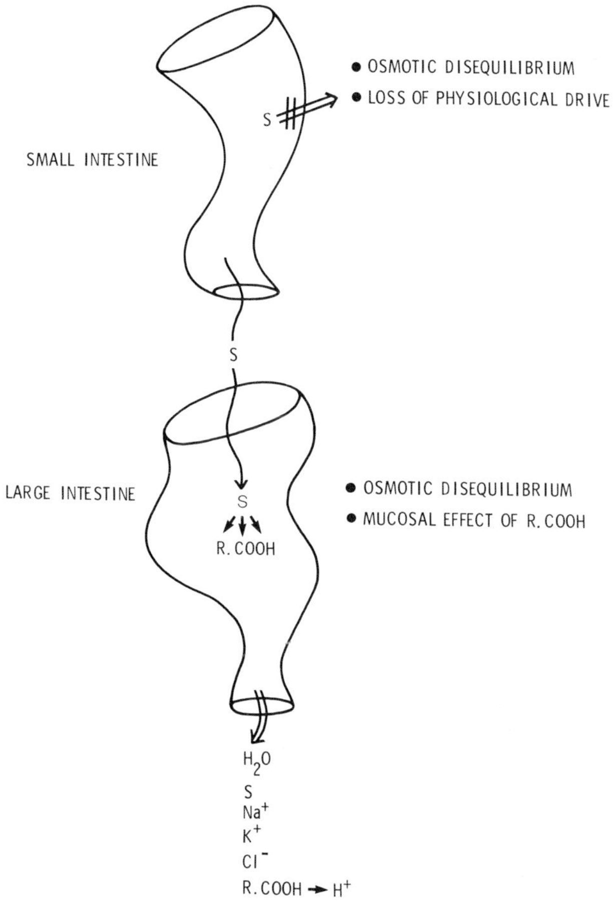

Fig. 10.3 Pathophysiological mechanisms which result in the clinical features of sugar intolerance. S indicates the sugar

sugars. The pathophysiological mechanisms resulting in these features are summarised in Figure 10.3. Unabsorbed sugars accumulate within the small intestinal lumen and create osmotic gradients between the plasma and lumen which result in the bulk movement of fluid and electrolytes into the lumen. Normally, actively absorbed monosaccharides provide an important physiological 'drive' for water and electrolyte absorption in the jejunum, and this process is dependent on hydrolysis of the disaccharides (i.e. lactose, maltose, sucrose and isomaltose) which contain the actively transported monosaccharides, glucose and galactose. Thus, in addition to producing an osmotic disequilibrium, disaccharidase deficiency will also deprive the jejunum of a physiological process which increases its ability to absorb water and electrolytes. The net effect of disaccharide malabsorption is the passage of large amounts of fluid and electrolytes into the large intestine which exceed the colon's reabsorptive capacity, resulting in diarrhoea. The metabolism of the unabsorbed sugars to short-chain organic acids by colonic bacteria further increases the osmolality of colonic contents producing further movement of fluid into the colon; in addition, short-chain organic acids may have a direct 'toxic' effect on colonic mucosa inducing secretion of fluid and electrolytes into the lumen. Abdominal pain and distention result from distention of the intestine with fluid and gas; the gases are hydrogen and carbon dioxide which are products of the fermentative process in the colon and which account for the frothy appearance of the stools.

The diagnosis may be suspected on the basis of a historical relationship between symptomatology and intake of dietary sugars, and should be confirmed by appropriate tests. The Clinitest method (Kerry and Anderson, 1964) is simple and determines the amount of reducing substances in the stool. The method can be applied to immediate testing of stools in the ward or even in field conditions. The test must be performed on the fluid component of the stool and must be done promptly to avoid bacterial degradation of sugars. A value of greater than 0·5 per cent of stool-reducing sugars suggests sugar intolerance. Sucrose is a non-reducing sugar, and prior hydrolysis of the stool fluid with hydrochloric acid is necessary to detect sucrose. Paper chromatography of stool water provides a semiquantitative method for determining the individual sugars. Oral sugar tolerance tests involve the determination of serial blood glucose levels following the administration of the suspected sugar (1 to 2 g/kg). If intolerant of the sugar, the patient develops gastrointestinal symptoms as described above, a rise of blood glucose of less than 1·6 mmol/l (30 mg/100 ml) and loose acid stools containing excessive amounts of reducing substances. It should be stressed that sugar loading tests may precipitate severe gastrointestinal symptoms and dehydration in susceptible children, particularly if they are sick infants with protracted diarrhoea. In most instances a confident diagnosis of sugar intolerance can be made on the basis of the history, examination of the stools and the response to withdrawal of the offending sugar from the diet. Stool pH is an unreliable test and merely creates additional work for the ward staff.

Determination of mucosal enzyme activities is unnecessary since it does not influence clinical management.

Monosaccharide intolerance

Transient secondary intolerance to one or all of the three monosaccharides, glucose, galactose and fructose, is now recognised as a clinical entity (Harries and Francis, 1968; Lifshitz *et al.*, 1970a and 1970b). The clinical features and diagnosis are similar to those for disaccharide intolerance.

Cows' milk protein intolerance

It is likely that an acute infective insult can render the bowel intolerant to cows' milk protein, probably as a result of immune interactions. Intolerance to this protein is considered in more detail in Chapter 9.

Transient gluten intolerance

As an entity, transient gluten intolerance has not been unequivocally established. It is our clinical impression, however, that certain infants with protracted diarrhoea benefit from temporary withdrawal of dietary gluten.

Bacterial overgrowth of the small intestine

Bacterial overgrowth of the small intestine in infants with protracted diarrhoea is common in both the developing (Coello-Ramirez and Lifshitz, 1972; Gracey and Stone, 1972; Heyworth and Brown, 1975) and developed (Challacombe *et al.*, 1974; Challacombe, Richardson and Edkins, 1974; Gracey, Burke and Anderson, 1969) parts of the world. Both aerobic (particularly *E. coli*) and anaerobic (particularly bacteroides) species may be found. Using an *in vitro* tissue culture technique a toxigenic strain of *E. coli* was identified in one infant (H. Holzel, personal communication).

The relationship between the bacterial overgrowth and the persistent diarrhoea and malnutrition is not at present clear and may well be multifactorial. The bacteria or their toxins may have a direct effect on mucosal function or, alternatively, an indirect effect secondary to the metabolism of certain intraluminal substrates as discussed below.

Intraluminal metabolism of substrates

Anaerobic bacteria contain enzymes which catalyse the deconjugation and 7-α-dehydroxylation of conjugated bile salts leading to the production of free dihydroxy bile acids such as deoxycholate and chenodeoxycholate. Deoxycholate has been shown to inhibit absorption of fluid and electrolytes in both the small and large bowel and, in the jejunum, to inhibit monosaccharide absorption and mucosal (Na^+-K^+)-ATPase activity; at high concentrations the bile acid produces gross structural abnormalities of the jejunal mucosa (Harries and Sladen, 1972; Sladen and Harries, 1972; Guiraldes *et al.*, 1975). Deoxycholate and other free bile acids have been shown to be present in the duodenal contents of some infants with protracted diarrhoea (Gracey *et al.*, 1969; Challacombe, Richardson and Edkins, 1974; Schneider and Viteri, 1974); the three infants reported by Gracey *et al.* (1969) were also intolerant of monosaccharides. Thus unconjugated bile acids may have an effect on small intestinal function and structure in some infants with protracted diarrhoea. Morphological abnormalities of the ileal mucosa have been reported in infants dying during the acute phase of gastroenteritis (Walker Smith, 1972), and it is likely that similar lesions may be present in some patients with protracted diarrhoea; this could result in bile salt malabsorption followed by bacterial degradation in the colon, the free bile acids inducing colonic secretion of fluid and electrolytes. Cholestyramine is a non-absorbable anion-exchange resin which is capable of binding bile acids and bacterial endotoxins. In this context it is of some interest that successful treatment of infants with intractable diarrhoea with this resin has been reported in an uncontrolled study (Tamer, Santora and Sandberg, 1974).

In addition to free bile acids, bacterial production of hydroxy fatty acids and short-chain organic acids may also result in inhibition of fluid absorption and contribute to the pathophysiology of the diarrhoea.

Differential diagnosis

The more important conditions which must be considered in the differential diagnosis of any child with protracted diarrhoea, particularly if the response to

Table 10.7 Differential diagnosis of protracted diarrhoea in infancy

Causes	Examples
Idiopathic (i.e. cause undetermined)	
Acquired sugar intolerance	Lactose intolerance
Coeliac disease	
Acquired protein intolerance	Cows' milk protein intolerance
Enterocolitis	
Surgical causes	Midgut malrotation
	Hirschsprung's disease
	Blind-loops
Selective inborn errors of absorption	Congenital chloridorrhoea
	Glucose-galactose malabsorption
	Lactase deficiency
Extraintestinal infections	Urinary tract infections
Antibiotics	Ampicillin
Immune deficiency states	Combined immune deficiency
	Defective opsonisation
Chronic inflammatory bowel disease	Ulcerative colitis
Tumours	Neuroblastoma
	Ganglioneuroma
	Lymphoma
Intrauterine infections	Cytomegalovirus
Miscellaneous	Histiocytosis X
	Intestinal lymphangiectasia

treatment is poor, are shown in Table 10.7. Surgical conditions such as midgut malrotation and Hirschsprung's disease must always be borne in mind.

Management

The management of infants with protracted diarrhoea depends on the cause and the general condition of the infant when first seen and can pose major therapeutic problems. If the infant's condition is reasonable appropriate investigations can be performed to provide a logical basis for treatment. Often, however, the child's condition limits the time available for diagnostic investigations, and empirical treatment based on theoretical assumptions is necessary.

Dietetic

The basis of management is dietetic, to which most patients respond. A skilled dietitian is a key member of any team involved in the care of infants with protracted diarrhoea.

Cause determined. If investigation reveals that the infant is intolerant to one or more of the dietary constituents listed in Table 10.6, then a rational approach is possible. A wide variety of commercial food products are available for the treatment of various sugar and protein intolerances, and for detailed information the reader is referred to the excellent monograph by Francis (1974). Generally speaking, preparations containing fat in the form of medium-chain triglycerides (MCT) and nitrogen as amino acids or peptides are unnecessary, and most infants respond to more physiological preparations. Moreover, the high osmolality of many preparations containing MCT may in itself exacerbate the

Table 10.8 Constituents of the full-strength feed for the treatment of protracted infantile diarrhoea of undetermined cause

Constituents	Amount in 100 ml
Protein (contained in comminuted chicken[a])	3·75 g
Fat (contained in chicken)	1·65 g
Gastrocaloreen[b]	5·0 g
Sodium[c]	1·85 mmol
Potassium[c]	2·32 mmol
Calcium[c]	1·75 mmol
Other minerals[c]	—
Total energy provided:	approximately 211 kJ

[a] See Appendix B for further details of composition.
[b] Gastrocaloreen is a glucose polymer; Scientific Hospital Supplies, England.
[c] Sodium, potassium, calcium and other minerals derived from the comminuted chicken and the metabolic mineral mixture; further details in Appendix B and Table 10.9.

diarrhoea. The management of infants who are unable to tolerate all three monosaccharides deserves special mention. Successful treatment depends on the complete elimination of all carbohydrates from the diet and such therapy makes these infants extremely susceptible to develop severe hypoglycaemia, which may be fatal (Lifshitz *et al.*, 1970a and 1970b). Limited hepatic glycogen stores may be a predisposing factor particularly if the infant is malnourished. Whilst receiving carbohydrate-free feeds frequent determination of blood glucose levels is essential, and hypothermia may be a sign of severe hypoglycaemia. Preventive measures include daily infusions of glucose, and ephedrine and epinephrine have also been successful in some patients. Details of the diets for such patients can be obtained from Francis (1974).

Cause undetermined. When the cause of the protracted diarrhoea cannot be established or when the infant's condition precludes detailed investigation, we have found that a diet free of disaccharides, cows' milk protein and gluten gives excellent results. Protein is provided as comminuted chicken (which contains some long-chain triglycerides), carbohydrate as glucose and Gastrocaloreen (a glucose polymer) and fat as Prosparol (an emulsion of long-chain triglycerides); carbohydrate can also be given solely as glucose or a mixture of glucose and fructose, up to a maximum concentration of 8 to 10 per cent. The basic constituents of a 100 ml of the full strength feed are shown in Table 10.8. Comminuted chicken (50 g), Gastrocaloreen (5 g) and the metabolic mineral mixture (0·8 g) are made up to 100 ml with water. Initially this formula is given as a quarter-strength feed with added sugar (5 per cent dextrose), from which the added fat (Prosparol) is omitted, in a suitable volume as small frequent feeds (e.g. one or two hourly feeds) together with disaccharide free complete vitamin supplements (e.g. three Ketovite tablets and five ml Ketovite liquid per day; see Appendix B); a metabolic mineral mixture is included (see Table 10.9 and

Table 10.9 Details of the full-feeding regime in the treatment of protracted infantile diarrhoea of undetermined cause

Constituents	Amounts in feeds
Comminuted chicken	Not more than 10 g protein/kg[b]/day
Gastrocaloreen	10 g/100 ml of feed
Fat (from prosparol[a] and comminuted chicken)	4 g/100 ml of feed
Metabolic mineral mixture	1·5 g/kg[b]/day (provided quantities do not exceed 1 g/100 ml of feed, or a total of 8 g/day)
Calcium (from comminuted chicken, metabolic mineral mixture and added calcium gluconate)	At least 1·25 mmol/100 ml of feed or a minimum of 12·5 mmol/day
Feed volume	200 ml/kg/day
Total energy provided:	750 or more kJ/kg/day

[a]Prosparol is a 50 per cent arachis oil emulsion of long-chain triglycerides; Duncan, Flockhart & Co. Ltd., London, England.
[b]Units of weight refer to actual not expected body weight. Vitamin supplements are given as Ketovite tablets (× 3/day) and liquid (5 ml/day)—see Appendix B for composition of Ketovite.

Appendix B), and any orally administered drugs must be free of disaccharides. The feeds are then slowly built up over a period of 10 to 30 days. This is achieved by first increasing the feeds to full strength and then by adding Prosparol in 2 to 5 ml increments; Gastrocaloreen and calcium gluconate are also added to the feeds during this build-up period to finally provide the requirements shown in Table 10.9. If this feeding regime is tolerated and the patient begins to thrive, then the following modifications are implemented prior to discharge home: (1) the intervals between feeds are increased (e.g. four hourly × 5); (2) introduction of suitable weaning solids (e.g. Robinson's baby rice mixed with 5 per cent dextrose; milk-free mashed potato and puree meat). The dietitian then spends two to three sessions with the mother teaching her the diet. Following a period of protracted diarrhoea infants often become ravenously hungry and there is a real danger of their becoming overweight. This should be discussed with the mother during the dietary teaching sessions.

We have used this feeding regime for several years at The Hospital for Sick Children, Great Ormond Street, in infants with protracted diarrhoea who have failed to respond to other dietary manipulations and have been impressed by the excellent response which has been achieved in the majority of patients.

Intravenous feeding

In patients who are severely malnourished or who fail to respond to dietetic management, a period of intravenous feeding may be life-saving (Harries, 1971).

Other approaches

No other form of treatment has been conclusively shown to be of value in the management of protracted diarrhoea. If, however, there is evidence of bacterial overgrowth of the small intestine and bile salt degradation, cholestyramine and/or antimicrobial agents are worth trying. Anticholinergic agents have no place in treatment.

Duration of treatment

After a period of two to three months the patient is readmitted and reintroduction of disaccharides and cows' milk protein is attempted according to the following scheme:

Day 1: Lactose replaces the feed carbohydrate, initially in a concentration of 1 per cent. If this is tolerated the concentration of lactose is increased on days 2, 3 and 4, to 3, 5 and 7 per cent respectively.

Day 5: If lactose is tolerated, a challenge (5 ml) of fresh pasteurised cows' milk is given.

Day 6: If the milk challenge does not precipitate any symptoms, the volume of a suitable low solute cows' milk formula is slowly increased over the next four days so as to completely replace the chicken feeds. Sucrose is added to the diet (e.g. as fruit puree) prior to discharge. If lactose is tolerated then almost invariably sucrose will also be tolerated, since lactose intolerance usually persists for longer periods of time than sucrose intolerance.

Day 10: The patient is discharged home on a temporary gluten-free diet.

After two to three months of treatment the majority of infants are able to tolerate disaccharides and cows' milk protein, but occasionally this is not the case. In those circumstances a further period of dietetic treatment is indicated, and one of the many commercially available disaccharide-free milk formulae containing soy protein or hydrolysed protein should be considered.

Assuming disaccharides and cows' milk protein are tolerated, the patient is followed up and growth and development checked at regular intervals. Failure to thrive may indicate persistent cows' milk protein intolerance, and a peroral intestinal biopsy may be helpful in confirming the diagnosis (see Ch. 9). If the infant continues to thrive a gluten-free diet is continued for approximately six months. Following the reintroduction of a gluten-containing diet follow up is continued for a year or more; the development of any biochemical or clinical abnormalities suggestive of gluten-intolerance is an indication for biopsy. If there is a family history of coeliac disease or a clinical suspicion that the initial cause of the protracted diarrhoea was due to coeliac disease, a gluten-free diet is continued for at least two years when a formal gluten challenge is performed, as outlined in Chapter 9.

PROGNOSIS

The infant mortality from gastroenteritis in the United Kingdom remains appreciable, and the likelihood of death as a result of any single episode is of the order of 0·4 per cent (from Kuzemko, 1969). Three-quarters of all deaths occur in children under the age of 6 months. Hypernatraemic dehydration carries a mortality of between 2·5 and 20 per cent and accounts for an appreciable

Table 10.10 Maintenance requirements of water, sodium and potassium

Age (months)	Requirements/kg/24 hours Water (ml)	Sodium (mmol)	Potassium (mmol)
0–6	120–150	1·0–2·5	1·0–2·5
6–12	100–120	2·5	2·5
12–24	80–100	2·5	2·5
>24	70–90	1·5–2·5	1·5–2·5

proportion of all deaths from gastroenteritis. Individual epidemics, particularly when caused by virulent strains of enteropathogenic *E. coli* in the newborn period, may be associated with mortality rates of as high as 25 per cent. In the absence of gastrointestinal, renal or other on-going complications and when the prognosis is that of the complicating disorder, the morbidity following acute gastroenteritis is low and almost confined to those patients who have had an episode of hypernatraemia. In two follow-up studies slightly less than 10 per cent of patients who survived an episode of hypernatraemic dehydration had neurological or intellectual deficits that could be attributed to the hypernatraemia (Morris-Jones *et al.*, 1967; Macaulay and Watson, 1967). It is possible that more subtle long-term neurological or intellectual deficits could follow acute gastroenteritis or protracted diarrhoea, particularly if the illness occurred in early infancy, but there are no reported studies to substantiate this.

APPENDIX A

CALCULATION OF THE INTRAVENOUS REQUIREMENTS IN THE MANAGEMENT OF DEHYDRATION

Table 10.10 lists the maintenance requirements of water, sodium and potassium for different age groups.

In the examples below a hypothetical patient will be considered. The infant weighed 3·72 kg on admission, was estimated to be 7 per cent dehydrated (7 per cent dry) and received half normal saline at a rate of 60 ml per hour for the first four hours.

Example 1—Hyponatraemia (plasma sodium = 115 mmol/l)

(1) Estimated rehydrated weight (WR)
WR = Admission weight × 100 ÷ (100 − % dry)
= 3·72 × 100 ÷ 93 = 4 kg.

(2) Water required (ml)
Deficit = WR × 1000 × % dry ÷ 100
= 4 × 1000 × 7 ÷ 100 = +280
Maintenance = 4 × 150 = +600
Less ½ normal saline given = 4 × 60 = −240
Total +640

(3) Sodium required (mmol)

Deficit = WR × 0·6 × (140 − plasma sodium)		
= 4 × 0·6 × (140 − 115)	=	+60
Maintenance = 4 × 2·5	=	+10
Less ½ normal saline given (0·24 × 75)	=	−18
Total		+52

(4) Potassium required (mmol)

Deficit = sodium deficit ÷ 2		
= 60 ÷ 2	=	+30
Maintenance = 4 × 2·5	=	+10
Total		+40

An intravenous infusion of half normal saline with 2·5 per cent dextrose and potassium chloride (40 mmol/l) at a rate of 32 ml/hour for 20 hours would provide:

		Amounts provided	Requirements	Difference to requirements
Water (ml)	= 20 × 32 =	640	640	0
Sodium (mmol)	= 0·64 × 75 =	48	52	− 4
Potassium (mmol)	= 0·64 × 40 =	25	40	−15

Note that though water and sodium requirements are met, only just over half the potassium requirements are given.

Example 2—Normonatraemia (plasma sodium = 135 mmol/l)

Rehydrated weight and water requirements as for Example 1 and equal 4 kg and 640 ml, respectively.

(1) Sodium required

Deficit = fluid deficit as ½ normal saline		
= 0·28 × 75	=	+21
Maintenance = 4 × 2·5	=	+10
Less ½ normal saline given	=	−18
Total		+13

(2) Potassium required

Deficit = sodium deficit ÷ 2		
= 21 ÷ 2	=	+10·5
Maintenance = 4 × 2·5	=	+10
Total		+20·5

An intravenous infusion of one-fifth normal saline with 4 per cent dextrose and potassium chloride (30 mmol/l) at a rate of 32 ml/hour for 20 hours would provide:

		Amounts provided	Requirements	Difference to requirements
Water	= 20 × 32	= 640	640	0
Sodium	= 0·64 × 30	= 19	13	+6
Potassium	= 0·64 × 30	= 19	21	−2

Example 3—Hypernatraemia (plasma sodium = 164 mmol/l)

Water required

Total required = 150 ml/kg	
= 4 × 150	= +600
Less ½ normal saline given (4 × 60)	= −240
Total	+360

An infusion of one-fifth normal saline with 4 per cent dextrose and potassium chloride (40 mmol/l) at a rate of 18 ml/hour would provide 460 ml water, 14 mmol sodium and 18 mmol of potassium.

APPENDIX B

COMPOSITION OF COMMINUTED CHICKEN*
(Cow & Gate Baby Foods, England)

Constituents	Amount in 100 g
Protein	7 to 8 g
Fat	2·5 to 4 g
Carbohydrate	Nil
Sodium	10 mg
Potassium	50 mg
Calcium	9 mg
Magnesium	8 mg
Iron	0·4 mg
Phosphorus	45 mg

*Minced chicken can also be simply prepared in the home (see Francis, 1974); sterility is extremely important because of the not infrequent endogenous bacterial contamination of poultry (e.g. Salmonellae).

COMPOSITION OF METABOLIC MINERAL MIXTURE
(Scientific Hospital Supplies, England)

Constituents	Amount (mg) in 1 g
Calcium	82
Potassium	83
Phosphorus	59
Sodium	39·6
Magnesium	9·7
Iron	0·5
Copper	0·063
Zinc	0·11
Manganese	0·057
Iodine	0·007
Aluminium	0·0002
Molybdenum	0·0015

COMPOSITION OF KETOVITE (Paines & Byrne Ltd., England)

Tablets	Content per tablet (mg)
Aneurine hydrochloride	1·0
Riboflavine	1·0
Pyridoxine hydrochloride	0·33
Nicotinamide	3·3
Calcium pantothenate	1·16
Ascorbic acid	16·6
α-tocopherol acetate	5·0
Inositol	50·0
Biotin	0·17
Folic acid	0·25

Liquid	Contents per 5 ml
Vitamin A	2500 units
Vitamin D	400 units
Choline chloride	150 mg
Cyanocobalamin	12·5 μg

References

Adler, J. L. & Zickl, R. (1969) Winter vomiting disease. *Journal of Infectious Diseases*, **119,** 668.

Bannister, A. (1975) Treatment of hypernatraemic dehydration in infancy. *Archives of Disease in Childhood*, **50,** 179.

Banwell, J. G. & Sherr, H. (1973) Effect of bacterial enterotoxins on the gastrointestinal tract. *Gastroenteroloy*, **65,** 467.

Bishop, R. F., Davidson, G. P., Holmes, I. H. & Ruck, B. J. (1973) Virus particles in epithelial cells of duodenal mucosa from children with acute non-bacterial gastroenteritis. *Lancet*, **2,** 1281.

Blacklow, N. R., Dolin, R., Fedson, D. S., Dupont, H., Northrup, R. S., Hornick, R. B. & Chanock, R. M. (1972) Acute infectious nonbacterial gastroenteritis: etiology and pathogenesis. *Annals of Internal Medicine,* **76,** 993.

British Medical Journal (1972) Acute infective gastroenteritis. *British Medical Journal,* **2,** 668.

British Medical Journal (1975) Susceptibility to cholera. *British Medical Journal,* **4,** 423.

Brown, W. R., Savage, D. C., Dubois, R. S., Alp, M. H., Mallory, A. & Kern, F. (1972) Intestinal microflora of immunoglobulin-deficient and normal human subjects. *Gastroenterology,* **62,** 1143.

Bryant, M. P. (1972) Interactions among intestinal microorganisms. *American Journal of Clinical Nutrition,* **25,** 1485.

Bullen, C. L. & Willis, A. T. (1971) Resistance of the breastfed infant to gastroenteritis. *British Medical Journal,* **3,** 338.

Bullen, J. J., Rogers, H. J. & Weigh, L. (1972) Iron-binding proteins in milk and resistance to Escherichia coli infection in infants. *British Medical Journal,* **1,** 69.

Center for Disease Control (1970) *Foodborne Outbreaks: Annual Summary 1969.* U.S. Department of Health, Education and Welfare/Public Health Service, Atlanta, Georgia.

Challacombe, D. N., Richardson, J. M. & Edkins, S. (1974) Anaerobic bacteria and deconjugated bile salts in the upper small intestine of infants with gastrointestinal disorders. *Acta Paediatrica Scandinavica* **63,** 581.

Challacombe, D. N., Richardson, J. M., Rowe, B. & Anderson, C. M. (1974) Bacterial microflora of the upper gastrointestinal tract in infants with protracted diarrhoea. *Archives of Disease in Childhood,* **49,** 270.

Chrispin, A. R. (1972) Medullary necrosis in infancy. *British Medical Bulletin,* **28,** 233.

Coello-Ramirez, P. & Lifshitz, F. (1972) Enteric microflora and carbohydrate intolerance in infants with diarrhea. *Pediatrics,* **49,** 233.

Cramblett, H. G., Azimi, P. & Haynes, R. E. (1971) The etiology of infectious diarrhea in infancy, with special reference to enteropathogenic *E. coli. Annals of New York Academy of Science,* **176,** 80.

Davidson, G. P., Bishop, R. F., Townley, R. R. W., Holmes, I. H. & Ruck, B. J. (1975) Importance of a new virus in acute sporadic enteritis in children. *Lancet,* **1,** 242.

Dingle, J. H., Badger, G. F., Feller, A. E., Hodgers, R. G., Jordan, W. S. & Rammelkamp, C. H. (1953) A study of illness in a group of Cleveland families. I. Plan of study and certain general observations. *American Journal of Hygiene,* **58,** 16.

Dixon, J. M. S. (1965) Effect of antibiotic treatment on duration of excretion of Salmonella typhimurium by children. *British Medical Journal,* **2,** 1343.

Donowitz, M., Keusch, G. T. & Binder, H. J. (1975) Effect of Shigella enterotoxin on electrolyte transport in rabbit ileum. *Gastroenterology,* **69,** 1230.

Drasar, B. S., Shiner, M. & McLeod, G. M. (1969) Studies on the intestinal flora. I. The bacterial flora of the gastrointestinal tract in healthy and achlorhydric persons. *Gastroenterology,* **56,** 71.

DuPont, H. L. & Hornick, R. B. (1973) Adverse effect of Lomotil therapy in Shigellosis. *Journal of the American Medical Association,* **226,** 1525.

Field, M. (1974) Intestinal secretion. *Gastroenterology,* **66,** 1063.

Fifth Caribbean Health Ministers Conference (1973). Strategy and plan of action to combat gastroenteritis and malnutrition in children under two years of age. *Journal of Paediatric and Environmental Child Health* (1975), **21,** 23.

Finberg, L. (1970) The management of the critically ill child with dehydration secondary to diarrhea. *Pediatrics,* **45,** 1029.

Finberg, L. (1973) Hypernatraemic (hypertonic) dehydration in infants. *New England Journal of Medicine,* **289,** 196.

Flewett, T. H., Bryden, A. S. & Davies, H. (1975) Epidemic viral enteritis in a long stay children's ward. *Lancet,* **1,** 4.

Francis, D. E. M. (1974) *Diets for Sick Children.* 3rd edition. Oxford: Blackwell.

Gerrard, J. W. (1974) Breast-feeding: second thoughts. *Pediatrics,* **54,** 757.

Giannella, R. A., Gots, R. E., Charney, A. N., Greenough, W. B. & Formal, S. B. (1975) Pathogenesis of Salmonella-mediated intestinal fluid secretion. *Gastroenterology,* **69,** 1238.

Gorbach, S. L. (1975) Intestinal microflora in acute diarrhoea. *Medicine,* **2,** 64.

Gorbach, S. L., Kean, B. H., Evans, D. G., Evans, D. J. & Bessudo, D. (1975) Travelers' diarrhea and toxigenic Escherichia coli. *New England Journal of Medicine,* **292,** 933.

Gordon, J. E. (1971) Diarrhoeal disease of early childhood: worldwide scope of the problem. *Annals of the New York Academy of Sciences,* **176,** 9.

Gracey, M., Burke, V. & Anderson, C. M. (1969) Association of monosaccharide malabsorption with abnormal small intestinal flora. *Lancet,* **2,** 384.

Gracey, M. & Stone, D. E. (1972) Small intestinal microflora in Australian Aboriginal children with chronic diarrhoea. *Australian and New Zealand Journal of Medicine,* **3,** 215.

Grady, G. F. & Keusch, G. T. (1971a) Pathogenesis of bacterial diarrhoeas. Part I. *New England Journal of Medicine,* **285,** 831.

Grady, G. F. & Keusch, G. T. (1971b) Pathogenesis of bacterial diarrhoeas. Part II. *New England Journal of Medicine,* **285,** 891.

Gray, G. M., Walter, W. M. & Colver, E. H. (1968) Persistent deficiency of intestinal lactase in apparently cured tropical sprue. *Gastroenterology,* **54,** 552.

Guiraldes, E., Lamabadusuriya, S. P., Oyesiku, J. E. J., Whitfield, A. E. & Harries, J. T. (1975) A comparative study on the effects of different bile salts on mucosal ATPase and transport in the rat jejunum in vivo. *Biochimica et Biophysica Acta,* **389,** 495.

Gyles, C. L. (1972) Plasmids in intestinal bacteria. *American Journal of Clinical Nutrition,* **25,** 1455.

Harries, J. T. (1971) Intravenous feeding in infants. *Archives of Disease in Childhood,* **46,** 855.

Harries, J. T. & Francis, D. E. M. (1968) Temporary monosaccharide intolerance. *Acta Paediatrica Scandinavica,* **57,** 505.

Harries, J. T. & Sladen, G. E. (1972) The effects of different bile salts on the absorption of fluid, electrolytes, and monosaccharides in the small intestine of the rat in vivo. *Gut,* **13,** 596.

Heese, H. De V., Tonin, C., Bowie, M. D. & Evans, A. (1966) Management of metabolic acidosis in acute gastroenteritis. *British Medical Journal,* **2,** 144.

Heyworth, B. & Brown, J. (1975) Jejunal microflora in malnourished Gambian children. *Archives of Disease in Childhood,* **50,** 27.

Hogan, G. R., Dodge, P. R., Gill, S. R., Master, S. & Sotos, J. F. (1969) Pathogenesis of seizures occurring during restoration of plasma tonicity to normal in animals previously chronically hypernatremic. *Pediatrics,* **43,** 54.

Hurst, A. F. (1934) The clinical importance of achlorhydria. *British Medical Journal,* **2,** 665.

Jones, G. W. & Rutter, J. M. (1972) Role of the K88 antigen in the pathogenesis of neonatal diarrhoea caused by Escherichia coli in piglets. *Infection and Immunity,* **6,** 918.

Kerry, K. R. & Anderson, C. M. (1964) A ward test for sugar in faeces. *Lancet,* **1,** 981.

Kimberg, D. V. (1974) Cyclic nucleotides and their role in gastrointestinal secretion. *Gastroenterology,* **67,** 1023.

Kingston, M. E. (1973) Biochemical disturbances in breastfed infants with gastroenteritis and dehydration. *Journal of Pediatrics,* **82,** 1073.

Kuzemko, J. A. (1969) Gastroenteritis in infancy. *Postgraduate Medical Journal,* **45,** 731.

Lancet (1975a) Rotaviruses of Man and Animals. *Lancet,* **1,** 257.

Lancet (1975b) Oral glucose/electrolyte therapy for acute diarrhoea, *Lancet,* **1,** 79.

Lifshitz, F., Coello-Ramirez, P. & Gutierrez-Topete, G. (1970a) Monosaccharide intolerance and hypoglycemia in infants with diarrhea. I. Clinical course of 23 infants. *Journal of Pediatrics,* **77,** 595.

Lifshitz, F., Coello-Ramirez, P. & Gutierrez-Topete, G. (1970b) Monosaccharide intolerance and hypoglycemia in infants with diarrhea. II. Metabolic studies in 23 infants. *Journal of Pediatrics,* **77,** 604.

Mata, L. J., Mejicanos, M. L. & Jimenez, F. (1972) Studies on the indigenous gastrointestinal flora of Guatemalan children. *American Journal of Clinical Nutrition,* **25,** 1380.

Macaulay, D. & Watson, M. (1967) Hypernatraemia in infants as a cause of brain damage. *Archives of Disease in Childhood,* **42,** 485.

McWeeney, P. M., & Emery, J. L. (1975) Unexpected postneonatal deaths (cot deaths) due to recognisable disease. *Archives of Disease in Childhood,* **50,** 191.

Mosley, W. H., Bevenson, A. S. & Barui, R. (1968) *A Serological Study of Cholera Antibodies in Rural East Pakistan.* Bulletin of World Health Organization, **38,** 327–346.

Morris-Jones, P. H., Houston, I. B. & Evans, R. C. (1967) Prognosis of the neurological complications of acute hypernatraemia. *Lancet,* **2,** 1385.

Peeters, T. & Vantrappen, G. (1975) The Paneth cell: a source of intestinal lysozyme. *Gut,* **16,** 553.

Puffer, R. R. & Serrano, C. V. (1973) Patterns of mortality in childhood. *Report of the Inter-American Investigation of Mortality in Childhood.* Scientific Publication PAHO No. 262.

Registrar General & Census Commissioner, New Delhi (1972) *Pocketbook of Population Statistics,* 1971.

Registrar General's Figures, 1958–1972.

Rout, W. R., Formal, S. B., Dammin, G. J. & Giannella, R. A. (1974) Pathophysiology of Salmonella diarrhea in the rhesus monkey: Intestinal transport, morphological and bacteriological studies. *Gastroenterology,* **67,** 59.

Rout, W. R., Formal, S. B., Giannella, R. A. & Dammin, G. J. (1975) Pathophysiology of Shigella diarrhea in the rhesus monkey: intestinal transport, morphological and bacteriological studies. *Gastroenterology,* **68,** 270.

Rutter, J. M., Burrows, M. R., Sellwood, R. & Gibbons, R. A. (1975) A genetic basis for resistance to enteric disease caused by E. coli. *Nature,* **257,** 135.

Sack, R. B., Hirschhorn, N., Brownlee, I., Cash, R. A., Woodward, W. E. & Sack, D. A. (1975)

Enterotoxigenic Escherichia coli-associated diarrhoeal disease in Apache children. *New England Journal of Medicine*, **292**, 1041.

Savage, D. C. (1972) Associations and physiological interactions of indigenous microorganisms and gastrointestinal epithelia. *Americal Journal of Clinical Nutrition*, **25**, 1372.

Schneider, R. E. & Viteri, F. E. (1974) Luminal events of lipid absorption in protein-calorie malnourished children: relationship with nutritional recovery and diarrhea. II. Alterations in bile acid content of duodenal aspirates. *American Journal of Clinical Nutrition*, **27**, 788.

Schreiber, D. S., Blacklow, N. R. & Trier, J. S. (1973) The mucosal lesion of the proximal small intestine in acute infectious nonbacterial gastroenteritis. *New England Journal of Medicine*, **288**, 1318.

Schultz, S. G., Frizzell, R. A. & Nellans, H. N. (1974) Ion transport by mammalian small intestine. *Annual Review of Physiology*, **36**, 51.

Sheehy, T. W., Artenstein, M. S. & Green, R. W. (1964) Small intestinal mucosa in certain viral diseases. *Journal of American Medical Association*, **190**, 1023.

Sladen, G. E. & Harries, J. T. (1972) Studies on the effects of unconjugated dihydroxy bile salts on rat small intestinal function in vivo. *Biochimica et Biophysica Acta*, **288**, 443.

Smith, H. W. (1966) The antimicrobial activity of the stomach contents of suckling rabbits. *Journal of Pathology and Bacteriology*, **91**, 1.

Smith, H. W. & Linggood, M. A. (1971) Observations on the pathogenic properties of the K88, HLY and ENT plasmids of Escherichia Coli with particular reference to porcine diarrhoea. *Journal of Medical Microbiology*, **4**, 467.

Stoliar, O. A., Pelley, R. P., Koniecki-Green, E., Klaus, M. H. & Carpenter, C. C. J. (1975) Secretory IgA against enterotoxins in breast milk. *Lancet*, **1**, 1258.

Tamer, M. A., Santora, T. R. & Sandberg, D. H. (1974) Cholestyramine therapy for intractable diarrhea. *Pediatrics*, **53**, 217.

Toivanen, P., Toivanen, A., Olkonen, L. & Aantaa, S. (1973) Hospital outbreak of Yersinia enterocolitica infection. *Lancet*, **1**, 801.

Waddell, W. R. & Kunz, L. J. (1956) Association of Salmonella enteritis with operations on the stomach. *New England Journal of Medicine*, **255**, 555.

Walker Smith, J. A. (1972) Uniformity of dissecting microscope appearances in proximal small intestine. *Gut*, **13**, 17.

Whitelaw, A. G. L., Dillon, M. J. & Tripp, J. H. (1975) Hypertension oedema and suppressed renin aldosterone system due to unsupervised salt administration. *Archives of Disease in Childhood*, **50**, 400.

Widerlite, L., Trier, J. S., Blacklow, N. R. & Schreiber, D. S. (1975) Structure of the gastric mucosa in acute infectious nonbacterial gastroenteritis. *Gastroenterology*, **68**, 425.

Williams, R. E. O. & Drasar, B. S. (1972) Alterations in gut bacterial flora in disease. In *Recent Advances in Gastroenterology*, eds. Badenoch, J. & Brooke, B. N., p. 31. Edinburgh: Churchill Livingstone.

Zen-Yoji, H. (1968) Vibrio parahaemolyticus: a newly identified source of diarrhea. *Symposium on Vibrio parahaemolyticus*. U.S. Dept. Agriculture, Consumer & Marketing Service, Beltsville, Maryland.

11. Selective inborn errors of absorption

J. T. Harries

Proteins and amino acids
Carbohydrates
Fat
Vitamins
Electrolytes
Minerals

The selective inborn errors of absorption are not commonly encountered in clinical practice but nevertheless represent an important group of disorders. Early recognition and treatment of entities such as glucose-galactose malabsorption and chloridorrhea may be life-saving to the young infant, as well as allowing for informed genetic counselling of parents. Because of the selective nature of the absorptive defects many important contributions to our understanding of the physiology of absorption have come from studies of affected patients.

This group of disorders may be classified according to the microlocalisation of the defect, or according to the dietary constituent(s) affected. For example, malabsorption may result from (1) a specific enzyme defect with impaired luminal hydrolysis of dietary substrates (e.g. isolated lipase deficiency); (2) impaired entry of the end-products of luminal hydrolysis into the absorptive cell (e.g. glucose-galactose malabsorption); (3) defective intracellular transport of the absorbed substance (e.g. selective B_{12} malabsorption); or (4) impaired exit out of the cell into the portal or lymphatic vessels (e.g. abetalipoproteinaemia). For clinical purposes, however, a more useful classification is that based on the dietary constituent(s) which are affected, as shown in Table 11.1.

Before considering each condition in more detail a few general statements can be made. Except for familial hypophosphataemic rickets and the non-Caucasian type of lactase deficiency, the mode of inheritance is autosomal recessive with a one in four risk of children being affected; clinically insignificant abnormalities can sometimes be detected in heterozygotes. Mucosal architecture is entirely normal, and by definition the absorptive defects are secondary to selective abnormalities of function. Although the transport defects are permanent, gastrointestinal symptoms improve with age in some of the entities such as in congenital chloridorrhea.

Each condition will now be considered in turn as listed in Table 11.1.

Table 11.1 Classification of the selective inborn errors of absorption

Dietary constituents	Disease entity
Proteins and amino acids	
Proteins	Trypsinogen deficiency
	Enterokinase deficiency
Cystine, lysine, arginine	Cystinuria
Proline	Iminoglycinuria
Tryptophan, histidine phenylalanine	Hartnup disease
Tryptophan	Blue diaper syndrome
Methionine	Methionine malabsorption
Lysine, arginine	Lowe's syndrome
Carbohydrates	
Lactose	Lactase deficiency
Sucrose, isomaltose	Sucrase-isomaltase deficiency
Trehalose	Trehalase deficiency
Glucose, galactose	Glucose-galactose malabsorption
Fat	
	Abetalipoproteinaemia
	Congenital lipase deficiency
Vitamins	
B_{12}	Gastric intrinsic factor deficiency
	Biologically inert intrinsic factor
	Selective B_{12} malabsorption
	Transcobalamin I deficiency
	Transcobalamin II deficiency
Folate	Congenital folate malabsorption
Electrolytes	
Chloride	Congenital chloridorrhea
Minerals	
Magnesium	Familial hypomagnasaemia
Calcium	Familial hypophosphataemic rickets

PROTEINS AND AMINO ACIDS

Protein digestion is initiated in the stomach by the enzyme pepsin and continued in the small intestine by the pancreatic enzymes. The end-products of this process are amino acids, dipeptides and oligopeptides. Prior to entering the portal vein the peptides are converted to their constituent amino acids by peptidases located at the brush border or within the absorptive cells. Amino acids, dipeptides and possibly small oligopeptides enter the absorptive cells by active carrier-mediated transport processes. The pancreatic enzymes are stored in the gland as inactive proenzymes (zymogens) and only become activated on arrival at the duodenum. The key enzyme in this activation process is enterokinase which is released from the proximal small intestinal mucosa and meets the pancreatic zymogens as they enter the duodenum. A sequence of activating events is initiated by the conversion of trypsinogen to trypsin by enterokinase, as shown in Figure 11.1. Trypsin then activates the remaining zymogens, procarboxypeptidase B, proelastase, chymotrypsinogens and procarboxypeptidase A. Recent evidence suggests that trypsin probably does not activate its own zymogen (B. Hadorn, personal communication) as previously reported.

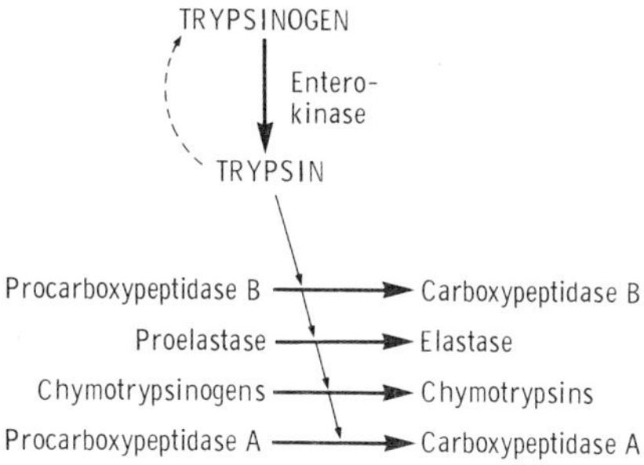

Fig. 11.1 Activation of pancreatic zymogens

Trypsinogen deficiency (Townes, Bryson and Miller, 1967)
The two patients described presented in early infancy with failure to thrive, oedema, hypoproteinaemia, anaemia and neutropenia. Feeding with a protein hydrolysate formulae resulted in rapid improvement. Addition of exogenous trypsin to the duodenal juice of the patients induced activation of all the proteolytic enzymes except trypsin.

Enterokinase deficiency (Tarlow, Hadorn, Arthurton and Lloyd, 1970)
The three reported infants presented in a very similar way to those with trypsinogen deficiency except for the presence of steatorrhoea; the mechanism of the steatorrhoea in enterokinase deficiency is not known. Treatment with pancreatic extract was highly effective. Addition of exogenous enterokinase to duodenal juice or incubation of juice with normal duodenal mucosa resulted in activation of all the proteolytic enzymes. Enterokinase was undetectable in both the mucosa and duodenal juice of the affected children.

Since exogenous trypsin may not activate trypsinogen, it is possible that the infants reported with trypsinogen deficiency were in fact lacking enterokinase and not the zymogen.

As can be seen from Table 11.1 six inborn errors of amino acid absorption have so far been described. The defective amino acid absorption in cystinuria (Morin, Thompson, Sanford and Sass-Kortsak, 1971), iminoglycinuria (Goodman, McIntyre and O'Brien, 1967), blue diaper syndrome (Drummond, Michael, Ulstrom and Good, 1964) and Lowe's syndrome (Bartsocas, Levy, Crawford and Thier, 1969) is of no clinical importance, and these conditions will therefore not be considered any further.

Hartnup disease (Navab and Asatoor, 1970)
Hartnup disease is characterised by a pellagrous rash, photosensitivity and neurological abnormalities such as cerebellar ataxia, fainting attacks and psychiatric disturbances. Stature is slightly reduced and the clinical manifestations tend to improve with age. There is a gross aminoaciduria and defective intestinal transport of tryptophan, histidine and phenylalanine. Tryptophan is an important precursor for the biosynthesis of nicotinamide, and the resultant nicotinamide deficiency accounts for all the clinical features; administration of

nicotinamide leads to a dramatic clinical improvement. Of great importance is the recent finding that absorption of these three amino acids from their dipeptides (e.g. carnosine—two constituent amino acids are L-histidine and β-alanine) is not impaired, and is probably the explanation why patients often remain asymptomatic on high protein diets.

Methionine malabsorption (Hooft *et al.*, 1965)
The reported patient presented at two years with generalised convulsions and intermittent diarrhoea. She was mentally retarded, had blue eyes and white hair and the urine had a sweetish smell. A primary defect of methionine absorption, with secondary malabsorption of branched-chain and certain other amino acids, was demonstrated. A low methionine diet resulted in colouring of the hair and an improvement in the diarrhoea and mental status; oral methionine loads precipitated diarrhoea. Bacterial degradation of the unabsorbed methionine in the colon resulted in the production of α-hydroxybutyric acid which was absorbed and excreted in the urine.

CARBOHYDRATES

A simplified representation of carbohydrate absorption is shown in Figure 11.2. The major dietary sources of carbohydrate are starch and the disaccharides sucrose and lactose. Starch is composed of two moieties, amylose and amylopectin; amylopectin constitutes 80 to 90 per cent of starch. The hydrolysis of starch is initiated by salivary α-amylase and continued by pancreatic α-amylase, the end-products being maltose, maltotriose and α-limit dextrins (5 to 6 glucose monomers linked to each other by α1-4 and α1-6 glycosidic linkages). Amylose is hydrolysed to maltose and maltotriose by the amylases, and the resultant di- and trisaccharides are hydrolysed to glucose by brush

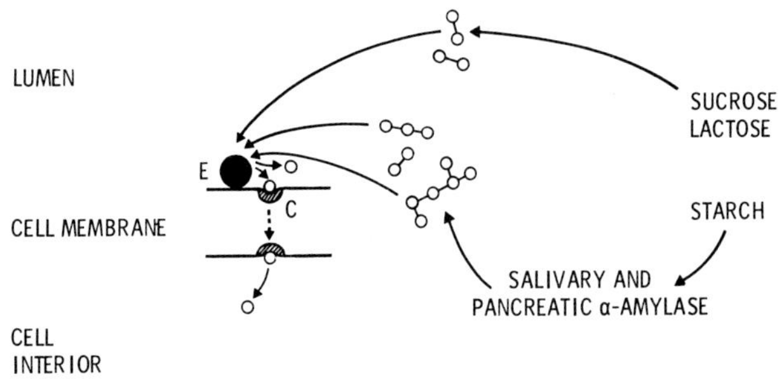

Fig. 11.2 Schematic representation of carbohydrate absorption
O = monosaccharides
O—O = disaccharides
O—O—O = maltotriose
O—O—O—O (with O branches) = α-limit dextrins

border maltases, of which there are at least four to five distinct types. Amylopectin is hydrolysed to maltose, maltotriose and α-limit dextrins by the amylases, and the α-limit dextrins are hydrolysed to glucose mainly by the brush border enzyme complex sucrase-isomaltase. The brush border enzyme lactase converts lactose to glucose and galactose, and sucrase converts sucrose to glucose and fructose. The monosaccharides glucose, galactose and fructose are then absorbed across the brush border into the absorptive cells of the small intestine. Glucose and galactose share the same active carrier-mediated transport process, which enables them to be absorbed across the brush border and against concentration gradients. Exit of monosaccharides from the cells into the portal vein is followed by hepatic uptake. The genetically determined errors of carbohydrate absorption are due either to impaired hydrolysis of disaccharides at the brush border (i.e. lactase, trehalase, and sucrase-isomaltase deficiency), or to defective uptake of monosaccharides into the cell (i.e. glucose-galactose malabsorption).

The clinical manifestations of carbohydrate malabsorption include vomiting, colicky abdominal pain and distention, and fluid stools of low pH containing excessive amounts of sugars.

Lactase deficiency

The age of presentation and the clinical manifestations of lactase deficiency differ in Caucasian compared with non-Caucasian races.

Caucasian type (Levin, Abraham, Burgess and Wallis, 1970)

Explosive watery diarrhoea follows the initiation of milk feeding at birth. Mucosal lactase activity is undetectable or grossly reduced whilst other disaccharidases are unaffected. Since monosaccharide absorption is unaffected, treatment with lactose-free formulae containing monosaccharides is highly effective. This rare condition must be distinguished from the temporary lactase deficiency which not uncommonly complicates enteric infections (see Ch. 10), and that found in various enteropathies (see Ch. 9).

Non-Caucasian type (Kretchmer, 1971)

This type is extremely common and occurs in a variety of ethnic groups throughout the world. Symptoms are relatively mild and do not occur until the age of 2 to 3 years, and lactase activity is not severely reduced; inheritance is autosomal dominant (Ransome-Kuti *et al.*, 1975).

Sucrase-isomaltase deficiency (Ament, Perera and Esther, 1973)

Since only a small proportion of the starch molecule is composed of isomaltose (i.e. α-limit dextrins), sucrase is the more important of the two disaccharides in precipitating symptoms. There is a wide spectrum in the severity of symptoms ranging from severe diarrhoea in infancy to intermittent, bothersome symptoms in the older child. A correct diagnosis may be delayed for several years, symptoms having been attributed to conditions such as 'irritable colon' or 'maternal anxiety'. Elimination of sucrose from the diet results in prompt improvement.

Table 11.2 Diagnostic features of abetalipoproteinaemia

Fat malabsorption
Neuropathy
Retinopathy
Acanthocytosis of red blood cells
Absence of β-lipoprotein in serum

Trehalase deficiency (Madzarovova-Nohejlova, 1973)
The only dietary source for trehalose in man is the young mushroom. Severe gastrointestinal symptoms were recently reported in a family following the ingestion of young mushrooms; trehalase activity was undetectable.

Glucose-galactose malabsorption (Wimberley, Harries and Burgess, 1974)
This condition is the only primary disorder of monosaccharide absorption so far reported. As with Caucasian lactase deficiency explosive watery diarrhoea secondary to osmotic shifts of fluid follows the institution of milk feeding. Glucose and galactose normally provide an important physiological drive for fluid absorption in the small intestine, and its absence in patients with this condition may be another factor contributing to the diarrhoea. Treatment consists of a diet containing fructose as the only source of carbohydrate and is highly effective. Differential diagnosis includes temporary monosaccharide malabsorption secondary to infection and/or mucosal damage. Tolerance to ingested glucose and galactose improves with age and some dietary relaxation is usually possible in the older child.

FAT

Abetalipoproteinaemia (Kayden, 1972)
Table 11.2 lists the diagnostic features of this rare condition. The patients present during early infancy with steatorrhoea and failure to thrive, and the ataxic neuropathy and pigmentary retinopathy do not develop until the end of the first decade. The diagnosis is confirmed by the demonstration of acanthocytes in a fresh wet blood film, complete absence of β-lipoprotein in serum and very low (20 to 40 mg/100 ml) concentrations of serum cholesterol. The fat malabsorption results from defective exit of fat from the mucosal cell into the lymphatics secondary to an inability of the cells to synthesise chylomicra; this is reflected by dense accumulation of intracellular lipid within the surface epithelial cells of the small intestine. The absorptive defect is not complete since some lipid can be absorbed via the portal vein. Hepatic abnormalities such as micronodular cirrhosis may occur (Partin *et al.*, 1974). Vitamin E is undetectable in the serum, and correction of the severe vitamin E deficiency with high oral doses (100 mg per kg body weight per day) of vitamin E may prevent the development of neurological and retinal lesions, or arrest their progression (Lloyd and Muller, 1972). Affected children thrive on a low fat diet which can be supplemented with medium-chain triglycerides; in addition to vitamin E, other fat soluble vitamin supplements are also necessary.

Table 11.3 Inherited defects of vitamin B_{12} absorption

Site of defect	Disease entity
Binding to gastric intrinsic factor	Congenital intrinsic factor deficiency Biologically inert intrinsic factor
Somewhere between uptake of B_{12} into ileal cells and exit into portal circulation	Selective B_{12} malabsorption
Exit from absorptive cell	Transcobalamin II deficiency Transcobalamin I deficiency

Congenital lipase deficiency (Sheldon, 1964; Figarella, Negri and Sarles, 1972)
Pale, bulky stools are present from birth, and a particularly characteristic feature is the leaking of free oil from the anus. Despite the complete absence of pancreatic lipase as much as 70 per cent of dietary fat may be absorbed. Studies in our patient suggest that gastric lipase compensates for the absence of pancreatic lipase and allows for the continued absorption of an appreciable percentage of dietary fat (Muller *et al.*, 1975). Physical development is normal and the prognosis is good with pancreatic extract therapy. Differential diagnosis lies between cystic fibrosis and Shwachman's syndrome (see Ch. 20).

VITAMINS

The nomenclature which describes vitamin B_{12} malabsorption states in childhood is somewhat confusing. For example, both autoimmune and non-autoimmune abnormalities of gastric intrinsic factor are often included under the term *juvenile pernicious anaemia*. For this reason the inherited abnormalities of B_{12} absorption have been classified according to the site of the defect, as shown in Table 11.3. Classical autoimmune pernicious anaemia must be excluded in any child with B_{12} deficiency and anaemia.

Gastric intrinsic factor deficiency (Arthur, 1972)
Intrinsic factor is secreted by the parietal cells of the gastric mucosa and binds to B_{12} in the stomach. The B_{12}-intrinsic factor complex passes down to the distal ileum where B_{12} is actively absorbed into the ileal cells. Intrinsic factor is necessary for the uptake of B_{12} into the ileum, and abnormalities of intrinsic factor result in B_{12} malabsorption and megaloblastic anaemia. Infants with intrinsic factor deficiency are normal at birth but develop megaloblastic anaemia in early childhood when maternally derived B_{12} stores become depleted. The diagnosis is made by demonstrating normal gastric acidity, reduced concentrations of intrinsic factor, histologically normal gastric mucosa, absence of intrinsic factor and parietal cell antibodies in the serum and malabsorption of B_{12} corrected by exogenous intrinsic factor.

Biologically inert intrinsic factor (Katz, Lee and Cooper, 1972)
To date there is one reported patient with this condition; a boy, whose parents were first cousins, presented at the age of 13 years with megaloblastic anaemia due to B_{12} deficiency. As judged by immunological techniques intrinsic factor was present in normal amounts but was shown to be biologically inactive.

Selective B_{12} malabsorption (Visakorpi and Furuhjelm, 1968; Bell *et al.*, 1973)
The precise site of the transport defect has not been defined but it lies somewhere between uptake of B_{12} into the ileal cells and exit into the portal circulation. Like patients with intrinsic factor deficiency the majority present in early childhood with megaloblastic anaemia; impaired physical development and gastrointestinal symptoms such as vomiting, anorexia and diarrhoea are common. As with all B_{12} deficiency states neurological manifestations may develop. An integral part of the syndrome is proteinuria, and this may be associated with renal tract abnormalities. In contrast to the two previously described abnormalities of B_{12} absorption, malabsorption of B_{12} cannot be corrected by exogenous intrinsic factor.

Several body fluids contain a group of glycoproteins which bind B_{12} and have been designated 'R' binders; transcobalamin I and II carry three-quarters and one-quarter, respectively, of circulating B_{12} in human serum.

Transcobalamin I deficiency (Hall, 1973)
Although serum B_{12} levels are reduced, tissue levels are normal and there are no haematological or clinical manifestations.

Transcobalamin II deficiency (Hall, 1973)
Transcobalamin II plays a critical physiological role in the transport of B_{12} from the absorptive cell to tissues of storage and from tissues of storage to tissues where it is utilised, such as the bone marrow. In contrast to other congenital defects in B_{12} absorption severe megaloblastic anaemia and gastrointestinal symptoms develop within a few weeks of birth and, since transcobalamin I is not affected, serum B_{12} levels may be normal. These patients probably survive intrauterine life and do not present until a few weeks after birth because of maternally derived transcobalamin II. The anaemia can be corrected by very large doses of parenteral B_{12}. The diagnosis is confirmed by the demonstration of deficient or absent transcobalamin II using electrophoretic techniques.

Congenital folate malabsorption (Lanzkowsky, 1970)
The three reported patients developed megaloblastic anaemia at about 3 months of age, were retarded and ataxic, and had convulsions and punctuate intracranial calcification.

ELECTROLYTES (Launiala, Perheentupa, Pasternack and Hallman, 1968; Bieberdorf, Gorden and Fordtran, 1972)

The only reported primary defect in electrolyte absorption is congenital chloridorrhea, and the typical clinical and biochemical features are listed in

Table 11.4 Diagnostic features of congenital chloridorrhea

Pregnancy complicated by hydramnios
Premature birth
Excessive weight loss in neonatal period
Hyperbilirubinaemia
Watery stools
Failure to thrive
Hypokalaemia, hyponatraemia, hypochloraemia
Metabolic alkalosis
Stool chloride concentration exceeds sum concentration of sodium and potassium

Table 11.4. Pregnancy is usually complicated by hydramnios and premature birth. Explosive watery stools are usually present from birth but may be delayed for several weeks. The absence of meconium and the extremely watery stools may suggest alternative diagnoses such as lower bowel obstruction and/or fistulae between the bowel and urinary tract. Similarly, abdominal distention secondary to ileus may be so pronounced (see Fig. 11.3) as to lead to an explorative laparotomy for suspected intestinal obstruction. In contrast to most other diarrhoeal states in infancy there is a metabolic alkalosis, which is associated with hyponatraemia, hypokalaemia and hypochloraemia; in the neonatal period, however, alkalosis is not a constant feature. Once the condition is suspected, diagnosis is simple, the pathognomonic finding being a stool chloride concentration which exceeds the sum concentrations of sodium and potassium. Treatment consists of oral supplements of potassium chloride and intravenous fluids when necessary; a low salt diet may dramatically reduce stool frequency and consistency (unpublished observations). Providing the patients survive the first few months of life, the long-term prognosis is good.

The absorptive error is confined to the ileum and colon, transport of fluid and electrolytes being entirely normal in the jejunum. Normally there is an active carrier mediated anion exchange system in ileum and colon, chloride being absorbed and bicarbonate secreted, and in the ileum this is linked to a cationic exchange system between sodium and hydrogen ions (Fig. 11.4). The primary abnormality in congenital chloridorrhea is a defect in anion exchange in the ileum and colon with secondary disturbances of cation exchange in ileum. This

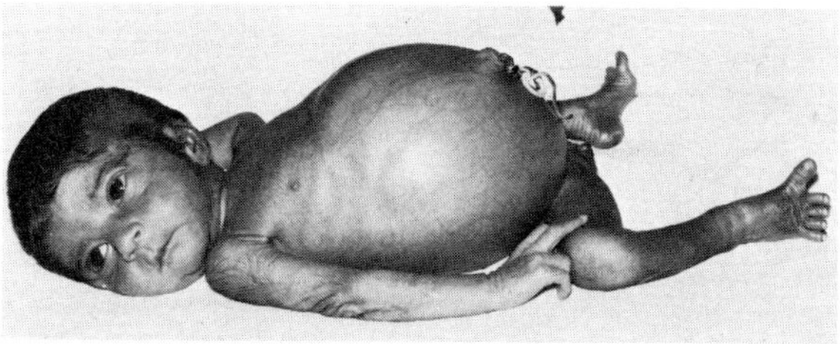

Fig. 11.3 Abdominal distention mimicking intestinal obstruction in congenital chloridorrhea

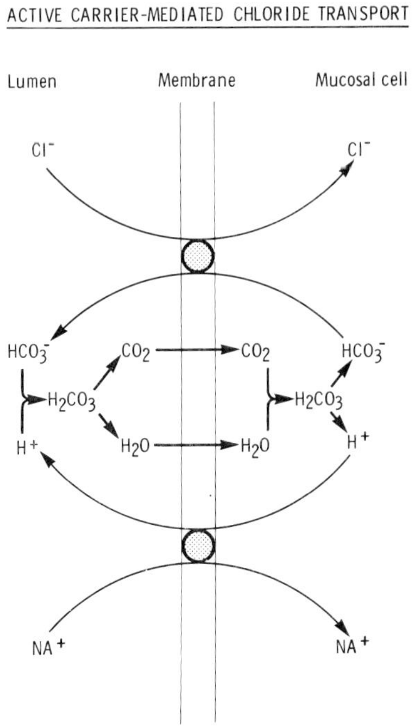

Fig. 11.4 Anionic and cationic exchange transport systems for electrolytes in ileum and colon

results in malabsorption and intraluminal accumulation of chloride and an osmotic diarrhoea. The alkalosis is due to retention of bicarbonate and hypokalaemia; the mechanism of the other electrolyte disturbances is controversial.

MINERALS

Familial hypomagnasaemia (Stromme *et al.*, 1969)
This condition presents within the first few weeks of life with tetanic convulsions resistant to calcium therapy; severe hypomagnasaemia is associated with hypocalcaemia and hyperphosphataemia. Initially the convulsions are treated with intravenous magnesium, and long-term control can be achieved with oral magnesium supplements. The precise site of the transport defect has not been defined.

Familial hypophosphataemic rickets (Hall, MacMillan and Bronner, 1969)
In contrast to the other inborn errors of absorption which have been discussed, this condition is inherited by a sex-linked dominant process. The patients present between the age of 1 and 2 years with vitamin D resistant rickets or osteomalacia; hypophosphataemia is due to impaired renal tubular reabsorption of phosphate. The skeletal abnormalities respond to large oral doses of vitamin D. The precise site of the defect in calcium absorption has not been defined.

References

Ament, M. E., Perera, D. R. & Esther, L. J. (1973) Sucrase-isomaltase deficiency—a frequently misdiagnosed disease. *Journal of Pediatrics,* **83,** 721–727.

Arthur, L. J. H. (1972) Juvenile pernicious anaemia. *Proceedings of the Royal Society of Medicine,* **65,** 728–729.

Bartsocas, C. S., Levy, H. L., Crawford, J. D. & Thier, S. O. (1969) A defect in intestinal amino acid transport in Lowe's syndrome. *American Journal of Diseases in Child Health,* **117,** 93–95.

Bell, M., Harries, J. T., Wolff, O. H., Dawson, A. M. & Waters, A. H. (1973) Familial selective malabsorption of vitamin B_{12}. *Archives of Disease in Childhood,* **48,** 896–900.

Bieberdorf, F. A., Gorden, P. & Fordtran, J. S. (1972) Pathogenesis of congenital alkalosis with diarrhea. *Journal of Clinical Investigation,* **51,** 1958–1968.

Drummond, K. N., Michael, A. F., Ulstrom, R. A. & Good, R. A. (1964) The blue diaper syndrome: familial hypercalcaemia with nephrocalcinosis and indicanuria. *American Journal of Medicine,* **37,** 928–948.

Figarella, C., Negri, G. A., and Sarles, H. (1972) Presence of colipase in a congenital pancreatic lipase deficiency. *Biochimica et Biophysica Acta,* **280,** 205.

Goodman, S. I., McIntyre, C. A. & O'Brien, D. (1967) Impaired intestinal transport of proline in a patient with familial iminoaciduria. *Journal of Pediatrics,* **71,** 246–248.

Hall, C. A. (1973) Congenital disorders of vitamin B_{12} transport and their contribution to concepts. *Gastroenterology,* **65,** 684–686.

Hall, B. D., MacMillan, D. R. & Bronner, F. (1969) Vitamin D resistant rickets and high fecal endogenous calcium output. *American Journal of Clinical Nutrition,* **22,** 448–457.

Hooft, C., Timmermans, J., Snoeck, J., Antener, I., Ayaert, W. & van den Hende, C. (1965) Methionine malabsorption syndrome. *Annales Paediatrici,* **205,** 73–104.

Katz, M., Lee, S. K. & Cooper, B. A. (1972) Vitamin B_{12} malabsorption due to a biologically inert intrinsic factor. *New England Journal of Medicine,* **287,** 425–429.

Kayden, H. J. (1972) Abetalipoproteinaemia. *Annual Review of Medicine,* **23,** 285–296.

Kretchmer, N. (1971) Memorial lecture: lactose and lactase—a historical perspective. *Gastroenterology,* **61,** 805–813.

Lanzkowsky, P. (1970) Congenital malabsorption of folate. *American Journal of Medicine,* **48,** 580–583.

Launiala, K., Perheentupa, J., Pasternack, A. & Hallman, N. (1968) Familial chloride diarrhea-chloride malabsorption. *Modern Problems in Pediatrics,* **11,** 137–149.

Levin, B., Abraham, J. M., Burgess, E. A. & Wallis, P. G. (1970) Congenital lactose malabsorption. *Archives of Disease in Childhood,* **45,** 173–177.

Lloyd, J. K. & Muller, D. P. R. (1972) Management of abetalipoproteinaemia in childhood. In *Protides of the Biological Fluids,* p. 331, ed. Peeters, H. Oxford: Pergamon.

Madzarovova-Nohejlova, J. (1973) Trehalase deficiency in a family. *Gastroenterology,* **65,** 130–133.

Morin, C. L., Thompson, M. W., Sanford, J. H. & Sass-Kortsak, A. (1971) Biochemical and genetic studies in cystinuria: observations on double heterozygotes of genotype I/II. *Journal of Clinical Investigation,* **50,** 1961–1966

Muller, D. P. R., McCollum, J. P. K., Trompeter, R. S. & Harries, J. T. (1975) Studies on the mechanism of fat absorption in congenital isolated lipase deficiency. *Gut,* **16,** 838.

Navab, F. & Asatoor, A. M. (1970) Studies on intestinal absorption of amino acids and a dipeptide in a case of Hartnup disease. *Gut,* **11,** 373–379.

Partin, J. S., Partin, J. C., Schubert, W. K. & McAdams, A. J. (1974) Liver ultrastructure in abetalipoproteinemia: Evolution of micronodular cirrhosis. *Gastroenterology,* **67,** 107–118.

Ransome-Kuti, O., Kretchmer, N., Johnson, J. D. & Gribble, J. T. (1975) A genetic study of lactose digestion in Nigerian families. *Gastroenterology,* **68,** 431.

Sheldon, W. (1964) Congenital pancreatic lipase deficiency. *Archives of Disease in Childhood,* **39,** 268.

Stromme, J. H., Nesbakken, R., Normann, T., Skjorten, F., Skyberg, D. & Johannessen, B. (1969) Familial hypomagnesemia. *Acta Paediatrica Scandinavica,* **58,** 433.

Tarlow, M. J., Hadorn, B., Arthurton, M. W. & Lloyd, J. K. (1970) Intestinal enterokinase deficiency. *Archives of Disease in Childhood,* **45,** 651.

Townes, P. L., Bryson, M. F. & Miller, G. (1967) Further observations on trypsinogen deficiency disease: report of a second case. *Journal of Pediatrics,* **71,** 220.

Visakorpi, J. K. & Furuhjelm, V. (1968) Selective malabsorption of vitamin B_{12}. *Modern Problems in Pediatrics,* **11,** 150.

Wimberley, P. D., Harries, J. T. & Burgess, E. A. (1974) Congenital glucose-galactose malabsorption. *Proceedings of the Royal Society of Medicine,* **67,** 755.

Acknowledgements. I am grateful to Professor J. K. Lloyd and Dr A. W. Ferguson for permission to include Figure 11.3.

12. Parasitic infections

G. J. Ebrahim

Roundworms
Tapeworms
Protozoa
Flukes

Many of the parasites affecting man have complex life cycles dependent upon the close proximity of one or more intermediate hosts. Hence geographic and ecologic conditions are important in the prevalence of the parasitic infestations. Activities which may affect the ecologic balance may produce an effect on the prevalence of parasites. Thus the construction of dams and irrigation canals in many parts of Africa has led to the spread of schistosomiasis. Dietary and personal habits as well as customs may also contribute to the spread of parasitic disease. For example, the eating of undercooked meat, common in many countries of the Middle East and in the Mediterranean regions, is responsible for taeniasis; on the other hand strong attachment to household pets like cats and dogs is held responsible for toxocara infestation.

Many of the common parasites of man inhabit the gastrointestinal tract, where pathological changes may occur in any of the following ways:

1. Loss of body constituents, e.g. blood loss in ankylostomiasis.
2. Interference with the absorption of nutrients, e.g. in taeniasis and giardiasis.
3. Tissue injury because of the invasive nature of the parasite, e.g. amoebiasis and fascioliasis.
4. Mechanical block, e.g. intestinal obstruction due to heavy infestation with ascaris.

In many of the affluent societies of Western Europe, socioeconomic improvement has resulted in a reduced prevalence of parasitic illnesses. In recent years, however, with increased travel and the arrival of immigrants from tropical and subtropical countries, the risk of reintroduction of parasitic illness has been considerably increased. In a survey of 4000 immigrant school children in Britain (Thompson, Hutchison and Johnston, 1972), 37 per cent had worms. Carriage rates were highest in children from the West Indies (51 per cent); those for children from India and Pakistan were in the range of 30 to 40 per cent and those for children from Kenya were lowest at 16 per cent. The commonest parasites were trichuris and ascaris. This chapter deals, in the main, with the gastrointestinal manifestations of parasitic infestation. The effects of parasites on liver function and structure are dealt with in more detail elsewhere (see Ch.

17). For further reading, the following excellent reviews on intestinal parasites are recommended: Knight *et al.,* 1973; Marsden and Hoskins, 1966; Marsden and Schultz, 1969.

ROUNDWORMS

Ascariasis

Ascaris lumbricoides

Infestation with *Ascaris lumbricoides* is widespread. In the United States it is more prevalent in southern than in northern states and is commoner in rural than in urban areas. In Europe the incidence in large cities varies from 1 to 5 per cent and is greater in rural areas, and in Kenya 58 per cent of children in rural families are infected (World Health Statistics Report, 1969). The soil is an important determinant of the rates of prevalence and transmission. For example, eggs placed in soil become infective when soil temperature reaches 20°C in summer months, and when placed 1 cm deep in the soil they are killed when soil humidity falls below 4 per cent (WHO Technical Report Series No. 379).

Life cycle. The life span of the adult worm is six months to one year and the fertile female deposits an average of 200 000 eggs daily. For optimal development the eggs need moist, shady soil with an environmental temperature of between 23°C and 33°C. Following ingestion the outer coats of the eggs dissolve in the stomach and hatched larvae pass into the small intestine where they penetrate the mucosa and enter portal venules along which they travel to the liver. The larvae travel to the right side of the heart and through the pulmonary circulation to the lungs where they penetrate capillary walls to enter the respiratory spaces. In experimental animals larvae can be seen in the lungs within 24 hours, although the majority arrive five to six days after ingestion of eggs. Growth of larvae in the lungs is accompanied by an inflammatory reaction in the alveoli and bronchial walls. The larvae travel up the bronchial tree to reach the hypopharynx where they are swallowed. In the small intestine they continue to grow, and about two to three months after ingestion of the ova the parasite attains sexual maturity.

Clinical features. In some cases, pulmonary symptoms such as cough, dyspnoea and asthmatic attacks occur about one week after ingestion of eggs. Rhonchi and rales may be present or rarely signs of consolidation occur; radiological findings include increased bronchial markings, diffuse mottling or areas of consolidation, depending upon the degree of parenchymal involvement. Spontaneous improvement occurs in about a week's time.

Abdominal symptoms depend on the parasitic load and vary from vague abdominal pains to serious complications. The latter are due to large numbers of parasites in the intestinal lumen and to their tendency to wrap themselves round one another into tight bundles; this may result in intestinal obstruction. In Capetown, South Africa, 12·8 per cent of all acute abdominal emergencies in children are caused by ascaris (Louw, 1966). Migration of adult worms from the intestinal lumen can result in bile duct obstruction, liver abscess and haemorrhagic pancreatitis. Appendicitis is a recognised complication and intestinal perforation with peritonitis has also been reported. Following abdominal surgery any existing ascaris infection is a potential hazard since the worms may penetrate suture lines and cause peritonitis.

Heavy infection may precipitate deficiency disorders particularly if the host's nutritional status is already impaired. In children infected with 13 to 40 worms (average 26) approximately 4 g of protein per day can be lost out of a daily intake of 35 to 50 g (Venkatachalam and Patwardhan, 1953).

Treatment. The presently available chemotherapeutic agents act only on adult worms in the intestinal lumen, and no drug is known to be effective against the larval stages in the body. Piperazine is the drug of choice. It acts by causing a neuromuscular block in the ascaris so that the worm loses its ability to maintain its position against peristalsis. A single dose of 3 to 4 g gives an 85 to 90 per cent cure rate and a considerable reduction of the worm load in the remainder.

Capillaria philippinensis

A newly discovered species of roundworm, *Capillaria philippinensis*, was the causal agent in an epidemic of severe and often fatal diarrhoea in the Philippines (Whalen *et al.*, 1969). In the epidemic 1000 cases were reported with more than a 10 per cent confirmed mortality. A survey in one village with a population of 700 showed that 32 per cent were clinically affected and that all those passing eggs in their stools subsequently became symptomatic. In untreated cases mortality rates varied from 19 to 35 per cent. The main clinical features were abdominal pain, diarrhoea, muscle wasting and oedema, leading to death in two to four months without treatment. Treatment with thiabendazole resulted in dramatic improvement.

Although the life cycle of *C. philippinensis* has not been fully elucidated, it is thought that it has a direct cycle with no intermediate hosts but may utilise certain fish and crustaceans as transport hosts. Most of the cases in the literature have been described from the northern Philippines where several outbreaks have been associated with a high mortality.

Strongyloides

The prevalence of strongyloides varies according to geography and climate. In warm semiarid areas the prevalence is seldom above 3 per cent, in the tropics rates vary from 35 to 40 per cent, and in the subtropics, with well-distributed yearly rainfall, prevalence rates can be as high as 85 per cent.

The adult female inhabits the crypts of the duodenum and first part of the jejunum, where eggs are deposited in the mucosa. The larvae hatch in the mucosa and gain access to the intestinal lumen, but occasionally they burrow in the opposite direction into the peritoneal cavity. In favourable conditions the larvae grow rapidly in the soil to become adult worms; copulation takes place and rhabditiform larvae emerge from the eggs which metamorphose into infective larvae. Under unfavourable conditions the larvae may metamorphose into infective larvae within the intestinal lumen and reinfect the host by penetrating the colonic mucosa. Infective larvae gain entry into the body of the host by

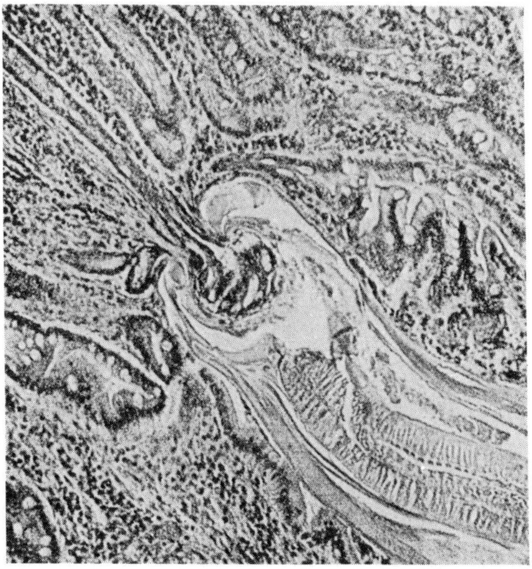

Fig. 12.1 Adult hookworm firmly attached to small intestinal mucosa

penetrating the skin and then travel to the lungs where they remain for several days growing into adults; the adult worms travel up the respiratory passages to the hypopharynx where they are swallowed.

Heavy infection gives rise to a duodenitis and jejunitis with malabsorption and steatorrhoea. The mucosa is damaged by the gravid female making burrows to lay eggs and by the larvae penetrating the epithelium to reach the lumen. Lesions vary from a mild enteritis to a severe ulcerative enteritis; healing of large ulcers may result in strictures and obstruction. The commonest presenting symptoms are anorexia, abdominal pain, nausea and vomiting, and loose stools which may contain blood. Pulmonary symptoms with pneumonitis and bronchopneumonia may dominate the clinical pictures, and in areas where strongyloides infection is prevalent it should be considered in the differential diagnosis of any patient presenting with gastrointestinal symptoms, particularly when accompanied by cough, dyspnoea and haemoptysis.

Treatment

Thiabendazole, a broad-spectrum anthelmintic, is the drug of choice (25 mg/kg twice daily for two days), and a mean cure rate of 96 per cent has been reported. Dizziness, nausea, vomiting and abdominal pain occur occasionally. Mebendazole (methyl-5-benzoyl-benzimidazole-2-carbamate), another broad-spectrum anthelmintic, is also effective and has virtually no side-effects.

Ankylostomiasis (hookworm)

Ankylostomiasis is a disease of hot humid regions; in temperate climates the prevalence of the disease depends upon the degree of atmospheric humidity and the temperature. In tropical countries, where the rainy season is clear cut, the most favourable transmission periods for the parasite are at the beginning and end of the rains. In areas with extensive irrigation systems or in the delta regions, the ground may be moist even in the absence of rain and hookworm transmission can occur all the year round. Agricultural practices such as the use of night soil as the main source of fertilisers help to facilitate transmission.

There are two distinct human hookworms, *Ankylostoma duodenale* and *Necator americanus*. Both are widespread throughout the tropics and subtropics and rigid demarcations are no longer possible.

The adult worm lives in the upper small intestine, firmly attached to the mucosa (Fig. 12.1) where it sucks the host's blood to obtain oxygen and nutrients. The amount of blood lost per day is approximately 0·03 ml per worm for *Necator americanus* and 0·015 to 0·02 ml per worm for *Ankylostoma duodenale* (Tasker, 1961). Eggs passed in the faeces hatch within a day under optimal conditions at 23°C to 30°C. In sandy soil and soil rich in organic matter the larvae can remain alive for up to six weeks. Man is infected by penetration of the exposed skin by the larvae, following which they enter the lymphatics and migrate to the lungs. The larvae then travel up the bronchial passages to the hypopharynx and are swallowed.

Heavy infections are accompanied by considerable blood loss, and hookworm infection is the commonest cause of iron deficiency anaemia in many tropical countries (Roche and Layrisse, 1966). Besides iron, albumin is also lost into the intestine in quantities proportional to the blood loss and may lead to hypoproteinaemia and oedema. Villous atrophy of the small intestinal mucosa may be accompanied by malabsorption in heavy infections (Tandon, Saraya and Deo, 1966).

Treatment

Tetrachlorethylene in a single dose of 0·12 ml per kg (maximum of 5·0 ml) is widely used in many countries because of its low cost. Treatment in the above dose can cure 80 per cent of *Necator americanus* and 25 per cent of *Ankylostoma duodenale* infections. A low fat diet is necessary to minimise drug absorption. Bephenium hydroxynaphthoate (Alcopar) is highly effective against both varieties of hookworm. A single dose of 2·5 g has been reported to cure 70 to 95 per cent of *Ankylostoma* infections and a daily dose of 5·0 g for three days has been reported to cure 55 per cent of *Necator* infections, with 80 to 90 per cent decrease in worm burden in the remainder. Fasting, dietary restrictions and other preparations of patients are unnecessary. Phenylene-di-isothiocyanate 1,4 (Jonit) is effective against both varieties of hookworm, though more effective against *Necator americanus*. Tetramisole, a broad-spectrum anthelmintic, gives cure rates of 90 per cent with ascaris and 80 per cent with hookworm. The availability of highly effective and non-toxic preparations with a broad spectrum of action has increased the possibility of regular mass treatments of defined rural communities in order to reduce the reservoir of the parasite in the community and thereby reduce transmission.

Trichuriasis

In a study of 9256 Puerto Rican children prevalence rates of 87 per cent were reported as compared to 40 per cent for ascariasis and 26 per cent for hookworm

(World Health Statistics Report, 1969), and similar high rates have been reported in Yugoslavia, Albania, rural France and Italy.

The adult worms are flesh-coloured, thin and hair-like at the anterior three-fifths, and thicker and fleshy in the posterior two-fifths. The usual habitat is the caecum but they may also be found in the appendix, any portion of the colon and in some cases even the ileum. The anterior hair-like part of the body of the worm is deeply attached to the mucosa. Freshly passed eggs must gain access to warm, moist and shaded soil where they become infective after about three weeks, and man is infected by ingestion of embryonated eggs. The larvae are set free in the small intestine, and later the mature larvae move to the large bowel where they develop further into adult worms. Mucosal lesions vary depending on the severity of the infection; in massive infections the mucosa shows degenerative changes with necrosis, inflammation and small subepithelial haemorrhages, and there may be lymphocytic or eosinophilic infiltration in the area adjacent to the worm.

Vague abdominal discomfort may be the only symptom in mild infection, whereas in massive infections there is diarrhoea with mucus and blood, tenesmus, loss of weight and, occasionally, rectal prolapse. The adult worm consumes about 0·005 ml of blood from the host each day (Layrisse *et al.*, 1967) and may precipitate an iron deficiency anaemia in children already undernourished.

Treatment

No fully satisfactory treatment is available. Stilbazium iodide in a dose of 20 mg/kg twice daily for three days results in cure rates of 80 per cent, but nausea, vomiting and abdominal cramps are common. A single oral dose of dichlorvos (6 to 12 mg/kg) produces cure rates of 85 to 90 per cent with only mild side-effects. Mebendazole (methyl-5-benzoylbenzimidazole-2-carbamate), a new broad-spectrum anthelmintic, has given encouraging results in preliminary trials; a single dose of 100 mg is effective with very few side-effects, and higher doses are also well tolerated.

Enterobiasis

Man is the only known host for the thread worm. There is no period of development outside the human body and no intermediate host, and transmission occurs from man to man. The normal habitat of the worm is the caecum and the appendix, but the ileum may also be affected in heavy infections. The male worm dies soon after copulation and is unimportant in pathogenesis. The gravid females descend to the rectum, pass through the anal sphincter at night and lay eggs in the perianal and the perineal region; they usually die after oviposition. The eggs are resistant to adverse environmental conditions and occur in dust, especially after bed-making when they may be found in bedclothes, pyjamas, on toys and furniture. The life cycle of the worm is completed by ingestion of its eggs. On reaching the duodenum, rhabditiform larvae are hatched which undergo several moults before becoming adult worms.

Lesions are commonly seen in the caecum, appendix and lower ileum and vary from mild inflammation to areas of mucosal erosions and, in some cases, large ulcers. In a histological study of 691 appendices removed from children, thread worms were found in 52 (Duran Jorda, 1957). Of these, eight showed abscess formation, 14 had early evidence of appendicitis and 30 had acute appendicitis. The most common presenting symptom is pruritis which can be intense and lead to skin changes. Mild gastrointestinal symptoms such as anorexia and abdominal discomfort are less common. Examination of stools does not show the presence of eggs and the diagnosis is made by swabbing the perineal region with sticky cellophane (Sellotape) followed by microscopic examination.

Treatment

Viprynium in a single dose of 5 mg/kg repeated in two weeks is the drug of choice. It is a cyanine dye and not always well tolerated, causing redness of the stools, diarrhoea, vomiting or abdominal discomfort; a smaller dose of 1·0 mg to 2·0 mg per kg may be satisfactory. Alternatively, piperazine 2·0 g daily for seven days may be used. Ideally the whole family should receive treatment.

Toxocariasis (viscera larva migrans)

Toxocara canis and *catis,* the common roundworm of dogs and cats, can occasionally give rise to serious illness in man (Woodruff, 1970; Lancet, 1972). Typically, symptoms occur in children 1 to 4 years old with a history of pica or close association with domestic animals. The characteristic features are persistent eosinophilia, hepatomegaly, fever, attacks of wheezing, hyperglobulinaemia, anaemia and leukocytosis. The disease is usually benign and improvement usually occurs spontaneously over a period of months, though fatalities have also been described. The occurrence of symptoms is related to the number of eggs ingested, and unless larvae invade vital organs like the brain or the eye, ingestion of a small number of eggs may go unnoticed. Toxocaral invasion of the eye occurs as an isolated lesion usually in older children who may show no other signs of visceral toxocariasis. It is nearly always unilateral. Pathologically, the lesion is a chronic endophthalmitis with or without retinal detachment. The presenting complaint is strabismus or contraction of the visual field. The natural history of ocular toxocariasis is one of resolution of the inflammatory mass leaving a residual scar and a degree of blindness which depends on the size of the scar and its proximity to the macula. Encephalopathy is another manifestation of toxocaral infection, and a wide spectrum of neurologic signs including convulsions may result.

The natural habitat of toxocara is the small intestine of cats and dogs. The eggs are passed in the faeces and are swallowed by mice, rats and a wide variety of animals in which they develop into larvae. If dogs or cats eat infected rats and mice these larvae develop into adults, in cats more readily than do those of *T. cani* in dogs. The most usual method of infection in dogs is during intrauterine life. When the dog swallows *T. cani* eggs the resulting larvae migrate into tissues and persist for long periods. From these tissues, particularly the retroperitoneal tissue in the pregnant bitch, they enter the fetus by a route the details of which are unknown.

When infective *T. canis* or *T. catis* eggs are swallowed by man, larvae emerge from the eggs in the human intestine, penetrate the bowel wall and travel in portal blood to the liver and thence to the lungs and beyond to other tissues of the body. The size and shape of the larvae determine the extent to which they can travel in the blood vessel, because they appear to leave the vessel at a point at which its diameter approaches that of the blood vessel. This fact may explain why ascaris larvae are filtered out of the circulation in man in the liver and lungs and do not pass beyond these organs to other tissues, since they are about twice the size of the *Toxocara* larvae.

Infection in man is widespread. In the United Kingdom *T. canis* infection in dogs may be as high as 21 per cent (Woodruff and Thacker, 1964), and *T. catis* infection in cats varies from 8 to 45 per cent (Lancet, 1972); in New York State 73 per cent of dogs examined passed eggs in their stools. In hospitalised patients in East Africa toxocara skin tests have been reported to be positive in 6 per cent of the population in Nairobi, and in 28 per cent in Dar es-Salaam (Wiseman and Woodruff, 1971).

Treatment

Diethylcarbamazine in a daily dose of 3 mg/kg administered three times daily for a period of 21 days causes death of the larvae in the tissues and amelioration of symptoms in some cases. Extensive endophthalmitis with or without retinal detachment often requires enucleation of the affected eye. Infected household animals should be dewormed with piperazine in doses of 200 mg/kg.

TAPEWORMS

Tapeworms (flatworms) are made up of three subunits: a scolex or 'head' which contains suckers or hooklets to facilitate attachment, a neck which is its region of growth and a series of segments (proglottids). The young immature proglottids arise from the distal part of the neck and reach maturity by the time they have arrived at the distal end of the worm. A mature proglottid contains a set of male and female genitalia, and a gravid proglottid acts as a store for the eggs which it contains. There are four stages in the life cycle of a tapeworm: egg, embryo, larva and the adult worm.

The distribution and prevalence of tapeworm infections depends on the dietary habit of eating undercooked or raw meat and fish. High incidence rates occur in many countries of tropical Africa, the Middle East and southern Mediterranean countries. The fish tapeworm, *Diphyllobothrium latum,* occurs among the Eskimos in Quebec, in Finland and in parts of Romania and Turkey.

Taeniasis

Gravid proglottids in human faeces are deposited on soil which infects cattle (*T. saginatum*) and pigs (*T. solium*). Following ingestion by these animals embryos emerge from the eggs in the proximal small intestine, penetrate the mucosa and migrate via vascular and lymphatic channels to other parts of the body (e.g. skeletal muscle, myocardium, diaphragm and tongue) where they encyst to produce a bladder-like structure containing fluid. The cells of the wall of this cyst give rise to the scolex and neck and become the cysticerus (i.e. larval stage). In the case of *Echinococcus granulosus,* the dog tapeworm, the cyst contains a germinal layer that gives rise to many scolices and is called a hydatid. Human infection results from the ingestion of raw or undercooked beef or pork. Following ingestion by man, the scolex evaginates and attaches itself to the intestinal wall of the host and grows into an adult parasite. The cycle is repeated by the faecal passage of gravid proglottids.

Taenia saginata

Taenia saginata, the beef tapeworm, has a length of 15 feet or more and contains 1000 to 2000 proglottids; the scolex has four suckers but no hooks. Following attachment to the mucosa they develop into adult worms over a period of two to four months. Occasionally the growing or adult worms may cause intestinal obstruction. Symptoms include dyspepsia, loose stools, abdominal pain (which may be due to inflammation of the appendix from detached proglottids) and rarely neurotoxic symptoms. The patient may be first alerted to the infection by the recognition of proglottids in the faeces. Diagnosis rests on finding eggs or proglottids in the faeces. Differentiation between *T. saginata* and *solium* can be made by examination of proglottids flattened between two slides; *T. saginata* has 15 to 21 main lateral arms whereas the pig tapeworm has seven to 13. The treatment of choice is quinacrine (Atabrine). The night before administration the bowels should be completely evacuated, preferably by purgation. In the morning oral Atabrine is administered (adult dose is 1·1 g and should be adjusted for a child according to his body weight); one hour later the worm is evacuated by purgation with castor oil.

Taenia solium

Taenia solium rarely grows to a length of more than eight feet and contains less than 1000 proglottids; it has four suckers and a ring of hooks. The clinical manifestations, diagnosis and treatment are as for *T. saginata* with one important exception. *T. solium* infection may be acquired by ingestion of eggs from the human host. The embryos emerge from the eggs, penetrate the mucosa and the resultant cysticerci become established in any soft tissue including the brain and eyeball; involvement of the brain may result in epilepsy.

Hydatid disease *(Echinococcus granulosus)*

The commonest hydatid-producing tapeworm is *Echinococcus granulosus*; other less important tapeworms are *E. multilocularis* and *E. oligarthus.* The mature tapeworm lives in the small intestine of the dog; almost all mammals can be intermediate hosts but the optimal one is the sheep. A cycle of transmission between livestock and dogs maintains the persistence of the worm. The eggs of the *Echinococcus* are remarkably resistant to environmental conditions. They can survive temperatures of $-16°C$ and viable eggs can be recovered after 35 days of exposure to sun. Human disease occurs when the eggs are swallowed by man (e.g. in communities where there is intimate contact with dogs); the eggs are digested releasing a free embryo in the duodenum which penetrates the mucosa to enter a venule which it travels along until it is arrested in a narrow capillary. Embryos develop into small bladder-like cysts, which grow to reach a diameter of 40 to 50 mm after three months. The fluid of the cyst contains granules called 'hydatid sand' which is actually brood capsules with developing scolices. When a hydatid cyst is ingested by the definitive host, e.g. dogs eating the flesh of dead livestock, the embryos are freed from the cyst and become attached to the intestinal mucosa to grow into adult worms. Thus the parasite reproduces itself in the final host by producing a large number of eggs and in the intermediate host by formation of numerous scolices.

A large majority of the embryos get trapped in the sinusoids of the liver, which is the organ most commonly affected in hydatid disease (see Ch. 17). Some embryos escape the hepatic vacular bed and are arrested in the pulmonary circulation, and the rest reach the systemic circulation. Hydatid cysts grow at the rate of 1 cm per year, and symptoms of a space-occupying lesion develop when they reach a size of 10 cm in diameter. Although the liver and/or lung are the commonest organs affected, other organs such as the spleen and kidney may occasionally be affected.

Treatment

The treatment of hydatid disease consists of surgical removal of the cysts from affected organs. Prevention of infection in dogs is an important public health measure and consists of regular administration of anthelmintics to dogs and destruction of affected viscera. The importation of livers and other offal for use as pet foods, and the use of meats for preparation of canned pet foods, must be under close health supervision.

Hymenolepiasis

Hymenolepiasis is produced by *H. nana* and *H. diminuta,* and the usual hosts are rats and mice, and rats and fleas, respectively. Eggs of *H. nana* passed in human faeces are directly infective to man, whereas eggs of *H. diminuta* undergo a period of larval development in certain insects, and ingestion of these intermediate hosts is the source of infection for man. Following ingestion, eggs of *H. nana* hatch and the resultant embryos penetrate the duodenal mucosa, transform into larvae, return to the intestinal lumen, become attached and grow into adults within a few weeks. Symptoms are absent or mild, and treatment is similar to that for taeniasis.

Diphyllobothrium latum

Diphyllobothrium latum is a fish tapeworm prevalent in certain parts of America, Europe and Japan, and infection in man results from eating raw or inadequately processed fish from endemic areas. Infection may cause vitamin B_{12} deficiency and megaloblastic anaemia. Treatment is as for taeniasis.

PROTOZOA

Amoebiasis

Amoebiasis is an endemic disease transmitted from man to man. Prevalence is highest in the tropics and subtropics but cases have been reported from practically every country. Different socioeconomic strata may show wide

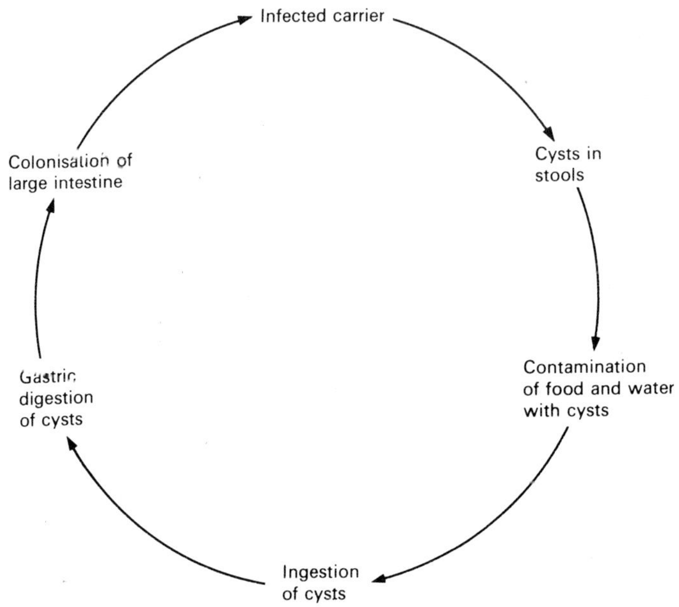

Fig. 12.2 Life cycle of *Entamoeba histolytica*

variations in the intensity of infection; for example, in South Africa amoebiasis is considered a nuisance in the white population but amongest the Bantu it presents as a serious illness. Autopsy data from Mexico City indicates that amoebiasis is the fourth commonest cause of death (Larracilla, Juarez and Resendiz, 1971). There is a high rate of symptomatic disease in children compared to adults, particularly between the ages of 1 and 4 years.

Entamoeba histolytica lives primarily as a commensal in the large intestine, feeding on bacteria and superficial mucosal cells. The factors which induce amoebae to become virulent and produce large intestinal ulceration have not been clearly defined. The life cycle of *E. histolytica* is shown in Figure 12.2. It is primarily a parasite of the large intestine affecting the caecum and the ascending colon predominantly; severe infections may involve the small intestine and the appendix. Dissemination to other tissues, particularly the liver, is common (see Ch. 17). Other common complications which may arise from intestinal amoebiasis are direct extension to the skin resulting in a painful and growing ulcer in the perianal area, and peritonitis with or without perforation. In different series the incidence of peritonitis has varied from 1·5 to 21 per cent (Kapoor, Nathwani and Joshi, 1972).

Diagnosis

This may present a problem, especially in countries where amoebic infection is not commonly seen. The mild attack presents with loose stools containing mucus and blood. In the absence of specific treatment there are recurrent relapses with intervening periods of quiescence, often leading to a mistaken diagnosis of ulcerative colitis. Treatment with corticosteroids can cause acute exacerbations in such cases. In the same way, hepatic or pleuropulmonary amoebiasis can be mistaken for other conditions, since cysts and trophozoites are frequently absent from the stools. In recent years the development of an indirect fluorescent antibody technique has improved the diagnostic capability. Serial dilutions of the patient's serum are tested against dried smears of *E. histolytica* grown in culture, and an antibody titre greater than 1 in 128 provides strong grounds for a diagnosis of active or recently active infection.

Treatment

Until recently all amoebicides were selective in their sites of action. Thus there were tissue amoebicides like emetine and chloroquin, predominantly luminal amoebicides like emetine bismuth iodide and furadantin, and indirect-acting, broad-spectrum antibiotics. With such selective action, therapy was not satisfactory and amoebiasis had achieved the reputation of being a chronic relapsing condition. The advent of metronidazole in recent years has greatly improved the prospect of effecting a cure. At a dose of 40 to 50 mg/kg daily, it is effective in amoebiasis of childhood. Good results are also obtained in chronic intestinal amoebiasis and in symptomless cyst passers. Metronidazole is rapidly absorbed from the intestine and is, therefore, more effective in hepatic than intestinal amoebic infections. Treatment results in rapid symptomatic improvement and disappearance of parasites from the stools and rectal ulcers in less than 24 hours. When the liver is involved, small abscesses resolve spontaneously, but large abscesses with tenderness require prompt surgical aspiration. Inadequate drainage is the commonest reason for treatment failure and relapse.

Giardiasis (see Yardley and Bayless, 1967)

Giardia lamblia is a flagellate protozoon which has both a trophozoic and a cystic stage. It inhabits the duodenum and jejunum (see Figs. 12.3 and 12.4) and is amongst one of the most common parasites of man. Incidence rates vary. A rate of 47 per cent was reported from hospital patients in Colombia (World Health Statistics Report, 1969) and a survey in primary school children in Rangoon, Burma, showed prevalence rates of 21 per cent for *Giardia* and 5·7 per cent for *E. histolytica* (World Health Statistics Report, 1969); a similar survey in Mexico City revealed rates of 13·7 and 14·3 per cent, respectively.

Transmission occurs mainly from person to person through ingestion of food and water contaminated with cysts, but flies may also play an important role in transmission. Many of the cases of so-called 'travellers' diarrhoea may be due to infection with this parasite.

Results of exposure to *G. lamblia* are variable depending upon variations in parasite or host factors, such as age, nutrition and immune status. In an experimental study (Rendtorff, 1954) 40 healthy volunteers were fed with a single strain of the parasite at different dose levels and only 21 became symptomatic. As few as 10 cysts were sufficient to cause infection in some individuals, though an average of 100 or more cysts were required to guarantee infection. It is likely that many individuals harbour this parasite in an essentially commensal relationship.

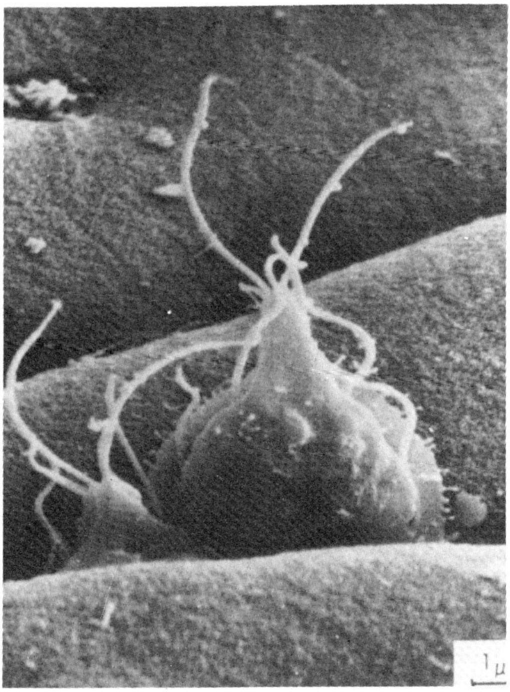

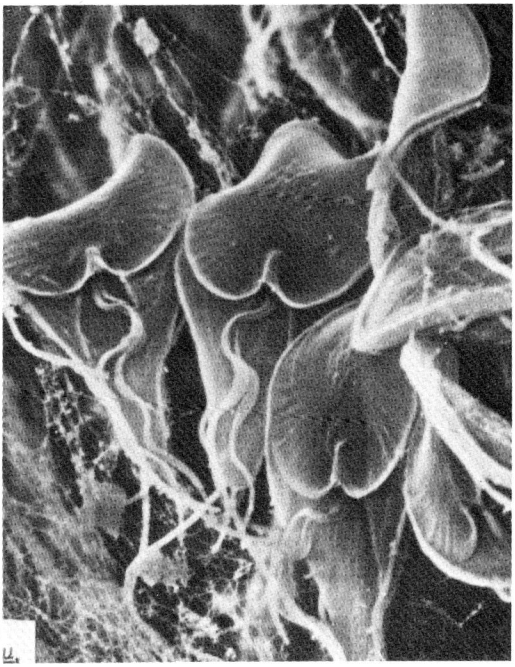

Figs. 12.3 and 12.4 Scanning electron microscopic appearances of the trophozoic stage of *Giardia lamblia* attached to the surface of small intestinal mucosa

Clinical symptoms vary from mild to severe diarrhoea. Diarrhoea may be acute and of short duration or may become prolonged and chronic; in the latter case malabsorption may lead to weight loss and failure to thrive. Unequivocal morphological abnormalities of the jejunal mucosa occur in some patients with giardiasis, particularly in patients with underlying immunodeficiency states (see Ch. 9). An immunodeficiency state should be suspected in any patient with giardiasis, particularly in the developed parts of the world, and appropriate investigations undertaken. It is likely that in such cases the defective immune mechanism leads to infection.

Diagnosis

In acute cases, examination of freshly voided stool may show trophozoites with their characteristic features and flagellar movements. The cysts, however, are more commonly found and can be seen even in well-formed stools. However, in many infected individuals several stool examinations may turn out to be negative. A definite periodicity of presence or absence of cysts in stools has been demonstrated in experimental infections (Rendtorff, 1954). Examination of duodenal juice or small intestinal mucosa for trophozoites is far more reliable as a diagnostic procedure than examination of stools for cysts.

Treatment

Metronidazole in a dose of 0·25 g two to three times a day for a period of five to 10 days is the drug of choice and has superseded mepacrine in the treatment of giardiasis. With the above regimen, a cure rate of 80 per cent or more can be expected from a single course of treatment.

FLUKES

Fascioliasis

Fascioliasis (liver fluke disease) is primarily a disease of cattle and the incidence in man is low, especially in Western countries because waterside plants are seldom eaten raw, except for watercress. The plant needs a flow of water, and infected snails may invade the beds from upstream or by migration from nearby pastures. In recent years outbreaks have been reported in France, England, Germany and Cuba. In all areas where the parasite is endemic in animals the possibility of human disease should be borne in mind.

The adult fluke lives in the liver of the host. Eggs are laid in the biliary passages and travel down the intestinal tract in the stools. They mature in a fortnight at an optimal temperature of 22°C to 25°C, and the emerging larvae (miracidium) must penetrate a snail of the genus *Lymnaea* in a few hours. Inside the snail it develops through several stages and free swimming cercariae burst out of the snail's body to encyst on water plants. Herbivores become infected by ingestion of the water plant. Following ingestion of the cysts by man, larvae emerge in the duodenum, penetrate the mucosa, migrate into the peritoneal cavity and penetrate Glisson's capsule to enter the liver. They burrow through the parenchyma to the biliary passages where they grow to adults. Penetration of the intestinal wall is associated with oedema, inflammation and haemorrhages. Invasion of the liver is associated with dyspepsia, fever, pain in the right hypochondrium and hepatomegaly. Other symptoms such as anorexia, myalgia, joint and bone pain, nausea and vomiting may also occur. A painful enlargement of the liver with fever and eosinophilia forms a characteristic clinical triad. Migration of flukes through hepatic tissue may rarely lead to massive haemorrhage and subcapsular haematomas, and fibrous adhesions between the liver and adjacent viscera may also occur. The flukes feed on hepatocytes and red blood cells, which accounts for the anaemia. Mechanical irritation and obstruction of biliary channels leads to progressive fibrosis and calcification, and may eventually result in biliary cirrhosis.

Treatment

The treatment of choice is intramuscular emetine hydrochloride given intramuscularly as a 6 per cent solution in a dose of 25 mg daily for seven to 10 days.

Fasciolopsiasis

Fasciolopsis buski is a fluke affecting man and pigs (Faust, Russell and Jung, 1970). Its life cycle is similar to that of the liver fluke, except that the adult lives attached to the duodenum producing inflammatory and ulcerative changes in the mucosa. The incidence of infection is directly proportional to the degree of water pollution where the aquatic plants grow and is higher in the rainy season, which favours multiplication and spread of the carrier snail. Hexylresorcinol crystoids in a dosage of 0·4 g in children 1 to 7 years of age, and 1 g in patients 13 or over, produce cure in 54 per cent of patients, and a 90 to 99 per cent reduction worm load in the remainder.

Schistosomiasis

Next to malaria, schistosomiasis is one of the most widespread parasitic infestations of man and occurs in most countries of tropical Africa, the Middle East, Central and South America, the Caribbean, and in the Far East. It is estimated that 200 million persons in the world are infected, and that of Egypt's 37 million people, 20 million have the disease. Developments involving major irrigation projects have resulted in an increase in the disease by facilitating the spread of the parasite and its intermediate host along irrigation canals to village communities.

The three main species are *S. haematobium,* which is found in the vesical venous plexus of man (occurs in Africa and the Middle East), *S. mansoni* which is found in the colonic venules (common in Africa and Central and South America), and *S. japonicum* also found in the colonic venules (occurs in the Far East). The adult worms are found in the vesical or colonic venules, and eggs pass through the vessel wall into the urine or faeces of the host, as the case may be, and find another host, the fresh water snail, in which they undergo many changes before emerging into the water as infectious cercariae. Man is infected by contact with surface water during washing or bathing or even wading through infected pools.

Schistosomiasis is one of those curious infections where many people get infected, some develop symptoms and only few have complications and die. The development of symptoms depends upon the worm load, the number of eggs laid and the reaction of the tissues to the parasite. In highly endemic areas virtually everyone is infected some time in life and infection rates of 100 per cent may occur. The host is protected against reinfection as long as some degree of infection by the parasite persists, and protection ceases soon after cure.

S. mansoni infection presents with bloody diarrhoea and must be distinguished from other dysenteric illnesses: Salmonella infections are relatively frequent in persons affected with *S. mansoni*. *S. haematobium* infection usually presents with haematuria and proteinuria, and long-standing infections can cause fibrosis and calcification of the bladder wall. Involvement of the ureteric orifices can lead to hydronephrosis even in comparatively recent infections. Many of these lesions are reversible with early treatment.

As the eggs are being laid many circulate to other organs, particularly the liver where they may induce fibrotic changes in adjacent tissue, and in advanced cases lead to portal hypertension with splenomegaly. Occasionally, eggs travel beyond the liver and become lodged in the pulmonary circulation causing pulmonary hypertension and cor pulmonale. *Schistosoma granuloma* have been described in the spinal cord causing cord pressure and paraplegia. Similar granuloma have also been reported in the introitus in females.

Treatment

In endemic areas treatment poses several problems. In a disease which may affect almost the entire population selection for chemotherapy is difficult, particularly since reinfection may occur soon after successful therapy. Antimonials remain the most effective in bringing about a parasitological cure, but treatment is prolonged, there are serious side-effects including cardiac toxicity and the drug has to be administered by the parenteral route. The commonly used antimonials are:

1. Intravenous sodium antimony tartarate beginning with a dose of 30 mg daily which is increased by 30 mg every 48 hours to a maximum dose of 120 mg until a total of 1·5 g has been administered.
2. Intramuscular stibocaprate in a total dose of 30 mg/kg body weight (to a maximum of 2·5 g) divided into five doses.

Oral niridazole is effective against *S. haematobium,* less effective against *S. mansoni* and has only a palliative action against *S. japonicum.* It is given in a daily dose of 25 mg/kg in two divided doses for a period of five days. Side-effects include anorexia, vomiting, headache and drowsiness, and central nervous system disturbances such as agitation, depression and major convulsions may occur in patients with portal hypertension with portosystemic communications. With lucanthone the best therapeutic effect is obtained by giving an intensive three-day course (10 to 20 mg/kg daily for three days). Side-effects such as nausea, vomiting and epigastric pain may occur, and convulsions and psychotic reactions have also been reported.

References

Duran Jorda, F. (1957) Appendicitis and enterobiasis in children. *Archives of Disease in Childhood,* **32,** 208.

Faust, E. C., Russell, P. F. & Jung, P. C. (1970) *Craig and Faust's Clinical Parasitology.* 8th edition. Philadelphia: Lea and Febiger.

Kapoor, O. P., Nathwani, B. N. & Joshi, V. R. (1972) Amoebic peritonitis—a study of 73 cases. *Journal of Tropical Medicine and Hygiene,* **75,** 4.

Knight, R., Schultz, M. G., Hoskins, D. W. & Marsden, P. D. (1973) Progress report: intestinal parasites. *Gut,* **14,** 145.

Lancet (1972) Editorial: toxocara. *Lancet,* **1,** 730.

Larracilla, A. J., Juarez, F. A. & Resendiz, Z. J. (1971) Amibiasis intestinal en los tres primeros meses de la vida. *Salud. publ. Mex.,* **13,** 79.

Layrisse, M., Aparcedo, C., Torres, M. & Roche, M. (1967) Blood loss due to infection with *Trichuris trichiura. American Journal of Tropical Medicine and Hygiene,* **16,** 613.

Louw, J. H. (1966) Abdominal complication of *Ascaris lumbricoides* infestation in children. *British Journal of Surgery,* **53,** 6, 510.

Marsden, P. D. & Hoskins, D. W. (1966) Intestinal parasites: a progress report. *Gastroenterology,* **51,** 701.

Marsden, P. D. & Schultz, M. G. (1969) Intestinal parasites. *Gastroenterology,* **57,** 724.

Rendtorff, R. C. (1954) The experimental transmission of human intestinal protozoan parasites. *American Journal of Hygiene,* **59,** 209.

Roche, M. & Layrisse, M. (1966) Nature and cause of hookworm anaemia. *American Journal of Tropical Medicine and Hygiene,* **15,** 1031.

Tandon, B. N., Das, B. C., Saraya, A. K. & Deo, M. G. (1966) Functional and structural studies of small bowel in Ankylostomiasis. *British Medical Journal,* **1,** 714.

Tasker, P. W. G. (1961) Blood loss from hookworm infection. *Transactions of the Royal Society for Tropical Medicine and Hygiene,* **55,** 36.

Thompson, R. G., Hutchison, J. G. P. & Johnston, N. M. (1972) Survey of intestinal pathogens from immigrant children. *British Medical Journal,* **1,** 591.

Venkatachalam, P. S. & Patwardhan, V. N. (1953) *Transactions of the Royal Society for Tropical Medicine and Hygiene,* **47,** 169.

Whalen, G. E., Rosenberg, E. B., Strictland, G. T., Gutman, R. A., Cross, J. H., Watton, R. H., Nylangco, C. & Dizon, J. J. (1969) Intestinal capillariasis—a new disease in man. *Lancet,* **1,** 13.

Wiseman, R. A. & Woodruff, A. W. (1971) Toxocariasis in Africa and Malta. The frequency of infection in host animals and its incidence and distribution in humans as revealed by skin sensitivity tests. *Transactions of the Royal Society for Tropical Medicine and Hygiene,* **65,** 439.

Woodruff, A. W. (1970) Toxocariasis. *British Medical Journal,* **3,** 663.

Woodruff, A. W. & Thacker, C. K. (1964) Infection with animal helminths. *British Medical Journal,* **1,** 1001.

World Health Organization Technical Report Series No. 379.

World Health Statistics Report (1969) **22,** 510.

Yardley, J. H. & Bayless, T. M. (1967) Giardiasis. *Gastroenterology,* **52,** 301.

13. Protein-losing enteropathies

W. L. Tift

Protein-losing enteropathies secondary to altered gut permeability
Protein-losing enteropathies secondary to lymph stasis

Catabolism of serum proteins by the gastrointestinal tract is a physiological process which accounts for a small percentage of the total daily turnover of albumin (Waldmann *et al.*, 1967a). Upon entering the gastrointestinal lumen, protein is broken down to its constituent amino acids, which are then reabsorbed and utilised for synthesis of new protein. In certain disease states, collectively referred to as protein-losing enteropathies, the magnitude of this protein loss becomes greatly increased. Since the rate of albumin synthesis by the liver can at best be doubled, and since immunoglobulin synthesis is triggered only by antigenic stimuli, this increased protein catabolism results in reduced serum concentrations of proteins.

The first demonstration of gastrointestinal protein loss was reported in 1957 by Citrin, Sterling and Halstead, who recovered intravenously administered ^{131}I-labelled albumin from the gastric juice of a patient with giant hypertrophy of the gastric mucosa. Since that time a number of other radioactive substances, including ^{131}I-polyvinyl pyrrolidone, ^{51}Cr-labelled albumin, ^{59}Fe-labelled iron dextran, ^{95}Nb-labelled albumin and ^{67}Cu-labelled ceruloplasmin, have been used to estimate the magnitude of the gastrointestinal loss of protein in both normal and abnormal states. The technique involves the intravenous injection of a labelled macromolecule followed by measurement of the amount of label appearing in a four-day stool collection, and results are expressed as a percentage of the administered dose. Details of the various methods, along with their relative merits, have been described by Waldmann (1972).

Disorders associated with excessive gastrointestinal loss of protein may be divided into two groups on the basis of the mechanism of protein loss (see Table 13.1). The first group consists of disease states with altered gut permeability, and the second group of conditions are associated with stasis in the intestinal and mesenteric lymphatics.

PROTEIN-LOSING ENTEROPATHIES SECONDARY TO ALTERED GUT PERMEABILITY

In ulcerative colitis and acute infective enteritis, excessive gastrointestinal loss of protein is related to altered permeability of an inflamed mucosa; a similar mechanism acts in the enterocolitis associated with aganglionic megacolon

Table 13.1 Conditions associated with excessive gastrointestinal loss of protein in childhood

Altered gut permeability
Ulcerative colitis
Acute infective enteritis
Aganglionic megacolon
Hypogammaglobulinaemia
Coeliac disease
Tropical sprue
Kwashiorkor
Cystic fibrosis
Allergic gastroenteropathies
Giant hypertrophy of the gastric mucosa
Crohn's disease
Nephrosis
Lymph stasis
Primary intestinal lymphangiectasia
Secondary intestinal lymphangiectasia
Congestive heart failure
Constrictive pericarditis
Mesenteric panniculitis
X-ray arteritis
Neuroblastoma
Lymphoma
Tuberculous adenitis
Crohn's disease
Nephrosis

(Schussheim, 1972). In hypogammaglobulinaemia the underlying defect in gamma globulin synthesis leads to secondary disorders of the intestinal tract, such as infective enteritis, which cause excessive leakage of protein into the intestinal lumen.

There are several conditions in which protein loss is part of a gross disturbance in mucosal function with altered permeability to a variety of substances. Coeliac disease, tropical sprue, kwashiorkor and cystic fibrosis are examples of these conditions whose major manifestations usually precede and overshadow the relatively unimportant protein loss.

Waldmann *et al.* (1967b) described a group of infants with a syndrome of oedema, hypoproteinaemia, iron deficiency anaemia, growth retardation, eosinophilia and allergic symptoms such as eczema, asthma and rhinitis; all had strong family histories of allergy. Although gastrointestinal symptoms were mild, excessive gastrointestinal protein loss was demonstrated in all cases. Radiology of the small intestine was either normal or showed mucosal oedema; jejunal biopsies showed a normal villous pattern with excessive eosinophilic infiltration of the lamina propria. The protein loss resolved following treatment with a cows' milk-free diet, and recurred when milk was reintroduced.

Giant hypertrophy of the gastric mucosa is a rare cause of excessive gastrointestinal protein loss in childhood. These patients present with hypoproteinaemia and oedema following an acute episode of diarrhoea and vomiting. Although the diagnostic radiological finding of prominent gastric rugae is identical to that seen in Menetrier's disease, the two conditions are quite distinct (Herskovic, Spiro, and Gryboski, 1968). In the adult form (Menetrier's disease), the hypoproteinaemia and oedema are persistent and may eventually lead to therapeutic gastrectomy. In the childhood disease, the hypoproteinaemia is transient and the gastric abnormalities are self-limited and completely reversible, and the radiological and histological abnormalities spontaneously resolve after several weeks of supportive management. While the aetiology of this condition is not known, there has been one report of cytomegalic inclusions in the hypertrophic gastric mucosa of a 3-year-old boy who demonstrated a rise in serum antibody titres against cytomegalovirus two months following the onset of oedema (Leonidas, Beatty and Wenner, 1973).

Both altered gut permeability and lymph stasis probably play a pathophysiological role in the intestinal protein loss which occurs in Crohn's disease and nephrosis. Lymphatic obstruction secondary to chronic inflammation is probably the main reason for protein loss in Crohn's disease (French, 1971). Similarly in nephrosis, de Sousa *et al.* (1968) have obtained jejunal mucosal biopsies consistent with intestinal lymphangiectasia in four of seven children with the nephrotic syndrome.

PROTEIN-LOSING ENTEROPATHIES SECONDARY TO LYMPH STASIS

Primary intestinal lymphangiectasia

Primary intestinal lymphangiectasia was first delineated as an entity by Waldmann *et al.* in 1961. In this condition the primary symptomatology is directly related to protein leakage, and the goal of management is to reduce the magnitude of protein loss.

Clinical and pathological features

It is characterised by the presence of dilated small intestinal lymph vessels which leak chyle into the lumen, and in severe cases the chyle leak can be demonstrated by lymphography (Mistilis, Skyring and Stephen, 1965). The disease probably represents a congenital disorder of the mesenteric lymphatics and is often associated with lymphatic anomalies elsewhere. Patients usually present with oedema and hypoalbuminaemia; the oedema is often asymmetrical, reflecting extraintestinal lymphangiectasia (Fig. 13.1). Ascites, pleural and pericardial effusions may be found both at the time of presentation and later in the course of the disease. These collections of fluid may be the direct result of hypoproteinaemia or may be chylous effusions resulting from leakage of chyle in localised areas of lymphangiectasia. Gastrointestinal symptoms are characteristically mild and consist of intermittent diarrhoea with minimal steatorrhoea. The diagnosis is usually established during the first or second decade of life (Waldmann, 1966), but in retrospect oedema is often noted to have been present from birth or early childhood (Tift and Lloyd, 1975).

The bulk leakage of chyle into the intestinal lumen results in the loss of proteins of all sizes together with lymphocytes. The degree of reduction in serum protein levels depends on the relative synthetic rates of the individual

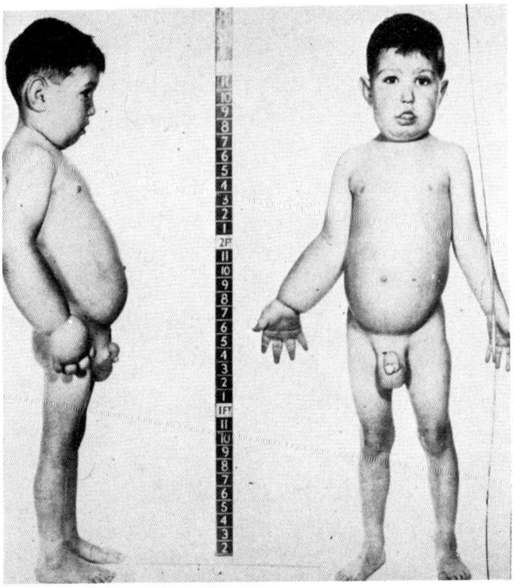

Fig. 13.1 Asymmetric distribution of peripheral oedema in a 5-year-old boy with primary intestinal lymphangiectasia

proteins. Thus albumin and globulin levels are markedly reduced, transferrin and ceruloplasmin are slightly reduced and fibrinogen is usually present in normal concentrations (Waldmann, 1966). Lymphopaenia (less than 1500/mm^3) is consistently present and is an important diagnostic feature. Reduced serum levels of calcium and magnesium are frequently observed and serum cholesterol may be normal or slightly reduced. Deficiencies of folic acid, vitamin B_{12}, vitamin E and iron are commonly found and can be corrected with oral supplements.

Radiological abnormalities of the small intestine are present in the vast majority of patients and consist of coarse mucosal folds through the small intestine without the dilatation seen in other malabsorptive states (Fig. 13.2). Dilution of barium in the ileum and puddling of barium may also be seen (Shimkin, Waldmann, and Krugman, 1970). Upper small intestinal biopsy, if taken from an affected area, shows dilated but intact lymphatics (Fig. 13.3); goblet cells may be markedly enlarged with liquefied granules being extruded into the lumen. Villous atrophy and cellular infiltration are absent (Ores *et al.*, 1966).

The diagnosis of primary intestinal lymphangiectasia can be made with confidence in patients who present with oedema, particularly if asymmetric, hypoalbuminaemia, lymphopaenia and the characteristic radiologic abnormalities. Measurement of labelled protein excretion, which is a difficult and non-specific investigation, and intestinal biopsy, which may miss the lesion, may not be necessary in children who show all of the above features (Tift and Lloyd, 1975).

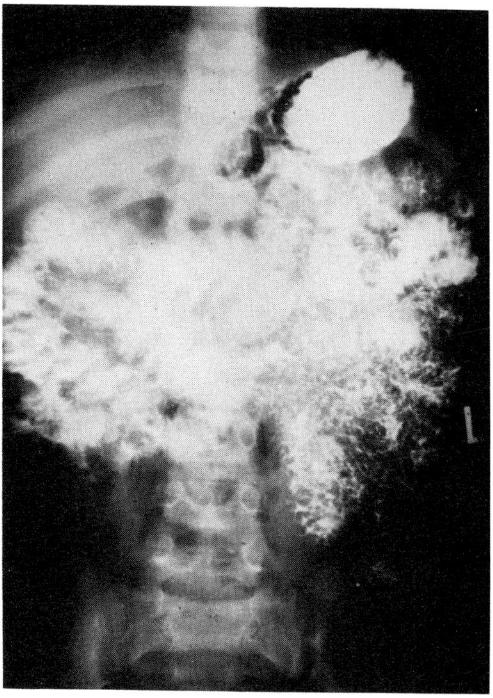

Fig. 13.2 Barium meal and follow-through in primary intestinal lymphangiectasia showing coarse mucosal folds

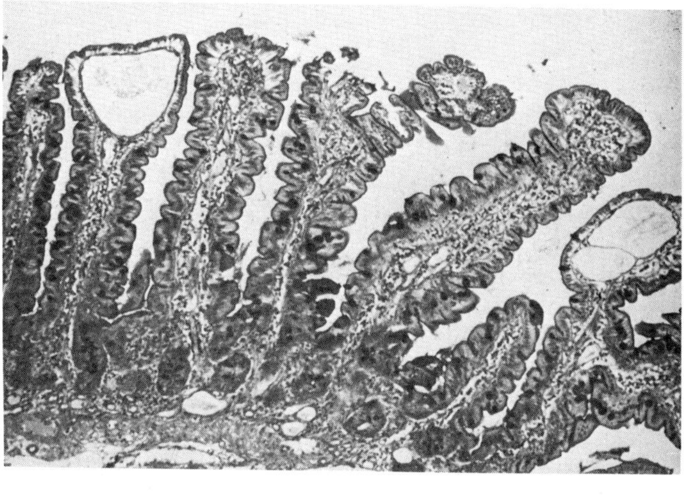

Fig. 13.3 Dilated jejunal lymphatics in primary intestinal lymphangiectasia

Immunological abnormalities

Intestinal lymphangiectasia can be regarded as a secondary immune deficiency state, with hypogammaglobulinaemia due to loss of protein and lymphopaenia due to loss of lymphocytes. Serum levels of IgG, IgA, and IgM are usually reduced to less than half the normal levels, and the fractional catabolic rate of the intravascular pool is increased to a similar degree for all three immunoglobulins (Strober *et al.*, 1967). This observation lends support to the theory that the protein leak in intestinal lymphangiectasia represents a bulk loss of lymph fluid. Antibody production (B lymphocyte function) is normal in response to stimulation by Vi and Tularemia antigens. T lymphocyte function in these patients, however, is abnormal as evidenced by prolonged allograft survival, a high percentage of negative skin tests for delayed hypersensitivity and impaired *in vitro* transformation of circulating lymphocytes in response to stimulation by mitogens and allogenic cells. Lymphocytes taken from chylous effusions show considerably greater transformation than normal when exposed to the same stimuli (Strober *et al.*, 1967). These observations can be explained by the relatively greater loss of long-lived T cells as compared with short-lived B cells in patients with intestinal lymphangiectasia. Since T cells circulate from the bloodstream to tissues and then via the lymphatic system back to the bloodstream, they are more vulnerable to gastrointestinal chyle leakage than are B cells which tend to remain in the peripheral circulation. Although impaired T cell function is a consistent feature, few patients develop serious infections. Of the 18 patients investigated by Strober *et al.* (1967), two (both under 6 years of age) died after prolonged periods of debilitation associated with recurrent bacterial infections, two had an increased frequency of mild respiratory tract infections and the remaining 14 patients had no increased incidence of infections. One of the six patients reported by Tift and Lloyd (1975) developed meningitis and recurrent episodes of pneumonia and had impaired lymphocyte transformation in response to PHA stimulation and a relative diminution in the number of circulating T cells.

Treatment

The lymphangiectasia is rarely sufficiently localised to permit cure by excision of the affected region of the small intestine. There has been one report of a surgical anastomosis between dilated lymphatics and the long saphenous vein which led to some improvement (Mistilis and Skyring, 1966). The basis of medical management is the restriction of dietary fat intake to the minimum possible so as to diminish mesenteric chyle flow and thereby reduce the intestinal leak of protein. The introduction of medium chain triglycerides (MCT), whose fatty acids are largely transported by the portal vein and whose absorption does not appreciably increase lymph flow, has enabled strict low-fat diets to be made more palatable and has also provided an additional source of high energy food (Leyland *et al.*, 1969). The intake of dietary fat is restricted to 5 to 10 g daily, while the use of MCT is unrestricted. All patients should receive oral vitamin supplements and some require long-term diuretics to control persistent oedema (Tift and Lloyd, 1975). Neither gamma globulin nor corticosteroid administration is beneficial.

The low-fat MCT-supplemented diet results in an improvement in the general well-being of patients despite laboratory evidence of a continuing chyle leak (i.e. persistent lymphopaenia, hypoalbuminaemia and abnormal ^{51}Cr-labelled albumin excretion). All six of the children reported by Tift and Lloyd (1975) showed a rapid and sustained improvement in dependent oedema, and it was possible to discontinue long-term diuretic therapy in two of four patients who had previously required it. The asymmetrical oedema, which results from peripheral lymphatic anomalies, was unaffected by dietary or diuretic therapy. Diarrhoea ceased to be a problem in the four patients who presented with that complaint. The most compelling evidence for the long-term benefit of the diet was the improvement in growth rates and the prompt clinical relapse which occurred when the diet was relaxed. These findings indicate a need for continued adherence to a strict diet, at least through puberty, in a disease whose ill-effects appear to be life long.

Secondary intestinal lymphangiectasia

Lymph stasis in secondary intestinal lymphangiectasia results from obstruction of chyle flow through mesenteric lymph channels. Impaired flow may be either functional, as in congestive heart failure and constrictive pericarditis, or the direct result of organic obstruction, as in mesenteric panniculitis, X-ray arteritis, retroperitoneal tumours and primary diseases of the mesenteric lymph nodes such as tuberculosis and lymphoma. The treatment is that of the underlying disorder and may be successful in eradicating the excessive gastrointestinal protein loss.

References

Citrin, Y., Sterling, K. & Halstead, J. A. (1957) The mechanism of hypoproteinemia associated with giant hypertrophy of the gastric mucosa. *New England Journal of Medicine,* **257,** 906.

de Sousa, J. S., Guerreiro, O., Cunha, A. & Araujo, J. (1968) Association of nephrotic syndrome with intestinal lymphangiectasia. *Archives of Disease in Childhood,* **43,** 245.

French, A. B. (1971) Protein-losing gastroenteropathies. *Digestive Diseases,* **16,** 661.

Herskovic, T., Spiro, H. M. & Gryboski, J. D. (1968) Acute transient gastrointestinal protein loss. *Pediatrics,* **41,** 818.

Leonidas, J. C., Beatty, E. C. & Wenner, H. A. (1973) Menetrier disease and cytomegalovirus infection in childhood. *American Journal of Diseases of Children,* **126,** 806.

Leyland, F. C., Fosbrooke, A. S., Lloyd, J. K., Segall, M. M., Tamir, I., Tomkins, R. & Wolff, O. H. (1969) Use of medium-chain triglyceride diets in children with malabsorption. *Archives of Disease in Childhood,* **44,** 234.

Mistilis, S. P. & Skyring, A. P. (1966) Intestinal lymphangiectasia. Therapeutic effect of lymph venous anastomosis. *American Journal of Medicine,* **40,** 634.

Mistilis, S. P., Skyring, A. P. & Stephen, D. D. (1965) Intestinal lymphangiectasia. Mechanism of enteric loss of plasma-protein and fat. *Lancet,* **1,** 77.

Ores, C. N., Ores, R. O., Denning, C. R. & Barker, H. G. (1966) Hypercatabolic hypoproteinemia with lymphangiectasia of the small bowel. *Journal of Pediatrics,* **69,** 439.

Schussheim, A. (1972) Protein-losing enteropathies in children. *American Journal of Gastroenterology,* **58,** 124.

Shimkin, P. M., Waldmann, T. A. & Krugman, R. C. (1970) Intestinal lymphangiectasia. *American Journal of Roentgenology,* **110,** 827.

Strober, W., Wochner, R. D., Carbone, P. D. & Waldman, T. A. (1967) Intestinal lymphangiectasia: a protein-losing enteropathy with hypogammaglobulinemia, lymphocytopenia, and impaired homograft rejection. *Journal of Clinical Investigation,* **46,** 1643.

Tift, W. L. & Lloyd, J. K. (1975) Intestinal lymphangiectasia. Long-term results with an MCT diet. *Archives of Disease in Childhood,* **50,** 269.

Waldmann, T. A. (1966) Protein-losing gastroenteropathy. *Gastroenterology,* **50,** 422.

Waldmann, T. A. (1972) Protein-losing enteropathy and kinetic studies of plasma protein metabolism. *Seminars in Nuclear Medicine,* **2,** 251.

Waldmann, T. A., Morell, A. G., Wochner, R. D., Strober, W. & Sternlieb, I. (1967a) Measurement of gastrointestinal protein loss using ceruloplasmin labeled with ^{67}copper. *Journal of Clinical Investigation,* **46,** 10.

Waldmann, T. A., Steinfeld, J. L., Dutcher, T. F., Davidson, J. D. & Gordon, R. S. (1961) The role of the gastrointestinal system in idiopathic hypoproteinemia. *Gastroenterology,* **41,** 197.

Waldmann, T. A., Wochner, R. D., Laster, L. & Gordon, R. S. (1967b) Allergic gastroenteropathy. A cause of excessive gastrointestinal protein loss. *New England Journal of Medicine,* **276,** 761.

Acknowledgement. I wish to thank Professor June K. Lloyd for permission to include Figure 13.1.

14. Gastrointestinal symptoms related to psychological disturbances

R. V. Howarth

Recurrent vomiting
Recurrent abdominal pain
Disorders of faecal elimination
Concluding remarks

Recurrent vomiting, abdominal pain and disorders of faecal elimination are common clinical problems encountered in paediatric practice. The pathogenesis of such symptoms is poorly understood, and the need for a critical approach in the exclusion of organic disease cannot be overemphasised. For example, recurrent abdominal pain and vomiting may occur in children with congenital malrotation of the intestine; Crohn's disease may have an insidious onset and lead to secondary psychiatric disturbances in the patient and family; congenital sucrase-isomaltase deficiency can be accompanied by mild gastrointestinal symptoms which may be attributed to an 'irritable bowel syndrome'. A careful history and physical examination and appropriate laboratory investigations are mandatory to exclude underlying organic disease. It is a salutary experience to diagnose symptoms as 'functional' in a child in the face of parental conviction to the contrary and to subsequently recognise that the parents were correct. Parents often have a sixth sense regarding the health of their children. In many instances a joint approach by the psychiatrist and paediatrician is necessary in the management of children with functional disturbances of the gastrointestinal tract.

Nevertheless, psychological factors need to be considered in children with recurrent vomiting and/or abdominal pain and in those with disorders of faecal elimination.

RECURRENT VOMITING

Recurrent vomiting occurs with a frequency of about 2 per cent in the middle childhood years (Rutter, Tizard and Whitmore, 1970; Cullen and MacDonald, 1963), and boys and girls are equally affected. Many present before the age of 6 with a duration of recurrent symptoms of from two to 13 years (Hoyt and Stickler, 1960); Hammond (1974), however, found seven out of 12 children who continued to have vomiting attacks in early adult life. The diagnosis, particularly of the first episode, is largely by exclusion of organic disease. Most diseases, within or outside the gastrointestinal tract, that cause vomiting declare themselves by the presence of other symptoms and signs or are revealed by laboratory investigation.

During the hours preceding an episode of vomiting prodromal symptoms such as a voracious appetite, irritability and other changes in temperament may be present. The vomiting attacks usually resolve within four days but occasionally persist for a week or two (Hoyt and Stickler, 1960); dehydration and ketosis are not uncommon. The attacks are often accompanied by headaches; whether the headache is an associated or secondary symptom is not known. The end of the vomiting, like the beginning, is presaged for some children by a lightening of mood and a recognition that it is all over; recovery is then rapid and the child remains well in between attacks (Smith, 1937). The recurrent nature of the symptoms becomes apparent, but the frequency and severity of the attacks are variable and there is no true cycle or periodicity. Of 44 patients with recurrent vomiting, 18 had three to five attacks per year, 21 had attacks every one to two months, and five had more than one attack each month (Hoyt and Stickler, 1960).

Recurrent vomiting and migraine may be expressions of the same underlying condition. A family history of migraine was first described by Smith (1937), who also showed that a proportion of children with recurrent vomiting went on to develop migraine. Similarly Hoyt and Stickler (1960), and Millichap, Lombroso and Lennox (1955) found that 25 and 39 per cent, respectively, of their patients had a family history of migraine. Farquhar (1956) reported a family history of migraine in 64 per cent of children with the periodic syndrome but not all of his patients vomited. Nine out of 38 patients developed recurrent headaches, five possibly migraine, in one study (Hoyt and Stickler, 1960). In a controlled study Hammond followed up 12 patients into early adult life and eight of these developed migraine compared to only one of the control group.

The form of the attacks, the absence of recognisable pathology and the recurrent timing of the symptoms, without a clear history of environmental precipitant factors, suggest a possible relationship to disturbances in central nervous function, in particular epilepsy. Millichap *et al.* (1955) found a family history of epilepsy in 15 per cent of affected children and claimed an improvement in their patients' vomiting with anticonvulsant therapy; this was an uncontrolled study, however, and there is doubt about the selection of cases. MacKeith and Pampiglione (1956) found no family history of epilepsy in 52 children with the periodic syndrome, many of whom were vomiters, and only one of 38 patients followed up by Hoyt and Stickler (1960) developed epilepsy. The consensus of findings is that although the central nervous system may be involved in the precipitation of attacks of vomiting, no link with epilepsy has been convincingly demonstrated.

The role of psychological factors is not yet clear either, but several authors consider them to be at least contributory. In the prospective study of Hammond (1974) eight of the patients showed significant handicapping psychiatric symptoms on reaching early adult life, compared with only three of the control subjects whose psychiatric symptoms were less troublesome. Seven of these adults had a history suggesting that stress was an important factor in precipitating gastrointestinal symptoms or migraine attacks; in contrast, stress was a precipitating factor in only one of the control subjects. Apley and MacKeith (1962) consider that recurrent vomiting and other periodic symptoms are reactions to stress and often form part of a family pattern. They emphasise the need for positive evidence of emotional disturbance, as well as an absence of organic disease, and the importance of establishing a relationship between the timing of attacks and emotional stress. Reduction in the frequency or severity of vomiting attacks by relieving emotional tension is also suggestive of stress being an important factor.

It is difficult to consider the role of psychological factors in isolation in children with recurrent vomiting since vomiting is so frequently associated with other symptoms, particularly headache and abdominal pain. Wyllie and Schlesinger (1933) brought together recurrent vomiting, abdominal pain, headache and fever to describe a periodic group of disorders in childhood and postulated a common aetiology. Since then it has become apparent that this poorly understood syndrome may be accompanied by other symptoms such as limb pains (Naish and Apley, 1951).

Improvement has been attributed to a wide variety of treatments: anticonvulsants (Millichap *et al.*, 1955), rectal administration of sedatives (Smith, 1937), phenobarbitone, chlorpromazine, antihistamines, removal of a normal appendix, a negative laparotomy, osteopathy, faith-healing and 'growing out of it'. Hoyt and Stickler (1960) suggest that all these have a non-specific psychotherapeutic or suggestive value, which supports the views of Apley and MacKeith (1962).

RECURRENT ABDOMINAL PAIN

It should be emphasised that recurrent abdominal pain may be an indicator not only of psychological disturbances but also of underlying organic disease, and the exclusion of organic disease is mandatory in children with this syndrome.

General features

The clinical features of patients with functional and recurrent abdominal pain (RAP) have been described by Apley and Naish (1958) and Apley (1959). Apley and Naish (1958) reported associated symptoms such as vomiting and headache in 20 per cent of patients, pallor in 38 per cent and fever in others; affected cases had a slightly lower mean body weight compared with control subjects but were physically and intellectually similar. Affected cases had more fears, sleep disturbances and disturbances of appetite, and they were rated as highly strung, fussy, excitable, anxious, timid and apprehensive or overconscientious. Apley and Naish (1958) have defined RAP as a child who has at least three episodes of pain over a period of not less than three months which affects the child's activities, with a history of attacks in the preceding year. On this basis they found an incidence of 10·8 per cent in a survey of 1000 school children, with a slight predominance in girls. The incidence varies with age and sex (Apley, 1959). In boys an incidence of 10 to 12 per cent between the ages of 5 and 10 years is followed by a reduced incidence, and then a further increase at about the age of 14 years. For girls the incidence is similar up to 8 years, but there follows a marked increase in incidence up to 9 years, which is followed by a reduction in the problem. Similar results have been reported by Oster (1972).

'Nervous breakdown', RAP, peptic ulcers and migraine are common in the parents and siblings of children with RAP compared with those without RAP (Apley and Naish, 1958). It is controversial whether children with RAP have children with similar symptoms (Conway, 1951; Christensen and Mortensen, 1975), but there is some evidence that the offspring of adults who complain of abdominal pain, whether or not they experienced abdominal pain in childhood, tend also to complain of abdominal pain (Apley, 1959; Oster, 1972; Christensen and Mortensen, 1975). This may indicate that environmental factors are important in pathogenesis.

The pain is localised at or around the umbilicus or epigastrium, and other localisations of pain should alert the paediatrician to the possibility of an underlying organic disease (Apley and Naish, 1958; Apley, 1959). Physical examination and investigation reveal an organic disease in a small proportion of children with RAP; this is the case in 6 to 7 per cent of children in England (Conway, 1951; Apley, 1959). The relationship between RAP and organic gastrointestinal disease in the developing countries and in immigrants to the developed parts of the world is more complex. For example, Gupta *et al.* (1974) showed that 76 per cent of children with RAP had associated intestinal infections; these observations cannot necessarily reflect a causal relationship between RAP and intestinal infestation since the incidence of bowel infestation in Indian children is particularly high.

As in recurrent vomiting, a relationship between RAP and epilepsy has been suggested. Apley (1959) found that 14 per cent of a group of children with epilepsy had abdominal pains, and there was a slightly higher incidence of convulsions in the families of children with RAP compared with the families of children without pains. Papatheophilou, Jeavons and Disney (1972) found abnormalities of the electroencephalogram in 22 per cent of 50 unselected children with RAP, but only one of these patients developed epilepsy. Apley (1959) reported a similar incidence of electroencephalographic abnormalities in his control groups as in his cases of RAP, and no patients developed epilepsy after follow-up for 20 years. The vast majority of children with RAP do not, therefore, seem to be at risk of developing epilepsy.

Diagnosis

Physical examination and laboratory investigations are usually unrewarding. Stone and Barbero (1970) studied 102 children with RAP who had been extensively investigated and in whom stress seemed to be an important precipitating factor in the development of abdominal pain; the main physical finding was abdominal tenderness on deep palpation at various sites. The proctoscopic findings in 88 of 90 patients investigated were rectal dilatation, mucosal hyperaemia and pallor, oedema and lymphoid hyperplasia. The authors suggest that these findings are compatible with a diagnosis of 'irritable colon syndrome'.

The diagnosis of a functional syndrome is based on the association between a physical complaint and emotional or behavioural symptoms, which include too little as well as too much expression of feelings for the given circumstances, the context in which the symptoms occur and the attitudes of the child and parents to the symptoms. The absence of physical disease can only be taken as a pointer towards stress being a possible alternative cause. To justify a diagnosis of RAP as an emotional or stress disorder, there should be evidence to eliminate organic disease, together with evidence of an emotional disturbance; in addition, a relationship in time between pain and stress and the relief of pain with the reduction in stress both lend weight to the diagnosis (Apley, 1959).

It should be emphasised that the stress is as perceived by the child, not necessarily as seen by the doctor or parent. What is seen as trivial through adult eyes may be interpreted as world-shattering to a child; also some innocent event may be misinterpreted as of worrying significance by a young child of limited experience and understanding. Thus, in addition to careful medical history, examination and investigation, evidence on these psychosocial aspects should be requested from as many sources as relevant, but always from parents, teachers, family doctor and, equally importantly, the child.

Abdominal pain is more likely to be due to organic disease in the preschool child and in those over the age of 10 years, and in children with pain which is localised elsewhere than at the umbilicus (Marshall, 1967). Urinary tract infections must always be excluded in patients with RAP.

Treatment

The basis of treatment is the removal of any stressful factors which may be discovered, and an approach to the whole child and family is required. When the stress results from interactions in the family, therapy aimed to help the whole group may provide indirect relief to the symptom (Berger, 1974). Simple explanatory models of the disorder given to both child and parents are sometimes helpful, though many patients continue to be symptomatic despite these simple measures (Apley and Hale, 1973; Christensen and Mortensen, 1975). A combined paediatric and psychiatric approach may offer longer lasting relief, though this is yet to be put to the test. The reader is referred to Green (1967) for a useful account of the diagnosis and management of recurrent non-organic abdominal pain in childhood.

Prognosis

Two important prospective studies have provided information on the prognosis in children with RAP. Apley and Hale (1973) followed up 30 children for 10 to 14 years who had been treated by simple reassurance and explanations of, and discussions about, their symptoms. This group was compared with 30 untreated patients who had been previously followed up for eight to 20 years (Apley, 1959). At the time of follow-up the patients were aged 15 to 28 years. Nine patients in each group lost their pain and did not develop other symptoms, and nine of the untreated and 10 of the treated groups lost their pain but developed other symptoms such as headaches, 'anxiety', other pains or somatic symptoms. Rather more than a third from each group continued to have abdominal pains and also developed other symptoms. Only three cases, all untreated, developed migraine in adolescence or early adult life. Persistence of pain occurred more often in boys than girls, but more girls developed other symptoms. The younger the child at the onset of symptoms and the longer the delay in treatment tended to worsen the prognosis.

Christensen and Mortensen (1975) studied 34 patients 30 years after they were first investigated and compared them with a randomly selected group of adult subjects who had not experienced RAP in childhood. They found abdominal pains to be a common complaint in the control group of adults (13 out of 45), but significantly less than in the group who had RAP in childhood (18 out of 34). Non-gastrointestinal complaints were also more frequent in the patient group (11 out of 34), especially headache, back pain, 'bad nerves' and gynaecological symptoms; in the control group six out of 45 had similar symptoms. The main difference between the adults who had RAP in childhood compared to those who did not was a tendency to complain more of physical or nervous symptoms generally, and only somewhat more of abdominal pain. Out of the 94 cases of RAP in childhood reported in these two studies only four were found to have organic abdominal disorders in adulthood; one had an ovarian cyst and the other three had duodenal ulcers. In general, therefore, there is a strong tendency for children with RAP to grow up to adults who complain of a variety of gastro-intestinal and other symptoms. When abdominal pain has been associated with vomiting there is a tendency to develop migraine or severe headaches, and a proportion of children with RAP grow up to develop irritable colon type of symptoms.

Pathophysiology

The pathophysiological mechanisms operating in RAP with or without associated vomiting are not known, but a variety of mechanisms may be tentatively postulated. For example, the early attacks may represent the transient somatic correlates of anxiety, depression or anger mediated by autonomic or endocrine systems, or simply physiological responses to ingested material. Local disorders of function such as spasm and associated distention of the gut may play a role. Changes in blood supply may lead to some of the symptoms of the 'periodic syndrome', and the link with migraine later in life supports this view. Symptoms may become conditioned somatic responses to stress; alternatively perpetuation of previously organically determined symptoms, or those with a psychological aetiology, may occur as a result of their reinforcement by the responses of parents or others. Hypochondrial concern by the child may be expressed by complaints of aches and pains, particularly if there are adult models of this type of behaviour in the family. In some children abdominal pain or vomiting can have the quality of hysterical conversion symptoms. In all cases, whatever the origin or mechanism, symptoms may achieve secondary and perhaps adaptive functions by diverting the attention, concern or interest of the child and those caring for him away from the external stress as perceived by the child and on to the physical complaint. The result is that the anxiety-provoking event for the child is curtailed or avoided and at the same time converted into a source of personal attention through the somatic symptom.

DISORDERS OF FAECAL ELIMINATION

Not only may abdominal pain be associated with recurrent vomiting as described earlier, but also with disturbances of large gut function (Dimson, 1971).

Functional disorders of the distal part of the alimentary tract present as faecal retention, diarrhoea or incontinence. In the absence of organic disease, the latter symptom is the one which is commonly considered to be associated with psychiatric problems. Lasting or repeated failure to control the time and place of evacuation of faeces is usually termed encopresis. Incontinence may or may not be accompanied by faecal retention. A careful history and physical examination are most important in deciding on management. Terms such as 'constipation', 'diarrhoea', 'soiling' and 'encopresis' are sometimes interpreted in different ways, not only by parents but also by doctors. For example, gross faecal retention with continuous perianal leaking of faecal-stained mucus may be attributed to 'diarrhoea', without performing a physical examination.

Diarrhoea

In childhood, the 'irritable colon' syndrome may result in a variety of symptoms depending on the child's age (Davidson, 1973). Thus, as well as recurrent abdominal pain in later childhood, colic in early infancy and chronic non-specific diarrhoea in the toddler period can be seen as manifestations of the irritable colon syndrome at various stages of development.

Davidson and Wasserman (1966) described 186 children with persistent diarrhoea having excluded the major organic diseases. The onset of diarrhoea was between the age of 6 and 20 months in 75 per cent of cases. Many of the patients were previously regarded as constipated and about a quarter had been colicky babies. The diarrhoea resolved by the age of 39 months in over 90 per cent of cases, many becoming constipated afterwards. Sixty-seven per cent of the parents and half of the siblings had functional bowel problems.

Typically the child had three to four bowel movements in the early part of the day, the first stool being large, formed or partly formed; subsequently motions were smaller, looser and contained more mucus and vegetable fibres if vegetable matter was in the diet. The presence of extracellular starch granules in the faeces was seen to be due to the rapid transit rather than a sign of starch intolerance. No evidence was found that diet played any part in this condition, nor were there any general or specific signs of malabsorption. The diagnosis is more or less given by the occurrence of three to six mucusy loose stools per day in an otherwise healthy 1- to 3-year-old child of normal growth and development, especially if there is a family history of functional disorders of the gastrointestinal tract. Davidson and Wasserman (1966) proposed that these functional symptoms in children should be identified as similar to the irritable colon syndrome in adults and suggested that the same diagnostic label be used. In those cases where there is doubt about the adequacy of weight, stature or rate of growth, tests for malabsorption should obviously also be carried out. The normality of simple routine investigations (e.g. stool microscopy and culture, haemoglobin and white blood count, and urine microscopy and culture) provides the necessary backing for the diagnosis. When there is doubt about the nutritional status of the child further investigations should be performed to exclude an underlying malabsorptive state.

Management is mainly by demonstration to the parents that no serious pathology is present, that the diarrhoea itself does not undermine the child's nutrition or health, and by reassurance that the condition is self-limiting. There is no evidence that dietary manipulations, anticholinergic agents or antibiotics provide symptomatic relief to children with this benign self-limiting disorder.

Encopresis

The prevalence of encopresis in patients treated in child psychiatric departments has varied from 2·9 to 10 per cent (Shirley, 1938; Vaughan and Cashmore, 1954; Olatawura, 1973); these figures are affected to some extent by the known interests of the clinic or psychiatrist. Shirley (1963) also gives a figure of 1·5 per cent for the incidence of encopresis in cases referred from a paediatric clinic to a Child Guidance Clinic. In a study of the general population in Stockholm, Bellman (1966) found an overall incidence of 1·5 per cent in children between 7 and 8 years of age; the incidence in boys (2·3 per cent) was greater than in girls (0·7 per cent) with a ratio of 3·4 to 1. These findings probably underestimate the magnitude of the problem, due to a reserve in reporting the symptom. Bellman (1966) also found a history of soiling in childhood in 15 per cent of fathers of the encopretic children, in 1·3 per cent of their mothers, and in four out of 77 siblings aged 4 years or more, all of whom were boys; none of the members of the families of the control group had been troubled.

The presence or absence of faecal retention and the association of other symptoms, personality characteristics, the parents' attitudes, and whether the encopresis is continuous with infancy soiling or not, are all factors which require different approaches and which have varying prognoses.

Aetiological factors and classification

In one of the first attempts to define the aetiological factors and to formulate a classification, Anthony (1957) considered some of the factors which might interfere with the successful learning of how to defaecate in an appropriate place in an acceptable manner, i.e. the level of intelligence, emotional disturbances, the occurrence of other and even apparently unrelated traumatic experiences, frequent changes of environment during the training period and organic gastrointestinal diseases, particularly those associated with diarrhoea. The patients were classified into one of three groups according to certain criteria:

Group 1 The continuity or discontinuity of the encopresis with the period of toilet training.
Group 2 The association or dissociation of the encopresis with enuresis.
Group 3 The presence or absence of faecal retention either as a persistent or an intermittent phenomenon

Out of a group of 76 patients with encopresis who had been referred to a psychiatric department, 30 had never been continent, 30 became incontinent following a period of continence during infancy and 16 had faecal retention. An attempt was made to relate the type of encopresis with the toilet training methods used and the personalities of the parents. For example in group 1 children with the continuous type of encopresis were described as 'a dirty child from a dirty family', whereas the discontinuous type tended to occur in the overcontrolled and inhibited child from a compulsive and obsessionally rigid family.

The association of encopresis with faecal retention was frequently associated with attempts at early or coercive toilet training regimes, and a 'battle of the bowel' struggle with the mother.

In contrast to these observations, others have found this classification too simple and inadequate in encompassing all their patients. For example, Olatawura (1973) found that 26 out of 32 cases referred to a psychiatric clinic because of soiling were of the discontinuous type, and these were predominantly from 'socially incompetent' and lower socioeconomic families; also in contrast to Anthony (1957) and Woodmansey (1972), this study did not find a relationship between coercive toilet training and encopresis.

Woodmansey (1972) includes a developmental category of faecal incontinence in infants with the continuous type of encopresis and suggests that this may be secondary to an immaturity of sphincter control; this may be due to the manifestations of an anxiety state which may be of two main types, 'reactive incontinence' which is part of a non-specific fear response, or 'paradoxical incontinence' due to a specific fear of incontinence engendered by exhortation, coercion and punishment of soiling. It is suggested that the mechanism of the incontinence may be related to anxiety factors and increased colonic motility. Woodmansey (1967) describes four stages of severity in the development of faecal retention in association with incontinence:

1. 'Respite soiling', i.e. stools of normal consistency passed at 'care-free' times and situations, often away from the mother and/or toilet.
2. Inhibition of defaecation generalised to all places with subsequent exigency soiling.
3. 'Displacement soiling', i.e. rectum never empty with the involuntary passage of small amounts of faeces.
4. Faecal retention (constipation) with overflow, i.e. firm faeces impacted in the rectum with perianal leaking of faecal-stained mucus around the faecal masses.

Berg and Jones (1964) reviewed 78 children with encopresis and describe four classified groups:

1. Training problems without severe faecal retention.
2. A 'pot refusal retention syndrome', i.e. similar to group 1 but the faecal retention resulting in rectal and colonic distention as in 'psychogenic megacolon' (Richmond, Eddy and Garrard, 1954); this group of patients often had a history of attempted coercion by the parents.
3. Progressive or severe faecal retention with overflow; this group often attempted to use the toilet but were unsuccessful for mechanical reasons.
4. Faecal incontinence in the absence of retention, i.e. the passage of normal stools at inappropriate times and places. This group was further subdivided into (i) children in whom there seemed to be a causal relationship between stress and incontinence, and (ii) children in whom there seemed to be an instability of neuromuscular control which was related to faecal incontinence.

Differential diagnosis

The exclusion of organic disease is particularly important in children with faecal retention. Tobon and Schuster (1974) reviewed 100 consecutive patients with a diagnosis of megacolon and found that 40 had Hirschsprung's disease and 60 had idiopathic megacolon. On clinical examination anal sphincter tone was usually normal or increased in those with Hirschsprung's disease, whereas in idiopathic megacolon tone was normal or decreased. Encopresis occurred in 45 per cent of cases with idiopathic megacolon, and not at all in Hirschsprung's disease. The most discriminating investigation was rectal manometry; the histological appearances of the rectum and barium enema were most useful when they provided positive findings (i.e. the demonstration of ganglion cells or a contracted segment of gut). Many of the children with idiopathic megacolon had personality disorders in contrast to those with Hirschsprung's disease.

Lawson and Clayden (1974) describe a group of children with a history of constipation dating from birth ('congenital constipation') in whom no organic disease could be demonstrated; anorectal manometry studies showed an exaggerated rhythmic activity, with inhibition occurring only in response to supranormal distention of the rectum in association with a reduced sensation of the wish to defaecate. In this type of constipation reduced colonic transit of faeces with increased fluid absorption may result in firm faeces and retention (Devroede and Soffie, 1973). An increase in colonic transit time also occurs in children with recurrent abdominal pain (Dimson, 1971).

Treatment

Woodmansey (1967, 1972) suggests that parents should be dissuaded from 'training', coercion or punishment. Toilet training is probably unnecessary and a normal child who is on good terms with his parents will wish to adopt their toilet habits when his sphincter control is mature. The continuation of infantile incontinence beyond the age of 3 to 4 years may require only simple discussion. Berg and Jones (1964) found that simple explanations of why the child was not using the toilet often sufficed, and suggested that this may be partly because of the child's recognition that the parents were sufficiently concerned to seek outside advice. Some children, however, come from chaotic families and in these circumstances some regular training is necessary (Anthony, 1957). In some of these families there may be long-standing stresses, and there may be other associated psychiatric symptoms in the child and other members of the family (Bemporad *et al.*, 1971; Hoag *et al.*, 1971); management involves advice on the family interactions as a whole, sometimes combined successfully with a toilet training programme.

Those children who have a period of bowel control in their preschool years but later become incontinent as a result of some acute or chronic stress in the family or school, hospitalisation, or specific illness will usually also show other signs of an emotional or behavioural disturbance. These disturbances include a fear of the toilet, separation anxieties sometimes associated with school refusal, regressive behaviour, tension, aggression or depression particularly when there are embittered, separating or separated parents. These children are usually deeply disturbed and in need of psychotherapy (Anthony, 1957). Woodmansey (1967, 1972) regards anxiety as the predominant emotional state in these patients and advocates a 'rescue approach', i.e. rescuing the child from whatever is already happening to him (e.g. coercion, exhortation and punishment over toilet training). In older children psychotherapy is the treatment of choice, with some form of psychotherapeutic approach to the parents as well (Berg and Jones, 1964; Woodmansey, 1972).

Mechanical emptying of the rectum may be necessary in patients with severe faecal retention. In less severe cases, when chronic distention of the rectum has not become established, a combination of a faecal softening agent and a laxative is often sufficient (Berg and Jones, 1964). Lawson and Clayden (1974) claim that anal dilatation under general anaesthesia leads to improvement in the majority of children with 'congenital constipation'. Nixon's regime (1961) includes manual evacuation under general anaesthesia in severe causes of megacolon and daily rectal washouts with saline followed by aperients and regular toilet training. The reader is referred to Neale (1963) and Young (1973) for accounts of toilet training programmes.

Prognosis

The prognosis in children with encopresis is generally good, and only a few patients remain symptomatic after puberty, and these usually have severe psychiatric disorders. Berg and Jones (1964) found that 87 per cent of their cases went into permanent remission after only a few months' treatment. Bellman (1966) reported that 56 per cent of patients were symptom-free for over six months after the discontinuation of treatment two years previously.

CONCLUDING REMARKS

Several lines of evidence suggest that autonomic reactivity patterns are established in early infancy, but it is not clear what effects mechanical factors or emotional stress have on the developing control systems of the infant's alimentary tract. It is possible that functional disorders of the gastrointestinal tract may start insidiously and be concurrent with the setting up of a deviant balance in the autonomic control of the infant's tract. Subsequently some of these minor deviations of function may be more prone to become exaggerated and develop into lasting symptomatic disorders as a result of the influence of environmental circumstances or events.

It is not coincidental that the major functional disorders affect the ends of the gastrointestinal tract. Although changes in autonomic balance may occur throughout the tract, it is at the proximal and distal ends that such changes have their impact on the external environment. It is likely that the responses of the key people in that environment play an important part in determining the course of these functional disorders. Similarly, abdominal pain, whatever its origins, is a complaint to the important people in the child's environment, and the responses of those people need to be considered carefully when the symptom is recurrent.

References

Anthony, E. J. (1957) An experimental approach to the psychopathology of childhood: encopresis. *British Journal of Medical Psychology*, **30**, 146.

Apley, J. (1959) The child with abdominal pains. Oxford: Blackwell Scientific Publications.

Apley, J. & Hale, B. (1973) Children with recurrent pain. How do they grow up? *British Medical Journal*, **3**, 7.

Apley, J. & MacKeith, R. (1962) The child and his symptoms. Oxford: Blackwell Scientific Publications.

Apley, J. & Naish, J. M. (1958) Recurrent abdominal pains: a field survey of 1000 school children. *Archives of Disease in Childhood*, **33**, 165.

Bellman, M. (1966) Studies on encopresis. *Acta Paediatrica Scandinavica* suppl. 170, 1.

Bemporad, J. R., Pfeifer, C. M., Gibbs, L., Cortner, R. H. & Bloom, W. (1971) Characteristics of encopretic patients and their families. *Journal of American Academy of Child Psychiatry*, **10**, 272.

Berg, I. & Jones, K. V. (1964) Functional faecal incontinence in children. *Archives of Disease in Childhood*, **39**, 465.

Berger, H. G. (1974) Somatic pain and school avoidance. *Clinical Pediatrics* (Philadelphia), **13**, 819.

Christensen, M. F. & Mortensen, O. (1975) The long term prognosis in children with recurrent abdominal pain. *Archives of Disease in Childhood*, **50**, 110.

Conway, D. J. (1951) A study of abdominal pain in childhood. *Great Ormond Street Journal*, **1**, 99.

Cullen, J. J. & MacDonald, W. B. (1963) The periodic syndrome: its nature and prevalence. *Medical Journal of Australia*, **50**, 167.

Davidson, M. (1973) Irritable colon in children. In *Gastrointestinal Disease*. Chap. 101, p. 1289. Ed. Sleisenger, M. H. and Fordtran, J. S. Philadelphia, London, Toronto: W. B. Saunders Co.

Davidson, M. & Wasserman, R. (1966) The irritable colon of childhood. *Journal of Paediatrics*, **69**, 6.

Devroede, G. & Soffie, M. (1973) Colonic absorption in idiopathic constipation. *Gastroenterology*, **64**, 552.

Dimson, S. B. (1971) Transit time related to clinical findings in children with recurrent abdominal pain. *Pediatrics*, **47**, 666.

Farquhar, H. G. (1956) Abdominal migraine in children. *British Medical Journal*, **1**, 1082.

Green, M. (1967) Diagnosis and treatment. Psychogenic recurrent abdominal pain. *Pediatrics*, **40**, 84.

Gupta, S., Agarwal, H. C., Bhardwaj, O. P. & Gupta, J. P. (1974) Recurrent abdominal pain in children. *Indian Pediatrics*, **11**, 115.

Hammond, J. (1974) The late sequelae of recurrent vomiting of childhood. *Developmental Medicine and Child Neurology*, **16**, 15.

Hoag, J. M., Norriss, N. C., Himeno, E. T. & Jacobs, J. (1971) The encopretic child and his family. *Journal of the American Academy of Child Psychiatry*, **10**, 242.

Hoyt, C. S. & Stickler, G. B. (1960) A study of 44 children with the syndrome of recurrent (cyclic) vomiting. *Pediatrics*, **25**, 775.

Lawson, J. O. N. & Clayden, G. S. (1974) Physiological aspects and treatment of severe chronic constipation. *Archives of Disease in Childhood*, **49**, 245.

MacKeith, R. & Pampiglione, G. (1956) Recurrent syndrome. Clinical and E.E.G. observations. *Electroencephalography and Clinical Neurophysiology*, **8**, 161.

Marshall, D. G. (1967) Recurrent abdominal pain in children: a surgeons viewpoint. *Pediatrics*, **40**, 1024.

Millichap, J. G., Lombroso, C. T. & Lennox, W. G. (1955) Cyclic vomiting as a form of epilepsy in children. *Pediatrics*, **15**, 705.

Naish, J. M. & Apley, J. (1951) 'Growing pains': a clinical study of non-arthritic limb pains in children. *Archives of Disease in Childhood*, **26**, 134.

Neale, D. H. (1963) Behaviour therapy and encopresis in children. *Behaviour Research and Therapy*, **1**, 139.

Nixon, H. H. (1961) Discussion on megacolon and megarectum with the emphasis on conditions other than Hirschsprung's disease. *Proceedings of the Royal Society of Medicine*, **54**, 1037.

Olatawura, M. O. (1973) Encopresis. Review of 32 cases. *Acta Paediatrica Scandinavica*, **62**, 358.

Oster, J. (1972) Recurrent abdominal pain and other pains. *Pediatrics*, **50**, 429.

Papatheophilou, R., Jeavons, P. M. & Disney, M. E. (1972) Recurrent abdominal pain: a clinical and electroencephalographic study. *Developmental Medicine and Child Neurology*, **14**, 31.

Richmond, J., Eddy, E. & Garrard, S. (1954) The syndrome of fecal soiling and megacolon. *American Journal of Orthopsychiatry*, **24**, 391.

Rutter, M., Tizard, J. & Whitmore, K. (1970) *Education, Health and Behaviour*, p. 206, London: Longman.

Shirley, H. F. (1938) Encopresis in children. *Journal of Pediatrics*, **12**, 367.

Shirley, H. F. (1963) *Pediatric Psychiatry*. Cambridge: Harvard University Press.

Smith, C. H. (1937) Recurrent vomiting in children. *Journal of Pediatrics*, **10**, 719.

Stone, R. T. & Barbero, G. J. (1970) Recurrent abdominal pain in childhood. *Pediatrics*, **45**, 732.

Tobon, F. & Schuster, M. M. (1974) Megacolon special diagnostic and therapeutic features. *The Johns Hopkins Medical Journal*, **135**, 91.

Vaughan, G. F. & Cashmore, A. A. (1954) Encopresis in childhood. *Guys Hospital Reports*, **103**, 360.

Woodmansey, A. (1967) Emotion and the motion: an enquiry into the causes and prevention of functional disorders of defaecation. *British Journal of Medical Psychology*, **40**, 207.

Woodmansey, A. (1972) Emotional problems in childhood and adolescence. Wetting and soiling. *British Medical Journal*, **3**, 161.

Wyllie, W. G. & Schlesinger, B. (1933) The periodic group of disorders in childhood. *British Journal of Childrens Diseases*, **30**, 1.

Young, G. C. (1973) The treatment of childhood encopresis by conditioned gastro-ileal reflex training. *Behaviour Research and Therapy*, **11**, 499.

PART 3

15. Inborn errors of hepatic metabolism

R. J. West and June K. Lloyd

Disorders of amino acid metabolism
Lipid storage disorders
Disorders of carbohydrate metabolism
Familial disorders of bilirubin metabolism
Abnormalities of metal metabolism
Hepatic porphyrias

Many metabolic processes are carried out in the liver and several inborn errors involving hepatic enzymes are known. In this chapter only those which result in clinical evidence of disturbed liver function or present with gastrointestinal symptoms will be considered. Most of the 'storage' disorders are not included even though considerable hepatomegaly may be a feature, as individually they are rare, and the main features are not primarily gastrointestinal. No attempt has been made to give a comprehensive review of the biochemical and genetic basis of the disorders, but some biochemistry has been included for comprehension of the essential diagnostic tests and rationale of treatment.

DISORDERS OF AMINO ACID METABOLISM

Defects of tyrosine metabolism

Biochemistry

Free tyrosine in plasma and other body fluids is derived mainly by conversion from dietary or endogenous phenylalanine and from the peptide-bound tyrosine in proteins. It is oxidised in the tissues, particularly in the liver; the main steps in the catabolic pathway are shown in Figure 15.1. Tyrosine filtered through the renal glomerulus is almost completely reabsorbed in the proximal tubule and very little free amino acid appears in the urine. Tyrosine metabolites, however, are rapidly secreted by the renal tubule and accumulation of tyrosine in the blood will result in their appearance in the urine. The urinary excretion pattern of metabolites varies in the different disorders of tyrosine metabolism. The subject has been comprehensively reviewed by Scriver and Rosenberg (1973a).

Defects of tyrosine oxidation may result from genetically determined deficiencies of specific enzymes or be secondary to hepatic damage. Hereditary tyrosinaemia is itself associated with liver damage, and the distinction between this disorder and tyrosinaemia secondary to liver disease may be difficult but is important for both genetic and therapeutic reasons. Disturbances of tyrosine

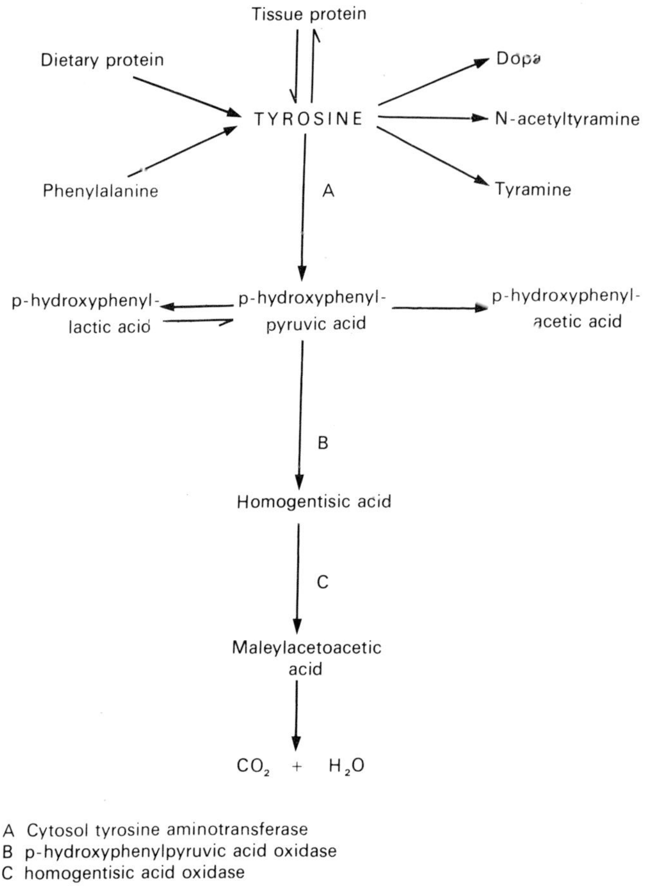

Fig. 15.1 Metabolism of tyrosine

metabolism can also occur in a variety of other disorders such as scurvy, hyperthyroidism and cystic fibrosis. Only neonatal tyrosinaemia and hereditary tyrosinaemia will be considered in further detail.

Neonatal tyrosinaemia

This is probably the most common amino acid disorder in man. It is due to partial impairment of p-hydroxyphenylpyruvic acid oxidase (PHPPA) activity and occurs in up to 30 per cent of preterm infants and in up to 10 per cent of full-term infants (Avery *et al.*, 1967; Levy *et al.*, 1969). Males are more likely to be affected than females.

The diet of the newborn infant with a protein intake greater than 5 g/kg/day contains a relatively large amount of tyrosine, and in affected infants plasma tyrosine reaches its peak towards the end of the first week of life and may exceed 2 mM (36 mg/100 ml) in concentration (normal $< 0{\cdot}07$ mM). In most affected babies hypertyrosinaemia is a transient phenomenon, but in a few may persist for several weeks. The urine contains excessive amounts of p-hydroxyphenyl-acetic, -lactic and -pyruvic acids as well as tyrosine and n-acetyl tyrosine. Neonatal tyrosinaemia can usually be easily distinguished from other forms of tyrosinaemia, as a prompt reduction in plasma tyrosine will occur in most infants by reducing protein intake to 2 to 3 g/kg/day or by giving ascorbic acid 50 to 100 mg/day.

The prognosis is generally considered to be excellent, but lethargy has been noted in some premature infants (Avery *et al.*, 1967), and impaired mental development in later childhood has been reported (Menkes *et al.*, 1972). Affected infants should certainly be treated with additional ascorbic acid and/or reduced protein intake, and premature infants should routinely receive adequate ascorbic acid supplements.

Hereditary tyrosinaemia

The term hereditary tyrosinaemia is now used in preference to that of 'tyrosinosis' as it seems certain that the condition originally described as 'tyrosinosis' by Medes (1932) was a disorder of tyrosine transaminase activity with a benign prognosis (Scriver and Rosenberg, 1973a).

Clinical features. Two clinical patterns occur, an acute and a chronic form; both may be found within the same family and it is thought that the mutant allele is the same (Bodegard *et al.*, 1969). Inheritance is autosomal recessive.

The acute form (Larochelle *et al.*, 1967) presents within the first six months of life. Hepatomegaly occurs in the majority, and fever, anorexia, vomiting, diarrhoea, oedema and bleeding episodes are common early features. In some children a peculiar cabbage-like odour has been reported. About one-third of patients are jaundiced, but this symptom occurs relatively late. Liver failure is usually rapidly progressive and about 90 per cent of untreated children die.

The chronic form presents in later infancy or childhood with nodular hepatic cirrhosis and a renal tubular lesion which results in hypophosphataemic rickets. Hepatic carcinoma develops in some patients.

Laboratory findings. Plasma concentrations of tyrosine and phenylalanine are raised; high levels of methionine may also occur, especially in the acute form, and are due, at least in part, to liver damage. The urine contains excessive amounts of tyrosine metabolites with p-hydroxyphenylacetic and -lactic acids predominating. Tests of liver function are abnormal. The prothrombin and partial thromboplastin times are grossly prolonged as is the bleeding time. Generalised aminoaciduria, glycosuria, proteinuria and phosphaturia reflect renal tubular damage, and plasma inorganic phosphorus may be low. Hypoglycaemia is common and may be severe. There is usually a normocytic anaemia and polymorphonuclear leucocytosis. In the chronic form X-rays may show rickets.

Differential diagnosis. Failure to respond to ascorbic acid distinguishes the disorder from neonatal tyrosinaemia. Differentiation from tyrosinaemia secondary to liver disease may be difficult, but renal tubular lesions and severe haemorrhages are less likely in primary liver disorders. Galactosaemia and hereditary fructose intolerance may present with similar features but are usually easily differentiated.

Treatment and prognosis. Dietary phenylalanine, tyrosine and if necessary methionine should be restricted (Hill, Nordin and Zaleski, 1970). Frequent feeding may be needed to prevent hypoglycaemia and vitamin D given if rickets is manifest. Vitamin K should be administered, but it usually fails to correct totally the haemorrhagic diathesis and blood transfusions may be required.

Clinical improvement in the acute form usually occurs rapidly, but severe relapses with intercurrent infections are to be expected. Treatment in the chronic form can reverse the nephropathy. Dietary treatment probably has to be continued indefinitely; in cases in which cessation of treatment has been possible (Harries *et al.*, 1969) it is likely that the disorder had a different basis.

Disorders of the urea cycle

Biochemistry

The biosynthesis of urea from ammonia involves five steps (Table 15.1). The liver is the only organ containing the complete urea cycle, though individual enzymes are found in other tissues, such as the small intestine which contains some ornithine transcarbamylase. All defects in the urea cycle result in hyperammonaemia, and ornithine, citrulline, arginosuccinic acid or arginine may accumulate in the plasma depending upon the site of the block. Five inherited disorders have so far been described (Table 15.1) and are comprehensively reviewed by Shih and Efron (1972) and Scriver and Rosenberg (1973b). Hyperammonaemia also occurs in inherited disorders not primarily involving the urea cycle such as hyperornithinaemia, proprionicacidaemia, methylmalonicacidaemia, lysine dehydrogenase deficiency and familial protein intolerance. In addition hyperammonaemia is also found in severe acquired liver

Table 15.1 Urea cycle disorders

Biochemical step	Enzyme	Disorder	Genetics
Ammonia + bicarbonate + 2ATP → carbamyl phosphate + 2ADP + Pi	Carbamyl phosphate synthetase (CPS)	CPS deficiency (congenital hyperammonaemia type I)	?
Carbamyl phosphate + ornithine → citrulline + Pi	Ornithine carbamyl transferase (OCT)	OCT deficiency (congenital hyperammonaemia type II)	? X-linked dominant
Citrulline + aspartate + ATP → arginosuccinic acid + AMP + PP	Arginosuccinic acid synthetase	Citrullinaemia	Autosomal recessive
Arginosuccinic acid → arginine + fumaric acid	Arginosuccinase	Arginosuccinicaciduria	Autosomal recessive
Arginine + H_2O → urea + ornithine	Arginase	Hyperargininaemia	Autosomal recessive

disease where it is due partly to hepatocellular failure and partly to portal systemic vascular shunting.

Clinical features

Symptoms common to all the urea cycle disorders include vomiting in infancy and a dislike of protein foods, irritability, lethargy, convulsions and coma, episodes of ataxia, and mental retardation. There is a wide variation in severity and age of onset of symptoms. In all types a rapidly fatal course may occur in the neonatal period.

Laboratory findings

The highest blood levels of ammonia occur in carbamylphosphate synthetase (CPS) and ornithine carbamyl transferase (OCT) deficiencies. In CPS deficiency ketoacidosis and cyclic neutropaenia have also been reported. Plasma and urinary glutamine are usually raised in OCT deficiency. In the other disorders the appropriate amino acid is found in excess in plasma and urine. Blood urea concentration is usually normal in all the disorders. The diagnosis can usually be suspected by estimation of blood ammonia and plasma and urine amino acid analyses, but since hyperammonaemia can occur in a variety of other disorders, assay of the urea cycle enzymes is necessary to establish the definitive diagnosis, especially in CPS and OCT deficiency.

Treatment

Dietary protein restriction (1·0–1·5 g/kg/day) may control the hyperammonaemia, gastrointestinal and neurological features. Peritoneal dialysis and exchange transfusion have been used in acutely ill children who have gross hyperammonaemia.

LIPID STORAGE DISORDERS

Hepatomegaly resulting from storage of lipid may occur due to a number of specific inherited enzyme defects. However, only in Wolman's disease are gastrointestinal symptoms prominent.

Wolman's disease (acid esterase deficiency)

Biochemistry

The disorder is due to deficiency of lysosomal acid esterase resulting in accumulation of cholesteryl esters and triglycerides in many organs, especially in the liver and intestinal mucosa (Patrick and Lake, 1973). The esterase can be estimated in leucocytes. Prenatal diagnosis can be made from fibroblasts in aminotic fluid (Patrick, personal communication). The mode of inheritance is autosomal recessive and heterozygotes can be identified by leucocyte enzyme estimations.

Clinical features

Patients usually present within the first few months of life with vomiting, diarrhoea, failure to gain weight and progressive abdominal enlargement with hepatomegaly (Wolman *et al.*, 1961); most have a rapidly downhill course and die in the first year. Some patients may present in later childhood with hepatomegaly only (Patrick and Lake, 1973).

Laboratory findings

Peripheral blood films show lipid droplets in lymphocytes. The bone marrow may contain foamy histiocytes, and the intestinal mucosa shows gross lipid deposition in histiocytes in the lamina propria. Liver biopsy should not be necessary since a definitive diagnosis can be made by leucocyte enzyme assay.

X-rays may show adrenal calcification. Abnormalities of the serum lipids and lipoproteins may occur but are non-specific; malabsorption of fat and fat-soluble vitamins is likely if there is much intestinal involvement; tests of liver function may be abnormal in the later stages of the disease.

Treatment

No specific treatment is yet available, but symptomatic treatment of the malabsorption may improve the nutritional state. We are treating one boy, whose brother died at 14 months, with general supportive measures together with an increased dietary cholesterol intake (in the form of eggs) in an attempt to cut down endogenous hepatic cholesterol synthesis. At the age of 8 years he is of short stature and still has gross hepatomegaly but is symptom-free and attends a normal school (unpublished observations).

DISORDERS OF CARBOHYDRATE METABOLISM

Hepatic glycogen storage diseases

Biochemistry

Glycogen is normally formed from glucose postprandially and is stored principally in the liver and muscles. Hepatic glycogen is broken down during periods of fasting to liberate glucose into the blood. Many enzymes are involved in glycogen synthesis and breakdown, and the glycogen storage diseases can be classified into types depending on which enzyme is deficient (Table 15.2). Glycogen storage diseases are the commonest storage disorders causing

Table 15.2 Glycogen storage disease with hepatic involvement

Type[a]	Biochemical step	Enzyme deficiency
1	Glucose-6-phosphate → glucose	Glucose-6-phosphatase
3	Glycogen → glucose, by hydrolysis of 1:4 glucose linkages in glycogen molecule	Debrancher enzyme
6	Glycogen → glucose, by splitting of 1:6 glucose linkages in glycogen molecule	Phosphorylase
4	Formation of 1:4 glucose linkages in glycogen synthesis	Brancher enzyme

[a] Types 1, 3 and 6 are concerned with breakdown of hepatic glycogen and type 4 with hepatic glycogen synthesis. Types 2 and 5 do not have significant liver involvement and are therefore not included in this table.

Table 15.3 Clinical features in 24 patients with hepatic glycogen storage disease seen at The Hospital for Sick Children, London 1970–1974

		Clinical features (No. affected)				
Type	No. of patients	Hepatomegaly	Short stature	Diarrhoea	Hypoglycaemia	Acidosis
1	5	5	2	2	4	3
3	8	8	7	0	3	1
6	2	2	0	1	0	0
not typed	9	9	6	4	6	6
Total	24	24	15	7	13	10

hepatomegaly. In types 1, 3 and 6, the breakdown of glycogen is defective, and glycogen accumulates in the liver. In type 4 an abnormal glycogen is formed because of brancher enzyme deficiency.

Clinical features

Types 1, 3 and 6 together are the commonest forms of hepatic glycogen storage disease. There is great variability in their clinical manifestations, and the principal features found in a series of patients seen at The Hospital for Sick Children, Great Ormond Street, London are shown in Table 15.3. Symptoms of hypoglycaemia may be the presenting feature in early infancy particularly in type 1. Acidosis, manifest clinically by vomiting and by deep and rapid respirations, occurs on fasting in some children and may accompany hypoglycaemia. Both hypoglycaemia and acidosis are likely to be exaggerated by intercurrent infection. In all children the liver is enlarged, smooth and firm, the enlargement being partly due to stored glycogen and partly to excess fat, and in many children hepatomegaly is the presenting feature. In infants and young children the enlargement may extend to the level of the iliac crest; during childhood the liver decreases in relative size, and enlargement may become inconspicuous by the time of adolescence. Splenomegaly rarely occurs; renal enlargement due to the deposition of glycogen is common and occasionally clinically evident. Most children with hepatic glycogen storage disease are short and many are obese. Short stature is most marked in children in whom control of hypoglycaemia or acidosis has proved difficult. Chronic diarrhoea during infancy has been a feature in several of our patients. The mechanism is uncertain; sugar malabsorption has not been detected but it is known that steatorrhoea may occur in glycogen storage disease occasionally (Spencer-Peet *et al.*, 1971). Eruptive xanthomata, most marked over extensor surfaces, are seen in occasional patients and are associated with hyperlipidaemia.

In type 4 glycogen storage disease, which is very rare, the abnormal glycogen induces a rapidly progressive cirrhosis with death in early childhood.

Laboratory findings

In those children with hypoglycaemia raised plasma levels of lactate, pyruvate and uric acid are commonly found. Secondary hyperlipidaemia occurs in most patients.

Diagnosis

Investigation can be considered in two stages: firstly, the demonstration of an abnormality in storage of glycogen and, secondly, the delineation of the enzyme defect present. Presumptive evidence of an abnormality in mobilisation of glycogen can often be obtained by showing that injected glucagon causes a subnormal rise in blood glucose in the fasting patient; in occasional patients a normal response is obtained. Red cell glycogen concentration is elevated in debrancher enzyme defects. Other biochemical tests, including response to glucagon after a carbohydrate meal, or a galactose load, may help to define the metabolic block (Cornblath and Schwartz, 1966a), but as there are often biochemical inconsistencies, typing should be by demonstration of the enzyme deficiency. Debrancher enzyme can be measured in leucocytes; if this is normal a liver biopsy should be obtained for histology and histochemistry, glycogen content and assay of glucose-6-phosphate and phosphorylase activity. In spite of full investigation a definite type cannot be ascertained in a significant proportion of children with glycogen storage disease (Table 15.3).

Treatment

In infancy the major management problems are usually due to hypoglycaemia and acidosis. Frequent feeds, sometimes as often as every two hours, of a high carbohydrate diet together with bicarbonate supplements will usually control these features. Gradual improvement can be expected after the first few years of life and prognosis for survival is good. Short stature is a continuing problem in many patients; experimental treatment with continuous intragastric or intravenous feeding (Folkman *et al.*, 1972; Greene *et al.*, 1975), portacaval shunt (Starzl *et al.*, 1973), and clofibrate (Greene *et al.*, 1975) have been reported to improve growth and decrease hepatomegaly.

Galactosaemia

Biochemistry

Galactose, formed from lactose in the diet, is normally phosphorylated in the body and converted to glucose by the action of the enzyme galactose 1-phosphate uridyl transferase. Galactosaemia is a rare autosomal recessive disorder in which uridyl transferase activity is deficient, and in consequence galactose and its metabolites accumulate in many tissues.

Clinical features

Affected children are normal at birth, only becoming unwell after milk feeding is started. There is wide variation in severity of presenting symptoms; the most commonly recognised features, which usually start in the first week of life, are vomiting and failure to thrive, hepatic enlargement and jaundice. If lactose ingestion continues there is progressive deterioration with wasting and liver failure. Splenomegaly and ascites may develop due to cirrhosis and portal hypertension. Most children develop cataracts; occasionally these may be an isolated feature. There is developmental delay. Untreated infants may have severe electrolyte disturbances and are prone to severe infection. Several cases have been reported in which the diagnosis of galactosaemia was established after the child had died of neonatal septicaemia (Shih *et al.*, 1971).

Laboratory findings
Provided the child is ingesting sufficient milk a reducing substance may be detected in the urine, which on further analysis is found to be galactose. As galactosuria may occur secondarily to liver disease this finding is not diagnostic. Proteinuria and aminoaciduria are common. Hyperbilirubinaemia, raised serum liver enzymes, abnormal clotting and hyperchloraemic acidosis frequently occur. Total blood sugar is normal or even high (due to galactose) but true glucose concentration may be reduced.

Diagnosis
Galactosaemia should be considered in a wide variety of clinical situations. Whenever the diagnosis is suspected estimation of erythrocyte uridyl transferase activity should be made. This investigation should also be carried out on cord blood of all infants in whom there is a positive family history. Milk feeds should be withheld until the result is known.

Treatment and prognosis
Dietary lactose and galactose must be excluded. In infancy treatment is relatively easy, as a proprietary lactose-free milk such as Galactomin or Nutramigen can be used. It must be remembered, however, that many medicaments including some vitamin preparations contain lactose. Once a mixed diet is begun it is more difficult to prevent the inadvertent consumption of lactose-containing foods and to provide a varied and balanced diet; the services of a dietitian are invaluable.

Although restriction of dietary lactose will be necessary for life, in later childhood it is usually possible to widen the diet by including small amounts of lactose-containing foods (Komrower and Lee, 1970). If detected early and adequately treated, children with galactosaemia should develop normally both physically and mentally. Untreated the majority die in early infancy.

Hereditary fructose intolerance

Biochemistry
Dietary fructose is converted in the liver to glucose, by the action of fructose-1-phosphate aldolase. Hereditary fructose intolerance is a rare autosomal recessive disorder in which there is reduced activity of this enzyme so that when fructose or sucrose is fed there is build up of fructose-1-phosphate, and fructosaemia and fructosuria may occur. Secondary hypoglycaemia results from inhibition of hepatic glucose release.

Clinical features
Symptoms do not occur in wholly breast-fed infants but date from the time of introduction of feeds containing sucrose, or the ingestion of fruit. Vomiting, abdominal pain and symptoms of hypoglycaemia may occur within a few hours of the ingestion of fructose-containing foods. If the infant continues to take the offending sugars there is failure to thrive and sometimes hepatomegaly, jaundice, proteinuria and aminoaciduria. As symptoms can be abolished by withdrawal of fructose and sucrose from the diet, some affected children, or

their mothers, voluntarily select a diet low in sugar so that the clinical presentation may be much delayed.

Diagnosis

If the diagnosis is suspected a fructose-loading test should be carried out (Cornblath and Schwarz, 1966b). The fructose is given intravenously (0·25 g/kg) to avoid nausea and abdominal pain. In hereditary fructose intolerance there is a rapid and prolonged fall in blood glucose and serum phosphorus. The test should be terminated by intravenous glucose if marked symptoms of hypoglycaemia occur. Fructosaemia is variable after the load, and fructosuria inconstant.

Treatment

Sucrose and fructose should be excluded from the diet.

FAMILIAL DISORDERS OF BILIRUBIN METABOLISM

Biochemistry

Bilirubin is formed by the breakdown of haem in cells of the reticuloendothelial system. This unconjugated bilirubin is transported in the blood largely bound to albumin and is taken up preferentially by the liver, where it is conjugated within the parenchymal cells to bilirubin glucuronide by the action of a microsomal enzyme UDP-glucuronyl transferase. Conjugated bilirubin is rapidly excreted into the bile and thence undergoes bacterial modification in the bowel before elimination in the faeces.

Inherited defects in the uptake, conjugation or excretion of bilirubin by the hepatocytes may give rise to chronic jaundice. Four main syndromes, representing defects at different stages of the bilirubin excretory pathway, can be recognised. In Gilbert's syndrome the defect is thought to be defective uptake of unconjugated bilirubin by the liver. In the Crigler–Najjar syndrome there is defective UDP-glucuronyl transferase activity in the liver, and in the Dubin–Johnson and Rotor syndromes the defect is in excretion of bilirubin from the hepatocyte into the bile canaliculi.

Gilbert's syndrome

Gilbert's syndrome is a common dominantly inherited condition in which there is a fluctuant mild jaundice. It is doubtful if any symptoms occur in childhood; in adult life some patients have presented with mild abdominal discomfort or malaise.

The disorder should be considered when a mild unconjugated hyperbilirubinaemia (<85 μmol/l [5 mg/100 ml]), is detected. Apart from elevation of serum bilirubin, tests of liver function are normal and there is no evidence of haemolysis. The diagnosis is largely by exclusion, and where doubt remains a provocative test may be useful. Both calorie restriction and nicotinic acid have been reported to exaggerate the jaundice, but it appears likely that administration of nicotinic acid is the more reliable test (Davidson *et al.*, 1975).

As Gilbert's syndrome does not cause any significant disability, both patient and relatives should be reassured and told of the excellent prognosis.

Crigler–Najjar syndrome

Two types of Crigler–Najjar syndrome can be recognised, the rare and severe type 1, and the more common but less serious type 2. Although the two types show some overlap clinically, they appear to be genetically distinct. In both forms autosomal recessive inheritance is likely.

In type 1 severe jaundice develops in the first few days of life. The level of unconjugated bilirubin in the serum increases rapidly and may rise as high as 850 μmol/l (50 mg/100 ml). Neurological symptoms due to kernicterus occur early in most children. The diagnosis may be suspected if parents are consanguineous or if there has been a previously affected child. Investigations show no other evidence of liver dysfunction or signs of haemolysis. Treatment is disappointing; exchange transfusion often fails to cause sufficient lowering of bilirubin concentration to prevent kernicterus, and the chronicity of the condition further limits the usefulness of this manoeuvre. Phenobarbitone is without effect on the jaundice, but phototherapy may result in slight lowering of serum bilirubin. Even if kernicterus does not develop in infancy, chronic severe jaundice persists, and kernicterus may develop later. Of the seven patients originally described (Crigler and Najjar, 1952) six died in infancy of kernicterus. The sole surviver subsequently developed progressive neurological disease and died at the age of 16 (Blumenschein *et al.*, 1968).

In type 2, unconjugated hyperbilirubinaemia is moderately severe (up to 340 μmol/l or 20 mg/100 ml) but kernicterus does not occur. Apart from the jaundice symptoms are unusual. Investigations show that the abnormality is limited to bilirubin metabolism. In mild cases it may be difficult to differentiate type 2 disease from chronic mild haemolysis, chronic hepatitis or Gilbert's disease. The administration of phenobarbitone has a marked effect in lowering the serum bilirubin (Arias *et al.*, 1969).

Dubin–Johnson syndrome

In the Dubin–Johnson syndrome there is wide variability in clinical expression. Icterus is usually mild with serum bilirubin not exceeding 85 μmol/l (5 mg/100 ml), although rarely it is more severe with bilirubin up to 340 μmol/l (20 mg/100 ml). Symptoms are inconstant and usually mild and less common in childhood than later in life. There may be abdominal pain, malaise, nausea, anorexia and diarrhoea, and hepatomegaly occurs in some patients.

Investigations show elevation of both conjugated and unconjugated bilirubin in the serum, and the urine may contain bile. Bromsulphthalein excretion is impaired and the gall bladder is not usually visible on cholecystography. Serum alkaline phosphatase is normal. Liver biopsy shows a characteristic greenish-black appearance macroscopically, and microscopically the cells contain brown pigment granules. The disorder may be suspected if a parent is affected, and unnecessary investigation and especially laparotomy should be avoided. The prognosis is benign and there is no specific therapy.

Rotor syndrome

Rotor syndrome clinically resembles Dubin–Johnson syndrome but there is no accumulation of pigment in the liver. Both syndromes may, however, be variants of the same basic disorder. The prognosis is equally good.

ABNORMALITIES OF METAL METABOLISM

Wilson's disease

Wilson's disease (hepatolenticular degeneration) is a rare, inherited disorder of copper metabolism in which copper is deposited in the tissues, especially in liver, brain, kidneys and cornea. It is inherited as an autosomal recessive; the enzyme defect is not yet known.

Clinical features

In childhood Wilson's disease commonly presents as hepatic cirrhosis with or without jaundice (Walshe, 1962). Symptoms are rare before the age of 6 years. Haematemesis from oesophageal varices may be the initial manifestation (Bearn, 1972). Haemolytic anaemia and hypersplenism with thrombocytopenia may also occur early.

The pathognomonic Kayser–Fleischer ring due to deposition of copper in the cornea is rarely present before the age of about 7 and may be absent when a child is first seen with hepatic cirrhosis. In most cases, however, careful slit lamp examination will reveal this sign. Very occasionally cataracts may occur.

Lenticular degeneration with spasticity, rigidity, tremor, dysarthria and dysphagia mainly occurs in later childhood and adolescence, and in such patients clinical signs of hepatic cirrhosis may be minimal or absent.

Other clinical features include psychiatric manifestations with behaviour disturbances and symptoms suggesting schizophrenia (Scheinberg, Sternlieb and Richman, 1968). Epileptiform fits may occur, and osteochondritis dissecans is a rare presenting feature (Walshe, 1962).

Laboratory findings and diagnosis

The majority of patients have low levels of serum copper and coeruloplasmin and increased urinary copper concentration. Abnormalities of liver function are variable depending upon the stage and severity of the hepatic lesion. Renal copper deposition results in progressive renal tubular failure with generalised aminoaciduria, glucosuria, proteinuria and phosphaturia. Only occasionally is it necessary to estimate the liver copper content.

Treatment and prognosis

Oral penicillamine is the most effective way of removing copper from the body and, if given early in the disease, marked clinical improvement can be produced. Affected but asymptomatic siblings of patients should also be treated. Toxic effects of penicillamine may limit treatment in some patients, and for these individuals BAL may be useful. With early and effective therapy the prognosis is good. Without treatment progressive deterioration occurs and hepatic failure usually supervenes.

Haemochromatosis

The term haemochromatosis signifies a widespread increase of tissue iron associated with characteristic pathological changes of tissue structure or function (Pollycove, 1972). Most frequently it occurs as a secondary manifestation due to repeated transfusions. Primary haemochromatosis is a rare, genetically determined disorder; neither the mode of inheritance nor the basic defect have yet been identified. Iron overload occurs as a result of persistently increased intestinal absorption of iron.

Because it takes many years to accumulate sufficient iron to give rise to symptoms, the disorder is seldom diagnosed until midadult life, when the classical triad of liver cirrhosis, skin pigmentation and diabetes mellitus occurs. Unequivocal cases below the age of 13 years have not been reported (Pollycove, 1972), but the disorder should be suspected if there is a family history. Clinical symptoms occur much more frequently in males because females are partially protected by greater physiological iron loss.

Investigations show raised plasma iron concentrations; transferrin is decreased and nearly completely saturated. Other findings reflect organ damage caused by the iron deposition, for example hyperglycaemia and glycosuria. Iron absorption and deposition can be reduced by chelating agents or venesection and, as organ damage may be irreversible, treatment should be started early.

HEPATIC PORPHYRIAS

Biochemistry

These disorders involve the formation of delta-aminolevulinic acid (ALA) which is the initial step in the biosynthesis of haem. Three main genetic types are recognised all of which are inherited as autosomal dominants; these are acute intermittent porphyria, variegate porphyria and hereditary coproporphyria. The genetic basis of a fourth type, porphyria cutanea tarda, is uncertain.

In all three main types acute attacks occur in which the synthesis of ALA and its immediate metabolite porphobilinogen (PBG) are increased due to excessive activity of ALA synthetase. This excess activity is thought to be due to interference in the negative feedback system for the synthesis of this enzyme; in acute intermittent porphyria there is probably a lack of uroporphyrinogen synthetase (Strand, Manning and Marver, 1971), and in the other disorders the defect is probably at other points in the pathway of haem production.

During the acute attacks there is excessive excretion of ALA and PBG in the urine in all three types, but the remainder of the excretion pattern of metabolites in faeces and urine varies between the different types (Marver and Schmid, 1972). During remission, ALA and PBG excretion are normal or only marginally raised; however, other porphyrins may be present in excess in urine and/or faeces.

Activity of ALA synthetase can be induced by a number of drugs such as barbiturates, sulphonamides and chloroquin, by other toxic agents and by some sex hormones. In individuals who only develop porphyria after the ingestion of such substances, the condition is usually designated as acquired, but it is likely that even in these cases there is a genetic basis, and no sharp distinction can be drawn between genetic and acquired porphyria.

Clinical features

Although occasional cases in early childhood have been reported, clinical manifestations are rare before puberty. Acute attacks of colicky abdominal pain, which may be severe and are usually accompanied by vomiting and constipation, are the commonest presenting feature, especially in acute intermittent porphyria. Neurological and psychiatric features are prominent in some patients. Attacks, with or without neurological symptoms, may be precipitated by infection, certain drugs, menstruation and other forms of stress. Hypertension occurs in about 50 per cent of patients (Eales, 1963). Cutaneous lesions, which are only found in variegate porphyria, hereditary coproporphyria and porphyria cutanea tarda, occur on exposure to sunlight and may also follow minor trauma.

Laboratory investigations

Red urine (due to uroporphyrin) is usually found only in patients with skin lesions. In acute visceral attacks the urine is often colourless at the onset and may or may not become red later. If the disorder is suspected, tests for PBG (which is colourless) must be performed on freshly passed urine. Examination of the various porphyrin excretion products in urine and faeces of patients and parents is necessary to establish the genetic type.

Severe hyponatraemia, hypomagnasaemia and decreased creatinine clearance are often found in the acute attacks. Hypercholesterolaemia occurs in some patients (Lees *et al.*, 1970).

Treatment and prognosis

Water and electrolyte disturbances require urgent treatment. All drugs known to exacerbate porphyria should be withdrawn and great care exercised in giving any drugs. Long-term management includes control of infection and avoidance of drugs and alcohol. Up to 25 per cent of patients with acute intermittent porphyria may die during an acute attack.

References

Arias, I. M., Gartner, L. M., Cohen, M., Ben Ezzer, J. & Levi, A. J. (1969) Chronic non haemolytic unconjugated hyperbilirubinaemia with glucuronyl transferase deficiency. *American Journal of Medicine*, **47**, 395.

Avery, M. E., Clow, C. L., Menkes, J. H., Ramos, A., Scriver, C. R., Stern, L. & Wasserman, B. P. (1967) Transient tyrosinemia of the newborn: dietary and clinical aspects. *Pediatrics*, **39**, 378.

Bearn, A. G. (1972) Wilson's disease. In *The Metabolic Basis of Inherited Disease*. 3rd edition. Ch. 43, p. 1033, ed. Stanbury, J. B., Wyngaarden, J. B. & Fredrickson. D. S. New York: McGraw-Hill.

Blumenschein, S. D., Kallen, R. J., Storey, B., Natzchka, J. C., Odell, G. B. & Childs, B. (1968) Familial non-haemolytic jaundice with late onset of neurological damage. *Pediatrics*, **42**, 786.

Bodegard, G., Gentz, J., Lindblad, B., Lindstedt, S. & Zetterström, R. (1969) Hereditary tryosinemia. III on the differential diagnosis and the lack of effect of early dietary treatment. *Acta Paediatrica Scandinavica*, **58**, 37.

Cornblath, M. & Schwartz, R. (1966a) Disorders of glycogen metabolism. In *Disorders of Carbohydrate Metabolism in Infancy*, ch. 7, p. 115. Philadelphia: Saunders.

Cornblath, M. & Schwartz, R. (1966b) Hereditary fructose intolerance. In *Disorders of Carbohydrate Metabolism in Infancy,* ch. 9, p. 177. Philadelphia: Saunders.

Crigler, J. F. & Najjar, V. A. (1952) Congenital familial non-haemolytic jaundice with kernicterus. *Pediatrics,* **10,** 169.

Davidson, A. R., Rojas-Bueno, A. Thompson, R. P. H. & Williams, R. (1975) Reduced calorie intake and nicotinic acid provocation tests in the diagnosis of Gilbert's syndrome. *British Medical Journal,* **2,** 480.

Eales, L. (1963) Porphyria as seen in Cape Town: a survey of 250 patients and some recent studies. *South African Journal of Laboratory and Clinical Medicine,* **9,** 151.

Folkman, J., Philippart, A., Tze, W. J. & Crigler, J. (1972) Portacaval Shunt for glycogen storage disease: value of prolonged intravenous hyperalimentation before surgery. *Surgery,* **72,** 306.

Greene, H. L., Burr, I. M. Slonim, A. E. & Vaughan, R. L., Jr. (1975) Medical treatment of type 1 glycogen storage disease. *Pediatric Research,* **9,** 303.

Harries, J. T., Seakins, J. W. T. Ersser, R. S. & Lloyd, J. K. (1969) Recovery after dietary treatment of an infant with features of tyrosinosis. *Archives of Disease in Childhood,* **44,** 258.

Hill, A., Nordin, P. M. & Zaleski, W. A. (1970) Dietary treatment of tyrosinosis. *Journal of the American Dietetic Association,* **56,** 308.

Komrower, G. M. & Lee, D. H. (1970) Long-term follow up of galactosaemia. *Archives of Disease in Childhood,* **45,** 367.

Larochelle, J., Mortezai, A., Belanger, M. Tremblay, M., Claveau, J. C. & Aubin, G. (1967) Experience with 37 infants with tyrosinemia. In Conference on hereditary tyrosinemia, eds. Partington. M., Scriver, C. R. and Sass-Kortsak, A. *Canadian Medical Association Journal,* **97,** 1051.

Lees, R. S., Song, C. S. Levere, R. D. & Kapas, A. (1970) Hyperbetalipoproteinaemia in acute intermittent porphyria. *New England Journal of Medicine,* **282,** 432.

Levy, H. L., Shih, V. E., Madigan, P. M. & MacCreay, R. A. (1969) Transient tyrosinemia in full-term infants. *Journal of American Medical Association,* **209,** 249.

Marver, H. S. & Schmid, R. (1972) The porphyrias. In *The Metabolic Basis of Inherited Disease.* 3rd edition, ch. 45, p. 1087, ed. Stanbury, J. B., Wyngaarden, J. B. & Fredrickson, D. S. Philadelphia: McGraw-Hill.

Medes, G. (1932) A new error of tyrosine metabolism: tyrosinosis. The intermediary metabolism of tyrosine and phenylalanine. *Biochemical Journal,* **26,** 917.

Menkes, J. H. Welcher, D. W., Levy, H. S., Dallas, J. & Gretsky. N. E. (1972) Relationship of elevated blood tyrosine to the ultimate intellectual performance of premature infants. *Pediatrics,* **49,** 218.

Patrick, A. D. & Lake, B. D. (1973) Wolman's disease. In *Lysosomes and Storage Disease,* ch. 20, p. 453, ed. Hers, H. G. & van Hoof, F. New York: Academic Press.

Pollycove, M. (1972) Hemochromatosis. In *The Metabolic Basis of Inherited Disease.* 3rd edition, ch. 44, p. 1051, ed. Stanbury, J. B., Wyngaarden, J. B. & Fredrickson, D. S. Philadelphia: McGraw-Hill.

Scheinberg, I. H., Sternlieb, I. & Richman, J. (1968) Psychiatric manifestations in patients with Wilson's disease. In *Birth Defects Original Article Series,* **4,** 85.

Scriver, C. R. & Rosenberg, L. E. (1973a) Tyrosine. In *Aminoacid Metabolism and its Disorders,* ch. 16, p. 338. Vol. X: *Major Problems in Clinical Paediatrics.* Philadelphia: Saunders.

Scriver, C. R. & Rosenberg, L. E. (1973b) Urea cycle and ammonia. In *Aminoacid Metabolism and its Disorders,* ch. 12, p. 234. Vol. X: *Major Problems in Clinical Paediatrics.* Philadelphia: Saunders.

Shih, V. E. & Efron, M. L. (1972) Urea cycle disorders. In *Metabolic Basis of Inherited Disease.* 3rd edition, ch. 17, p. 370, ed. Stanbury, J. B., Wyngaarden, J. B. & Fredrickson, D. S. New York: McGraw-Hill.

Shih, V. E. *et al.* (1971) Galactosaemia screening of newborns in Massachusetts. *New England Journal of Medicine,* **284,** 753.

Spencer-Peet, J., Norman, M. E., Lake, B. D., McNamara, J. & Patrick, A. D. (1971) Hepatic glycogen storage disease: clinical and laboratory findings in 23 cases. *Quarterly Journal of Medicine,* **40,** 95.

Starzl, T. E. *et al.* (1973) Portal diversion for the treatment of glycogen storage disease in humans. *Annals of Surgery,* **178,** 525.

Strand, L. J. Manning, J. & Marver, H. S. (1971) Acute intermittent porphyria; studies of the enzymatic basis of disordered haem biosynthesis. *South African Journal of Laboratory and Clinical Medicine,* 25 Sept., 108.

Walshe, J. M. (1962) Wilson's disease, the presenting symptoms. *Archives of Disease in Childhood,* **37,** 253.

Wolman, M., Sterk, V. V. Gatt, S. & Frenkel, M. (1961) Primary familial xanthomatosis with involvement and calcification of the adrenals. *Pediatrics,* **28,** 742.

16. Persistent neonatal jaundice

A. P. Mowat

Unconjugated hyperbilirubinaemia
Conjugated hyperbilirubinaemia

Persistent jaundice in the first months of life has many causes and may be classified according to whether the raised serum concentrations of bilirubin are predominantly conjugated or unconjugated. In unconjugated hyperbilirubinaemia the concentration of conjugated bilirubin is not raised, whereas in conjugated hyperbilirubinaemia the concentration of conjugated bilirubin is raised to usually more than 20 per cent of the total. In both types of jaundice the intensity and duration is accentuated by the temporarily increased production and ineffective hepatic excretion of bilirubin commonly called physiological jaundice. Since nearly all newborn infants have some degree of jaundice, the term 'hyperbilirubinaemia' in this age group is used to indicate a degree of jaundice which should alert the physician to further investigate the infant so that treatable causes of jaundice can be detected and kernicterus prevented. 'Hyperbilirubinaemia' is defined as serum concentrations of greater than 255 μmol/l (15 mg/100 ml) in the full-term infant, and greater than 204 μmol/l (12 mg/100 ml) in the preterm infant.

UNCONJUGATED HYPERBILIRUBINAEMIA

The unconjugated hyperbilirubinaemias can be classified according to the pathophysiological mechanisms which lead to the increased serum concentrations of bilirubin (Table 16.1).

Physiological jaundice

Serum unconjugated bilirubin exceeds 34 μmol/l (2 mg/100 ml) in the first week of life in over 90 per cent of normal full-term infants: maximum levels occur on the second to fourth day of life and rarely exceed 102 μmol/l (6 mg/100 ml). In preterm infants, levels of 204 to 238 μmol/l (12 to 14 mg/100 ml) are commonly reached by the fifth to seventh day. Jaundice may persist until the tenth day of life.

The physiology of bilirubin formation and excretion is discussed elsewhere (see Ch. 15) and has been extensively reviewed by Lathe (1974). Since many instances of persistent unconjugated hyperbilirubinaemia arise from accentuation of factors causing physiological jaundice, the imperfectly understood handicaps causing bilirubin retention in the human newborn infant must be briefly considered (Johnston, 1975).

Table 16.1 Pathophysiological mechanisms and causes of unconjugated hyperbilirubinaemia

Pathophysiological mechanism	Examples of causes
1 Increased haemolysis	
Blood group incompatibility	Rhesus and ABO incompatibility
Defects of RBC membrane	Hereditary spherocytosis
RBC enzyme deficiencies	Glucose-6-phosphate dehydrogenase deficiency
Haemolytic agents	Vitamin K
Infections	Septicaemia
Extravasated blood	Cephalhaematoma
2 Increased red cell mass	Placental transfusion Twin-to-twin transfusion
3 Defective hepatic uptake and/or conjugation of bilirubin	Prematurity Hypoxia Hypoglycaemia Dehydration Drugs sharing metabolic pathways of bilirubin Hypothyroidism Breast-milk jaundice Transient familial neonatal hyperbilirubinaemia Gilbert's syndrome
4 Increased enteric absorption	Meconium retention
5 Ill-understood; possibly involving some or all of above mechanisms	Hypothyroidism Pyloric stenosis and high intestinal obstruction Infants of diabetic mothers Down's syndrome Galactosaemia

In the newborn infant bilirubin production may be twice that of the adult as a result of shortened red blood cell survival, increased turnover of haem-containing enzymes and from ineffective erythropoiesis. There is impaired hepatic uptake of bilirubin due to a variety of factors, such as ineffective hepatic perfusion associated with the complex vascular changes occurring after birth, including persistent patency of the ductus venosus and inequality of the hepatic sinusoidal perfusion. In addition, it has been postulated that there may be inefficiency of hepatocyte uptake of bilirubin secondary to defective transport across the hepatocyte membrane, or lack of anion binding transport proteins such as ligandin in the hepatic cytoplasm. There is impaired ability to form bilirubin conjugates. Although xylose and glucose conjugates of bilirubin are formed in man, the major conjugate is thought to be glucuronide (Heirwegh, Meuwissen and Fevery, 1973). The reasons for the deficient glucuronidation are not clear; there may be transient deficiency of glucuronide donors such as UDPGA, which is derived exclusively from hepatic glycogen via glucose 1 phosphate; equally, deficiency of the enzyme UDP glucuronyltransferase may be rate-limiting. It is also postulated that hepatic excretion of bilirubin glucuronide may be transiently impaired, although there is no information on this in the human neonate. In primates bilirubin clearance may be inhibited by saturation of the excretion process between day two and day four after birth.

A major factor in physiological jaundice can probably be attributed to the intestinal reabsorption of unconjugated bilirubin; meconium contains 40 mg of bilirubin per 100 g and thus presents a total load of 200 mg of bilirubin to be excreted by the gut. To this must be added absorption of bilirubin released from bilirubin glucuronide by the action of the enzyme β glucuronidase which is present in high concentration in the intestine of the neonate, as well as the absence of bacterial degradation of bilirubin due to limited bacteriological colonisation.

Persistent jaundice with hyperbilirubinaemia

The many factors which cause neonatal hyperbilirubinaemia must be briefly considered since they are commonly followed by jaundice which persists beyond the tenth day of life. The most important are those which cause increased erythrocyte destruction. Blood group incompatibility between the infant and mother (isoimmunisation) must always be considered when jaundice occurs in the first 24 h of life and is associated with features of erythroblastosis. Rhesus isoimmunisation remains the most frequent cause in Western Europe, but this is falling with the successful use of anti-D-gammaglobulin which, when given in the puerperium following the birth of a Rhesus positive infant to a Rhesus negative mother, prevents sensitisation to the Rhesus factor. In other areas, incompatibility of the ABO blood groups and minor blood groups may be more important. Structural abnormalities of red cells such as hereditary spherocytosis and red cell enzyme deficiencies, such as glucose-6-phosphate dehydrogenase deficiency or pyruvate kinase deficiency, are rarer causes but in some parts of the world are important.

Bacterial infections and intrauterine viral infections are also important causes of hyperbilirubinaemia since they promote bilirubin production by haemolysis; they may, however, also impair bilirubin excretion. Bilirubin formation is also excessive where marked bruising has occurred. There are also many factors which singly or in combination add to the functional inefficiency of the liver in the newborn period and cause hyperbilirubinaemia and persistence of jaundice. These include prematurity, hypoxia, hypoglycaemia, dehydration, drugs which compete with bilirubin for the same excretory pathways and any circumstance which leads to meconium retention.

In many instances no definite cause for the hyperbilirubinaemia or persistent jaundice can be identified. Factors in pregnancy, induction of labour, the use of oxytocin infusions and the time of clamping of the cord have all been implicated (Chalmers, Campbell and Turnbull, 1975).

Persistent jaundice without hyperbilirubinaemia

Breast-milk jaundice syndrome

During the first week of life, jaundice is more commonly observed in breast-fed than in bottle-fed infants. The reasons for this are not clear, but possibly result from the combination of handicaps causing physiological jaundice aggravated by steroids in breast milk, possibly inhibition of bilirubin excretion by fatty acids, and contentiously by some action of prostaglandins. In most instances jaundice disappears within two weeks of birth. A rarer form of jaundice associated with breast feeding is that in which serum bilirubin concentrations of 255–360 μmol/l (15–20 mgm/100 ml) occur in the second or third week of life in infants who are entirely well. The jaundice may persist for as long as 10 weeks. If breast feeding is discontinued, however, the jaundice usually resolves within six days and may not recur if breast feeding is recommenced.

The aetiology of this syndrome is not known; 75 percent of the siblings of such infants are similarly affected. Breast milk from the mothers of affected infants competitively inhibits glucuronide formation *in vitro*; pregnane 3α–20β pregnanediol, a powerful inhibitor of glucuronide formation has been isolated from such milk in a few instances, but it is likely that this steroid is not the sole cause of the jaundice.

Although kernicterus has not been described, breast feeding should be discontinued for 24 to 48 h if serum bilirubin levels are greater than 290 μmol/l (17 mg/100 ml).

Transient familial hyperbilirubinaemia

Jaundice in this condition starts in the first few days of life and persists into the second or third week. Apparently healthy mothers give birth to infants all of whom develop jaundice. It is thought to be caused by an unidentified inhibitor of glucuronide formation which can be recovered from the serum of the mothers and their children.

Crigler–Najjar syndrome

This syndrome must always be considered in the differential diagnosis of any severe (type 1) or persistent (type 2) hyperbilirubinaemia (see Ch. 15).

Other causes

Hypothyroidism may be associated with prolonged jaundice lasting three to four weeks and should be considered in any infant in whom jaundice lasts more than two weeks; the precise cause of the jaundice is not certain. Jaundice may complicate any high intestinal obstruction such as pyloric stenosis; again the reasons are not certain, but the jaundice resolves when the obstruction is removed (Felsher *et al.*, 1974).

Kernicterus

Kernicterus is a disorder in which death or permanent neurological damage follows the deposition of unconjugated bilirubin in the brain, and occurs when the serum concentration of unconjugated bilirubin exceeds the capacity of serum proteins to bind bilirubin. It is not possible to measure unbound bilirubin. The accurate estimation of the reserve capacity of serum proteins to bind bilirubin may provide a more precise indication of the risk of kernicterus than serum bilirubin concentrations, but this has only been demonstrated for the salicylate saturation index method, which is technically difficult and available only in a limited number of laboratories (Odell, Storey and Rosenberg, 1970).

In full-term infants, a serum bilirubin of 340 μmol/l (20 mg/100 ml) or more is associated with a significant risk of kernicterus. There are several conditions in which kernicterus may occur at lower serum bilirubin concentrations because

Table 16.2 Laboratory investigation of unconjugated hyperbilirubinaemia

Serial determination of total and direct serum bilirubin
Haemoglobin
Red blood cell morphology, reticulocyte and normoblast count
Blood group in mother and child
Direct Coomb's test in saline and albumin
Maternal antibodies and haemolysins
Urine microscopy and culture
Urine-reducing substances
Blood culture and other appropriate bacteriological studies
Specific tests for abnormalities of red blood cells, e.g. G-6-PD deficiency
Serum T4 concentration
Breast-milk inhibitors of bilirubin conjugation *in vitro*

of diminished capacity of the serum proteins to bind bilirubin. These include prematurity, hypoalbuminaemia, asphyxia, acidosis and the administration of drugs which compete with bilirubin for albumin binding.

Management of unconjugated hyperbilirubinaemia

Identification and treatment of the cause of hyperbilirubinaemia and the prevention of kernicterus are dual objectives in management. Diagnosis will be established by careful history, together with scrutiny of the obstetrical case record, physical examination of the infant and appropriate laboratory investigations (Table 16.2).

General measures

In controlling unconjugated hyperbilirubinaemia and preventing kernicterus, the factors which cause aggravation of physiological jaundice must be identified and minimised. It is particularly important to prevent hypoxia and hypothermia and to maintain an appropriate intake of fluid and calories.

Exchange transfusion

Exchange transfusion is a most effective means of removing bilirubin when the risk of kernicterus is high and must be undertaken when the serum level of unconjugated bilirubin exceeds 340 μmol/l (20 mg/100 ml). It may be indicated at lower levels, e.g. 255 μmol/l (15 mg/100 ml), in premature infants particularly if they are acidotic or if serum albumin levels are low. In infants with haemolytic disorders a rise of serum bilirubin of greater than 8·5 μmol/l/h (0·5 mg/100 ml/h) usually indicates that bilirubin will accumulate more rapidly than it can be excreted, and exchange transfusion usually proves necessary. Administration of anti-D-gamma-globulin to Rhesus negative mothers following the birth of a Rhesus positive infant has markedly decreased the frequency of sensitisation to Rhesus factor in Britain. As a result, exchange transfusion is much less commonly performed in British newborn nurseries.

Phototherapy

In the last decade it has been unequivocally shown that exposing the jaundiced infant to artificial light of moderate intensity is effective in preventing hyperbilirubinaemia and in lowering elevated serum bilirubin. Light of a wavelength near 450 nm is perhaps most effective, but white light is to be preferred since observation of the patient is easier. Current evidence suggests that photodegradation of bilirubin occurs predominantly in the skin. The *in vivo* breakdown products remain ill characterised, but a well-documented effect is the excretion in the bile of bilirubin which reacts chemically like unconjugated bilirubin (Ostrow, 1972). It is not known whether this results from an action of phototherapy on the hepatocytes or from photobiochemical transformation of the bilirubin in the skin, nor is it known whether these photodegradation products are toxic to intact cells.

A number of side-effects have been recognised as complicating phototherapy. The most frequent is an increased insensible water loss which may lead to dehydration and aggravate hyperbilirubinaemia. Diarrhoea has been reported but where detailed observations have been made with appropriate controls the incidence of loose stools has not in fact increased. Skin reactions such as maculopapular rashes, tanning of Negro infants and bronzing of the skin with acute haemolysis in infants with liver disease occur rarely. Other possible biological effects of phototherapy must be considered. These include neuroendocrine functions mediated through the pineal gland and photoreceptors in the retina, which may possibly affect growth, diurnal rhythms, sexual maturation and direct photochemical reactions on other body tissues including the retina itself; with appropriate protection of the eye this last side-effect can be avoided. To date, no permanent abnormalities have been detected in human infants treated with phototherapy. Nevertheless this type of treatment should be limited to those infants who strictly need it and therapy should not be given for longer than is absolutely necessary.

It has yet to be shown that the widespread use of phototherapy in the management of non-haemolytic jaundice in low birth weight infants is in the patient's best interests. Although it is postulated that neonatal hyperbilirubinaemia may cause a continuum of brain damage extending from kernicterus to minor intellectual impairment, this has never been confirmed in careful studies (British Medical Journal, 1974).

Phenobarbitone

Phenobarbitone, particularly if given to the mother for some days before delivery of the infant, is effective in both premature and full-term infants in controlling neonatal hyperbilirubinaemia, even when caused by haemolysis due to ABO or Rhesus incompatibility. The mechanism of action of phenobarbitone is not clear. Animal studies suggest that the drug stimulates hepatic uptake, conjugation and excretion of bilirubin, as well as stimulating the bile salt-independent component of bile flow. If treatment is instituted at birth (8 mg/kg/day), the frequency of exchange transfusions in infants with Rhesus isoimmunisation and glucose-6-phosphate dehydrogenase deficiency is significantly reduced. Since the effect of phenobarbitone is not apparent until at least 48 h after the drug is commenced, it is of no value in treating established hyperbilirubinaemia. In addition to its effects on bilirubin, phenobarbitone influences other metabolic systems. It stimulates haem synthesis and may there-

Table 16.3 Causes of conjugated hyperbilirubinaemia

Hepatitis syndrome of infancy
infective
metabolic
idiopathic
Extrahepatic biliary atresia
Choledocal cyst
Ruptured bile duct
Intrahepatic biliary hypoplasia
Posthaemolytic
Neonatal hepatic necrosis
Gallstones
Microcystic disease

fore aggravate jaundice. It modifies the activity of many microsomal enzymes which are involved in the metabolism of drugs, vitamins, clotting factors and hormones; also, it influences the intracellular ratios of the reduced and oxidised forms of NAD(H) and NADP(H). The routine use of phenobarbitone in the management of hyperbilirubinaemia is thus to be discouraged. In circumstances, however, where optimal perinatal care cannot be achieved the small risks of phenobarbitone and phototherapy may be discounted if they increase the chance of survival with an intact neurological system.

CONJUGATED HYPERBILIRUBINAEMIA

The causes of the conjugated hyperbilirubinaemias are listed in Table 16.3.

Hepatitis syndrome of infancy

The clinical features of this syndrome are jaundice with a raised conjugated bilirubin, pale to clay-coloured stools, dark bile-containing urine and usually hepatomegaly. There is biochemical and pathological evidence of hepatocellular necrosis with hepatitis, i.e. inflammatory cell infiltrate in the portal tract and hepatic parenchyma. Splenomegaly, a mild haemolytic anaemia and failure to thrive are frequent features (Alagille, 1972). The onset in the vast majority of cases is in the first four weeks of life with a smaller number presenting between five and eight weeks and very few as late as four months of age.

Both clinically and pathologically there can be considerable difficulty in determining whether the lesion is primarily in the hepatic parenchyma, the portal tracts, the major intrahepatic bile ducts or the extrahepatic bile ducts. These difficulties may remain unresolved even with laparotomy, operative radiological investigations and at autopsy. There may be marked differences between the right and left hepatic lobes which accentuate the sampling errors of biopsies. Failure of hepatic bile secretion is accompanied by narrow extrahepatic bile ducts in which detection of the lumen is difficult without destroying them. Successful retrograde radiographic demonstration of intrahepatic ducts is difficult and failure does not necessarily indicate the ducts are abnormal. Obstruction of the extrahepatic bile ducts is most commonly associated with narrow, tortuous intrahepatic ducts which cannot be demonstrated by trans-hepatic cholangiography, a situation totally different from extrahepatic bile duct obstruction due to choledochal cyst in an older child or gall-stones in an adult. Marked portal tract changes with bile duct reduplication and increased fibrosis, together with hepatocellular abnormalities which may include giant cell transformation, are a constant feature in extrahepatic biliary atresia. These problems are enumerated in order to emphasise that although the small size of the structures involved account for some of the difficulties in classification, the unique histological response associated with hepatobiliary disease in this age group is a major factor. Further the term 'giant cell hepatitis' has little to recommend it, since giant cell transformation occurs in association with a wide range of known causes of liver disease in this age group, as well as in the idiopathic varieties (Landing, 1974).

Controversy exists as to the most appropriate terminology for such cases. Neonatal hepatitis, neonatal hepatitis syndrome, intrahepatic cholestasis, obstructive cholangeopathy of infancy and bile retention syndrome of infancy all have their advocates. Lack of agreement on terminology is a reflection of our ignorance of the aetiology and the many aspects of the pathophysiology of obstructive jaundice in this age group, and of the need to abandon rigid concepts (Emery, 1974). Thus, although 'hepatitis syndrome of infancy' has been used in this chapter, it must be emphasised that this syndrome has many possible causes. Priorities in management are the recognition of those causes which are amenable to specific therapy, recognition of genetically determined disorders and the identification of patients who require surgical intervention.

Infections

Generalised infection acquired *in utero*, during delivery, or early in the new-born period by agents such as toxoplasma gondi, treponema pallidum, listeria, mycobacterium tuberculosis, rubella, cytomegalovirus, herpes simplex virus, Coxsackie B and adenovirus may cause a marked hepatitis. The infecting agents, the screening and definitive investigations and the principal extrahepatic clinical manifestations are listed in Table 16.4; as can be seen, there is involvement of extrahepatic organs in many instances (Dommergues, 1973).

The diagnosis of these infections may be made by appropriate vir... cal and bacteriological tests, and it is particularly important that th... agents listed in Table 16.4 are excluded since specific antibio... ilable.

Hepatitis B antigen is responsible for a small... e mother has had hepatitis B antigen positive h... pregnancy or early in the puerperium ... incidence of hepatitis B antiger... mild with only moderate elevatic... in the serum, but it may be chron... have mild disease, however, and c... tory (Kattamis *et al.*, 1973). In inf... carriers of hepatitis B antigen, ther... and only about 5 per cent of the infant... er disease; in some instances liver disea... 972). Infants born to mothers

Table 16.4 Infectious causes of the hepatitis syndrome of infancy

Infecting agents	Scre[illegible]stigations	Definitive investigations	Principal extrahepatic clinical manifestations
Cytomegalovirus	[illegible]y in serum	Isolation from urine and liver with demonstration of virus in liver by IF	Small for dates; microcephaly; meningoencephalitis; intracranial calcification; neonatal thrombocytopaenic purpura; splenomegaly; retinitis, deafness
[illegible]	[illegible]nd HAI antibodies in [illegible]um	Specific IgM antibody, virus isolation from nasopharynx and liver	Small for dates; cataracts; retinitis; congenital heart defects; microphthalmia, buphthalmos and corneal oedema; myocarditis; neonatal thrombocytopaenic purpura; splenomegaly; osteopathy; lymphadenopathy
[illegible]	Antigen and antibody in mother	Hepatitis B antigen in infant Demonstration of Hepatitis B antigen in liver by IF and EM	None described
[illegible]	Perinatal herpes in mother	Isolation and demonstration of virus from superficial lesions and liver	Splenomegaly; heart failure, pneumonitis; skin vesicles; meningoencephalitis
[illegible] virus	Isolation from respiratory tract and faeces	Isolation from liver	Myocarditis; meningoencephalitis; pneumonitis
[illegible]a zoster	Demonstration of virus from superficial lesions	Demonstration of virus in the liver	Disseminated infection as in herpes simplex; skin lesions more obvious
[illegible]acterial infection		Blood culture, urine culture, CSF	Anaemia; any other system may be involved
Listeria		Isolation of organisms from blood culture, CSF or liver	Septicaemia; meningitis; pneumonitis; purpura
Treponema pallidum	VDRL or TPI, particularly in mother	Demonstration of *Treponema* by dark ground illumination	Rhinitis; skin rash; bone lesions; anaemia; lymphadenopathy; meningoencephalitis
Toxoplasma gondii	CF antibody in serum	Rising antibody titre in infant; specific IgM antibody; isolation of organisms from liver and CSF; visualisation of organism from liver and CSF	Microcephaly; macrocephaly; meningoencephalitis; intracranial calcification; choreoretinitis; thrombocytopaenia; purpura

CF = Complement fixing; HAI = Haem. agglutination inhibition; IF = Immunofluorescence microscopy; EM = Electron microscopy; CSF = Cerebrospinal fluid whose serum also contains the E antigen, a marker for infectivity, are particularly prone to become Hb sAg positive (Gerety and Schweitzer, 1977). The possible role of hepatitis A virus as a cause of hepatitis in young infants remains undetermined, since there is as yet no readily available means of detecting this infection.

Conjugated hyperbilirubinaemia associated with bile stasis and hepatocellular damage complicates many bacterial infections, particularly urinary *E. coli* infections, septicaemia and enteritis; the pathogenesis of the liver damage is obscure. Urine analysis, blood cultures and stool cultures are necessary investigations in any case of conjugated hyperbilirubinaemia.

Genetically determined disorders

Galactosaemia, fructosaemia and tyrosinosis are rare but important causes of hepatitis in infancy since they are amenable to dietary treatment. They are discussed elsewhere (see Ch. 15) and will not be considered further in this section.

Alpha-1-antitrypsin deficiency in serum. Genetic deficiency of the serum protein alpha-1-antitrypsin has in the last six years been shown to be an important factor in liver disease in childhood, equalling in incidence biliary atresia as a cause of obstructive jaundice in the newborn period (Cottrall, Cook and Mowat, 1974). Alpha-1-antitrypsin is a glycoprotein synthesised in the liver and is found in the serum in concentrations of approximately 250 mg/100 ml; it is present in much lower concentrations in other tissues and fluids. Its physiological role is unknown. Deficient individuals have approximately 10 to 20 per cent of the normal concentration of serum alpha-1-antitrypsin. Many genetically determined alleles of alpha-1-antitrypsin can be distinguished by acid starch-gel electrophoresis, the proteins moving as distinct bands labelled alphabetically according to their electrophoretic mobility. Normal individuals have clear M bands with a protease inhibitor (Pi) phenotype M, while deficient subjects have fainter, slower moving Z bands and a Pi phenotype Z. Less marked reduction of alpha-1-antitrypsin concentrations are found in subjects with Pi genotype MZ, SZ, with very low concentrations in Pi nil individuals. Deficient individuals may have liver disease or develop emphysema in early adult life, or escape either of these associated conditions; rarely both may coexist in the same patient. Only in individuals with a Pi Z phenotype has a close association with liver disease been established. In an on-going prospective study of 120 alpha-1-antitrypsin deficient infants, only seven were found to have liver disease (Svegar, 1974; Svegar, 1976). Sporadic case reports exist of cirrhosis in SZ individuals, but these may indicate a chance association (Wilkinson *et al.*, 1974). Just how the deficiency of this serum protein predisposes to liver disease is not known (Porter *et al.*, 1972).

Liver disease usually presents with acute hepatitis in the first four weeks of life. In one of 30 infants we have investigated with this condition, however, jaundice did not appear until the 60th day. Serum bilirubin concentrations vary from 34 to 272 μmol/l (2 to 16 mg/100 ml), eventually returning to normal values over periods varying from 10 days to 13 months. The clinical severity of the hepatitis is very variable. Some infants appear well, apart from icterus and slow weight gain, while in others the hepatitis is complicated by irritability, lethargy, inability to feed, vomiting, hypertension, and purpura with low platelet counts and prolonged prothrombin time, and septicaemia. In the acute stage asparate transaminase levels vary from 80 to 600 iu/l, and the alkaline phosphatase from 150 to 1300 iu/l; liver biopsy shows a variable degree of cholestasis, hepatocellular necrosis, glandular transformation of hepatocytes with an inflammatory cell infiltrate in the parenchyma and portal tracts and an increase in periportal fibrous tissue; giant cell transformation of hepatocytes is not a prominent feature. The clinical severity of the hepatitis is reflected by the degree of hepatocellular necrosis and fibrous tissue proliferation; cirrhosis develops during the first year of life in patients with severe hepatitis and protracted hyperbilirubinaemia (Cottrall *et al.*, 1974). We have subsequently documented an established cirrhosis in an infant aged 3½ months who had mild hepatitis at 2 months with jaundice lasting only 10 days. Occasionally cirrhosis is found in children and adults with alpha-1-antitrypsin deficiency who have had no history of acute hepatitis (Brunt, 1974). The cirrhosis may be macronodular, micronodular or take a so-called 'biliary' form, and there is no qualitatively unique histological feature using standard stains. Distinct diastase-resistant, PAS positive, magenta-coloured globules 2 to 20 microns in diameter are seen in the periportal hepatocytes of Pi ZZ infants, but only after 12 weeks of age (Talbot and Mowat, 1975). Although serum bilirubin levels return to normal, aspartate transaminase and alkaline phosphatase levels remain elevated throughout childhood, and the liver disease commonly progresses to cirrhosis with death from its complications in early adult life. Recent reports, however, suggest that cirrhosis is not inevitable (Sass-Kortsak, 1974). There is at present no effective treatment.

Other genetic disorders such as cystic fibrosis and Niemann–Pick disease may occasionally be complicated by jaundice in the newborn period. Obstructive jaundice occurs in 20 to 30 per cent of infants with chromosomal abnormalities such as trisomy 13 or 18 (Taylor, 1968); it may also occur in 45 X Turner's syndrome (Gardner, 1974). The occasional occurrence of familial cases of obstructive jaundice in the absence of any recognisable metabolic or chromosomal abnormalities is well known. Aagenaes (1974) reported from South-west Norway a group of children in whom obstructive jaundice in infancy was followed by recurrent episodes of jaundice throughout childhood, and who then developed unexplained oedema of the legs towards puberty. Familial neonatal liver disease with varying degrees of hepatic dysfunction and pulmonary stenosis has also been described (Watson and Miller, 1973).

Erythroblastosis

Transient conjugated hyperbilirubinaemia occurs during the recovery stage of erythroblastosis in which it appears that bilirubin is conjugated more rapidly than it can be excreted. When the unconjugated hyperbilirubinaemia has been protracted and severe, or when there has been marked anaemia at birth, elevated serum amino transferase levels, hepatocellular necrosis and giant transformation of hepatocytes may occur (Walker, 1971). The prognosis is good.

Acute neonatal hepatic necrosis

Neonatal hepatic necrosis is a rare condition presenting in the first four weeks of life with a haemorrhagic diathesis which usually precedes jaundice. There is a rapid downhill course, and at autopsy the liver is small with indistinct greyish-yellow streaks. Microscopically there is massive necrosis, collapse of liver reticulum, marked haemosiderin deposition and scanty giant cells are present. The aetiology is unknown. Vigorous supportive therapy with fresh blood transfusions, vitamin K and steroids is indicated (Reubner *et al.*, 1969; Philip and Larson, 1973; Dupuy, Frommel and Alagille, 1975).

Intrahepatic cholestasis of the newborn

This disorder is characterised pathologically by cholestasis without hepatocellular necrosis (Hass, 1968). The liver architecture is preserved, and variable inflammatory cell changes occur in the portal tracts. These findings may represent a resolving hepatitis, and the prognosis is considered to be good.

Idiopathic

In most cases none of the above can be sited as causes (Silverman, Roy and Cozzetto, 1971). In a recent analysis of an on-going study in South-east England which included 103 patients with intact extrahepatic bile ducts, we found that 57 cases were without an identifiable cause, and in a further 14 the association of liver disease with a possible cause could not be firmly established. In some instances parenchymal damage or intrahepatic cholestasis may be associated with exposure to agents such as Halothane, or drugs, but their association is tenuous and the frequency rare.

Other causes

Other rare causes of the hepatitis syndrome of infancy include choledocal cyst which may be responsible for 1 to 2 per cent of such cases; spontaneous perforation of the bile ducts, in which bile-stained ascites may occur, may add to the usual clinical features of the syndrome (Howard, Johnston and Mowat, 1976). In both cases surgical correction is necessary. Other causes are gallstones, microcystic disease of the liver and kidney and Rotor syndrome (Sass-Kortsak, 1974).

Course and prognosis

The course and prognosis of the hepatitis syndrome of infancy are determined by the underlying cause and by the degree of liver damage. In idiopathic cases the prognosis is variable; 10 to 20 per cent of hospitalised cases die from hepatocellular failure in the first six weeks of life, while in the remainder the acute hepatitis resolves four to 26 weeks from the onset. Between 15 and 30 per cent of survivors, however, are estimated to have chronic liver disease, and more than a third have developed cirrhosis within three to five years. These estimates for mortality and morbidity in idiopathic hepatitis may exaggerate the seriousness of the condition (Grand *et al.*, 1975) since the reported series may include patients with alpha-1-antitrypsin deficiency, which appears to carry a worse prognosis than the idiopathic variety of the disease (Cottrall *et al.*, 1974).

Management

No specific treatment is available for idiopathic or hepatitis of known viral cause. Bacterial infection, listeria, syphilis and toxoplasmosis can all be treated by specific agents. Vigorous supportive management, particularly of the haemorrhagic diathesis and any complicating bacterial infections, is necessary. Corticosteroids are often advised but are of no proven value and predispose the patient to the risks of overwhelming infection. Cholestyramine may improve liver function in some patients and is particularly helpful as a symptomatic measure if pruritus is a problem. A minority of patients will benefit from treatment with phenobarbitone. Parenteral fat-soluble vitamins A, D and K are occasionally necessary to prevent deficiency. Vitamin D requirements are very variable in this syndrome; close biochemical monitoring is required to avoid rickets, on the one hand, and the effects of hypercalcaemia on the other. Nutrition may be improved by a diet low in neutral fats and supplemented with medium-chain triglycerides.

Obstructive biliary disease

Extrahepatic biliary atresia

Extrahepatic biliary atresia is characterised by a complete inability to excrete bile and by obstruction, destruction or absence of the bile duct(s) anywhere between the duodenum and the first or second order of branches of the right and left hepatic ducts. In distal atresia the proximal ducts are dilated together with the gall bladder if the lesion is below the junction of the cystic duct and the hepatic duct; these dilated segments contain bile and are in continuity with the main intrahepatic ducts. Such cases are regarded as 'surgically correctable'. The extent and site of the obstruction or absence of the bile ducts is extremely variable. The most common finding, however, is complete destruction of all the extrahepatic bile ducts with obliteration of the lumen and their replacement by fibrous cords, and glandular proliferation (Gautier, Jehan and Odievre, 1976).

Within the liver the main histological abnormalities are in the portal tracts which show marked portal fibrosis with angulation, distortion and proliferation of bile ducts; also there is medial hypertrophy of the hepatic arteries and bile plugs within the bile ducts. Giant cell transformation occurs and intrahepatic cholestasis is common. Late in the course of the disease the intrahepatic bile ducts are no longer evident as in bile duct hypoplasia (Koop, 1975). There is a progressive increase in periportal fibrosis with encroachment on hepatic parenchyma until the full pathological features of cirrhosis are produced. The rate of pathological progression and the time of appearance of the complications of cirrhosis vary a great deal from patient to patient.

Aetiology. The bile duct abnormalities are now generally considered not to be true primary malformations, since hepatic parenchymal cells are derived from the primitive duct system. Distal lesions associated with stenosis of the duodenum may be attributed to vascular accidents occurring later in intrauterine life. For the remainder, the condition results from a destructive inflammatory lesion with degeneration of bile duct epithelium, luminal obliteration and periductal sclerosis, often associated with periportal lymph gland enlargement (Landing, 1974). Twenty-five per cent of affected infants have extrahepatic congenital malformations. Three of 29 patients who were subjected to liver transplantation were found to have a composite vascular abnormality including absence of the inferior vena cava, a preduodenal portal vein and an anomalous hepatic artery; a further five in this series had anomalous hepatic arterial vasculature (Lilly and Starzl, 1974).

Biliary atresia has been reported in association with congenital rubella, cytomegalovirus infection, listeriosis and hepatitis B antigenaemia. These observations and the many similarities in the hepatic pathology of these conditions have led to the suggestion that idiopathic neonatal hepatitis and biliary atresia may have a common aetiology (Alagille, 1972; Landing, 1974). It must be stressed, however, that the extensive hepatocellular changes which are seen in association with such infections are not found in typical idiopathic extrahepatic biliary atresia. Teratogenic agents interfering with different stages of pre- and postnatal development, and cholangitis with destruction of formed bile ducts, have been postulated as possible causes, but no agent has been implicated.

Clinical and laboratory features. Jaundice followed by pale stools and dark urine may start at birth, but in 50 per cent of cases it is delayed for two to three weeks. Serum bilirubin levels vary considerably from day to day, but are usually less than 200 μmol/l (12 mg/100 ml) during the first few months of life; later they rise to higher concentrations. The direct reacting bilirubin is almost always greater than 68 μmol/l (4 mg/100 ml). Stools contain no bilirubin, and urobilin is absent from both stools and urine. Bilirubin is of course present in the urine and this can easily contaminate stool specimens and is a possible reason for spurious investigative results. Liver function tests show raised aspartate aminotransferase and alkaline phosphatase levels, but are not helpful in distinguishing biliary atresia from hepatitis. Choledochal cysts may present in a similar fashion.

Diagnosis. Diagnosis must ultimately be established by laparotomy, operative cholangiography through the gall bladder if it is present and dissection of the portahepatis. Recent reports indicate that bile drainage and resolution of jaundice can be achieved in a high percentage of infants with biliary atresia, previously considered inoperable, if surgery is carried out by the age of 10 weeks. Unfortunately differentiation of biliary atresia from severe cholestasis due to any of the various forms of the hepatitis syndrome of infancy is particularly difficult. Clinical features and standard liver function tests are unhelpful unless a progressive fall in serum bilirubin can be demonstrated, indicating hepatitis. A major clinical problem is therefore the early preoperative identification of those infants who would benefit from surgery. Thaler and Gellis (1968) reported that cirrhosis was three times as common in patients with a primary intrahepatic cause of jaundice if they had been submitted to such surgical investigation, when compared to a similar group of infants who had not had surgery. Applying modern techniques it is possible that the results would not have been so deleterious. Nevertheless surgery should be avoided whenever possible and attempts made to discriminate between infants with extrahepatic biliary obstruction and those with intrahepatic disease.

Table 16.5 Histological features of the hepatitis syndrome of infancy and biliary atresia

Hepatitis	Biliary atresia
Hepatocellular necrosis Giant cell transformation Disorganisation of liver cords Inflammatory cell infiltrate in parenchyma and portal tracts Cholestasis Focal portal bile duct proliferation	Widened portal tracts with prominent, distorted, elongated and angulated bile ducts; increased fibrosis; inflammatory cell infiltrate Normal hepatic architecture Cholestasis with bile lakes Giant cell transformation

To distinguish between biliary atresia and hepatitis three lines of investigation must be initiated as soon as biliary obstruction is suspected: (1) investigations to identify known causes of the hepatitis syndrome of infancy, bearing in mind that bile duct lesions may occur in a number of systemic infections; (2) percutaneous liver biopsy; and (3) investigations to determine the degree of biliary obstruction.

The investigations which are necessary to identify the known causes of the hepatitis syndrome of infancy have already been discussed.

Percutaneous liver biopsy should not be performed if the platelet count is less than 40 000 and/or the prothrombin time is prolonged by more than five seconds. The careful histological evaluation of a percutaneous liver biopsy is an important part of the investigation of all children with persistent liver disease due to the hepatitis syndrome, providing invaluable information on the degree of liver involvement and the prognosis, as well as furnishing final proof of a metabolic abnormality, as for example in hereditary fructosaemia. Furthermore biopsy may help in differentiating the hepatitis syndrome from biliary atresia (Table 16.5); unfortunately there is no single histological feature which is specific to either, and there may be considerable histological overlap (Brough and Bernstein, 1969; Brough and Bernstein, 1974). Operative biopsies are no more informative (Hays *et al.*, 1967). In our experience of 84 infants with cholestatic jaundice without extrahepatic biliary atresia, only eight had histological features (percutaneous liver biopsy) consistent with atresia, and two of these had choledochal cysts; 15 of 20 percutaneous liver biopsies in patients with biliary atresia shaved the typical pathological features of extrahepatic biliary atresia. The frequency of correct histological diagnosis was not influenced by the timing of the percutaneous liver biopsy in the first three months of life.

The intravenous radioactive Rose Bengal faecal excretion test is the most reliable investigation for the demonstration of biliary obstruction (Mowat, Psacharopoulos and Williams, 1976). Three drops of Lugol's iodine solution are given for two to three days before the intravenous injection of an exactly measured amount of labelled Rose Bengal (^{131}I or ^{125}I), at a dose of approximately one μCi/kg body weight. Rose Bengal is rapidly taken up by the liver, secreted via bile into the intestine and excreted in the faeces. The amount of isotope recovered in the faeces over a three-day period is thus an estimate of bile flow. In obstructive jaundice much of the isotope is excreted in urine, and it is therefore important to collect stools that are uncontaminated by urine (Sass-Kortsak, 1974). An excretion of 10 per cent or less is indicative of marked biliary construction due to biliary atresia or severe intrahepatic disease. Excretion rates of above 10 per cent make biliary atresia unlikely; excretion of less than 10 per cent with biopsy features of extrahepatic biliary atresia are indications for immediate laparotomy. When the histological features are equivocal or suggestive of hepatitis, the Rose Bengal excretion test should be repeated after three weeks, during which time the infant is given cholestyramine in a dose of 1 g four times daily. If atresia is not present excretion may rise to above 10 per cent (Campbell *et al.*, 1974).

We have confirmed these observations in 12 patients with extrahepatic biliary atresia, but have found three patients with intact extrahepatic ducts who had excretion rates of less than 5 per cent even after three weeks of cholestyramine. However, by combining these two investigations (i.e. biopsy and the Rose Bengal excretion test), we have been able to advise against laparotomy in all but one of 96 infants with conjugated hyperbilirubinaemia in whom the jaundice subsequently cleared completely, and have correctly advised laparotomy in all cases of biliary atresia and in two cases of choledochal cyst seen in the last five years.

Over the years many tests on blood and serum have been advocated for the distinction of extrahepatic biliary atresia from hepatitis, but their value has subsequently not been confirmed in clinical practice. Standard tests of liver function do not distinguish the two conditions. We have been unable to confirm the observations of Javitt *et al.* (1973) that high concentrations of chenodeoxycholic acid indicate biliary atresia, or that cholic acid predominates in infants with other forms of obstructive liver disease in the newborn period. Although we have confirmed that the alpha-fetoprotein concentrations were higher in hepatitis than in biliary atresia, the overlap in concentrations between the two conditions during the first two months of life precludes the use of this test in prognosis (Johnston *et al.*, 1976). The serum concentrations of alphafetoprotein (Zeltzer *et al.*, 1974), lipoprotein X (Campbell *et al.*, 1974) and 5′-nucleotidase (Sass-Kortsak, 1974) have been reported as being useful, but further clinical evaluation of these tests will be required.

Surgical management. It is only possible to establish biliary drainage by anastomosing the gall bladder or distended bile duct to a Roux-en-**Y** loop from small bowel in less than 10 per cent of cases. Even when this procedure is possible associated intrahepatic abnormalities or established cirrhosis may prevent complete cure, but long-term survival has been reported (Berenson, Garde and Moody, 1974). For the remainder, hepatic portoenterostomy has been advocated with up to 40 per cent showing biliary drainage if the operation is performed early (Lilly, 1975); ascending cholangitis, however, is a frequent complication. Kasai, Watanabe and Ohi (1975) have recently reported 14 of 57 infants with 'non-correctable' biliary atresia operated on in this fashion who survived for more than two years after surgery. The survival period extended up to 18 years, with nine surviving five or more years; three, however, have cirrhosis and one has portal hypertension. This procedure appears to be successful in producing biliary drainage if carried out at a stage when microscopic lumina are still present within the biliary duct cords, despite the fact that these are not visible to the naked eye. This procedure has brought a welcome wave of enthusiasm for the active management of obstructive jaundice in infancy. It places a great responsibility, however, on the surgeon who has to decide whether the small bile ducts without discernible lumina seen at laparotomy represent ducts which are not being filled from above because of hepatocellular disease, or whether they are ducts which are being destroyed by a local lesion. The proponents of hepatic portoenterostomy advise the procedure to be performed by the age of 10 weeks, although Danks *et al.* (1974) and ourselves have seen occasional short-term successes when the operation has been performed later. Surgery should not be delayed when there are clear indications of total biliary obstruction and the histological features are those of extra-hepatic biliary atresia.

Supportive management involves close medical supervision to prevent vitamin and/or calorie deficiency, and the careful use of diuretics will minimise the effects of salt and fluid retention. Febrile illnesses deserve prompt investigation and vigorous treatment; if surgery has produced bile drainage, cholangitis must be considered.

Intrahepatic biliary hypoplasia

This disorder is characterised by complete absence or reduction in the number of bile ducts in the hepatic portal tracts. The diagnosis rests on the microscopic appearance of a number of portal tracks which contain normal portal vein and hepatic artery branches, but no accompanying bile ducts. This abnormality is seen in two circumstances; firstly, in patients with extrahepatic biliary atresia who have survived beyond the age of 12 months, and secondly, as an isolated, ill-understood syndrome in which the extrahepatic bile ducts are intact.

The latter condition commonly presents as a hepatitis syndrome in the new-born period, and the early pathological picture is dominated by cholestasis with variable changes in the portal tract; there is usually minimal fibrosis. Bile ducts may be absent or initially may proliferate, and there is a minimal to moderate polymorphonuclear inflammatory response; the extrahepatic ducts are patent but small. In some instances, severe fibrosis develops in the portal tracts to give the pathological features of so-called 'biliary cirrhosis', and portal hypertension and varices eventually develop. Pruritus and xanthoma are prominent, and may be presenting features in some patients.

The aetiology is unknown. Alagille *et al.* (1975) have recently described 15 of 30 infants who had in addition abnormal facies, mental retardation, cardiac murmurs and vertebral anomalies. Why some patients remain free of jaundice for much of their course despite the almost total absence of hepatic bile ducts remains a mystery. Survival into the teens is usual without very much systemic upset unless malabsorption occurs. Phenobarbitone and/or cholestyramine may result in clinical and biochemical improvement in some instances.

Recently an identical histopathological syndrome has been described in two siblings who had a defect in the liver's capacity to convert 3α, 7α, 12α-trihydroxy-5β-cholestan-26-oic acid (THCA) to cholic acid (Hanson *et al.*, 1975); this appeared to be due to a deficiency of the 24-hydroxylating enzyme system required to convert THCA to varanic acid, and the condition seemed to be transmitted in an autosomal recessive fashion. Both children developed cirrhosis and portal hypertension and died before the age of 3 years. These studies raise the possibility that a primary defect in bile acid synthesis may be responsible for the liver disease seen in some infants with so-called 'intrahepatic biliary hypoplasia', 'intrahepatic biliary atresia' and 'paucity of the intrahepatic bile ducts'.

References

Aagenaes, Ø. (1974) Hereditary recurrent cholestasis with lymphoedema. *Acta Paediatrica Scandinavica,* **63,** 465.

Alagille, D. (1972) Clinical aspects of neonatal hepatitis. *American Journal of Diseases in Children,* **123,** 287.

Alagille, D., Odievre, M., Gautier, M. & Dommergues, J. P. (1975) Hepatic ducular hypoplasia associated with characteristic facies, vertebral malformation, retarded physical, mental, and sexual development, and cardiac murmur. *Journal of Paediatrics,* **86,** 63.

Berenson, M. M., Garde, A. R. & Moody, F. G. (1974) Twenty-five years survival after surgery for complete extrahepatic biliary atresia. *Gastroenterology,* **66,** 260.

British Medical Journal (1974) Management of neonatal jaundice. *British Medical Journal,* **1,** 469.

Brough, A. J. & Bernstein, J. (1969) Liver biopsy in the diagnosis of infantile obstructive jaundice. *Paediatrics,* **43,** 519.

Brough, A. J. & Bernstein, J. (1974) Conjugated hyperbilirubinaemia in early infancy. *Human Pathology,* **5,** 507.

Brunt, P. W. (1974) Antitrypsin and the liver. *Gut,* **15,** 573.

Campbell, D. P., Poley, J. Rainer, Alaupovic, P. & Smith, E. I. (1974) The differential diagnosis of neonatal hepatitis and biliary atresia. *Journal of Paediatric Surgery,* **9,** 699.

Chalmers, I., Campbell, H. & Turnbull, A. C. (1975) Use of oxytocin and incidence of neonatal jaundice. *British Medical Journal,* **2,** 116.

Cottrall, K., Cook, P. J. L. & Mowat, A. P. (1974) Neonatal hepatitis and alpha-1-antitrypsin deficiency: an epidemiological study in South-east England. *Postgraduate Medical Journal,* **50,** 376.

Danks, D. M., Campbell, P. E., Murray Clarke, A., Jones, P. G. & Solomon, J. R. (1974) Extrahepatic biliary atresia: the frequency of potentially operable cases. *American Journal of Diseases in Children,* **128,** 684.

Dommergues, J. P. (1973) Hepatites infectieuses non virales du nourrisson. *La Revue du Practicien,* **23,** 55.

Dupuy, J. M., Frommel, D. & Alagille, D. (1975) Severe viral hepatitis type B in infancy. *Lancet,* **1,** 191.

Emery, J. L. (1974) Pathology with reference to the bile retention syndrome. *Postgraduate Medical Journal,* **50,** 344.

Felsher, B. F., Carpio, N. M., Woolley, M. M. & Asch, M. J. (1974) Hepatic bilirubin glucuronidation in neonates with unconjugated hyperbilirubinaemia and congenital gastrointestinal obstruction. *Journal of Laboratory and Clinical Medicine,* **83,** 90.

Gardner, L. I. (1974) Intrahepatic bile stasis in 45X Turner's syndrome. *New England Journal of Medicine,* **290,** 406.

Gautier, M., Jehan, P. & Odievre, M. (1976) Histologic study of biliary fibrous remnants in 48 cases of extrahepatic biliary atresia: correlation with postoperative bile flow restoration. *Journal of Pediatrics,* **85,** 704.

Gerety, R. J. & Schweitzer, I. L. (1977) Viral hepatitis type B during pregnancy, the neonatal period and infancy. *Journal of Pediatrics,* **90,** 368.

Grand, R. J., Watkins, J. B., Katz, A. J. & Lawson, E. E. (1975) Neonatal jaundice—recent developments. *New England Journal of Medicine,* **292,** 1028.

Hass, L. (1968) Intrahepatic cholestasis in the newborn. *Archives of Disease in Childhood,* **43,** 438.

Hanson, R. F., Isenberg, J. N., Williams, G. C., Hachey, D., Szczepanik, P. Klein, P. D. & Sharp, H. L. (1975) The metabolism of 3, 7, 12-trihydroxy-5β-cholestan-26-oic acid in two siblings with cholestasis due to intrahepatic bile duct anomalies. *Journal of Clinical Investigation,* **56,** 577.

Hays, D. M., Woolley, M. M., Snyder, W. H., Redd, G. B., Gwinn, J. L. & Landing, B. H. (1967) Diagnosis of biliary atresia; relative accuracy of percutaneous liver biopsy, open liver biopsy and operative cholangiography. *Journal of Pediatrics,* **71,** 598.

Heirwegh, K. P. M., Meuwissen, J. A. T. P. & Favery, J. (1973) Critique of the assay and significance of bilirubin conjugation. *Advances in Clinical Chemistry,* **16,** 239.

Howard, E. R., Johnston, D. I. & Mowat, A. P. (1976) Spontaneous perforation of common bile duct in infants. *Archives of Disease in Childhood,* **51,** 883.

Johnston, D. I., Mowat, A. P., Orr, H. & Kohn, J. (1976) Serum alpha-fetoprotein levels in extrahepatic biliary atresia, idiopathic neonatal hepatitis and alpha-1-antitrypsin deficiency (Pi Z). *Acta Paediatrica Scandinavica,* **65,** 623.

Johnston, J. D. (1975) Neonatal non-haemolytic jaundice. *The New England Journal of Medicine,* **292,** 194.

Javitt, N. B., Morrissey, K. P., Seigel, E., Goldberg, H., Gartner, L. M., Hollander, M. & Kok, E. (1973) Cholestatic syndromes in infancy; diagnostic value of serum bile acid pattern and cholestyramine administration. *Paediatric Research,* **7,** 119.

Kasai, M., Watanabe, I. & Ohi, R. (1975) Follow-up studies of long-term survivors after hepatic porto-enterostomy for 'non-correctable biliary atresia'. *Journal of Paediatric Surgery,* **10,** 173.

Kattamis, C., Demetrious, D., Karambula, K., Davri-Karamouzi, Y. & Matsaniotis, N. (1973) Neonatal hepatitis associated with Australia antigen (Au-1). *Archives of Disease in Childhood,* **48,** 133.

Koop, C. E. (1975) Progressive extrahepatic biliary obstruction. *Journal of Paediatric Surgery,* **10,** 169.

Landing, B. H. (1974) Consideration of the pathogenesis of neonatal hepatitis, biliary atresia, and choledochal cyst—the concept of infantile obstructive cholangeopathy. In *Progress in Paediatric Surgery,* **6,** p. 5. Munchen: Urban Schwarzenberg.

Lathe, G. H. (1974) Newborn Jaundice: bile pigment metabolism in the fetus and newborn infant. In *Scientific Foundation of Paediatrics,* ed. Davis, G. A. & Dobbing, J., p. 105. London: Heinemann.

Lilly, J. R. & Starzl, T. E. (1974) Liver transplantation in children with biliary atresia and vascular anomalies. *Journal of Paediatric Surgery,* **9,** 707.

Lilly, J. R. (1975) The Japanese operation for biliary atresia: remedy or mischief. *Pediatrics,* **55,** 12.

Manthorpe, D. J. & Mowat, A. P. (1976) Serum bile acids in the neonatal hepatitis syndrome. In *Liver Diseases in Children,* p. 57, ed. by Alagille, D. Paris: INSERM.

Mowat, A. P., Psacharopoulos, H. T. & Williams, R. (1976) Extrahepatic biliary atresia versus neonatal hepatitis: review of 137 prospectively investigated infants. *Archives of Disease in Childhood,* **51,** 763.

Odell, J. B., Storey, J. M. B. & Rosenberg, L. A. (1970) Studies in kernicterus III. Saturation of serum proteins with bilirubin during neonatal life and its relationship to brain damage at five years. *Journal of Paediatrics,* **76,** 12.

Odievre, M., Valayer, J., Razemon-Pinta, M., Habib, E. & Alagille, D. (1976) Hepatic porto-enterostomy or cholecystostomy in the treatment of extrahepatic biliary atresia. *Journal of Pediatrics,* **88,** 774.

Ostrow, J. D. (1972) Photochemical and biochemical basis of the treatment of neonatal jaundice. In *Progress in Liver Disease,* **4,** p. 447, ed. Popper, H. & Schaffer, F. New York: Grune and Stratton.

Philip, A. & Larson, E. (1973) Overwhelming neonatal infection with ECHO 19 virus. *Journal of Pediatrics,* **82,** 391.

Porter, C. A., Mowat, A. P., Cook, P. J. L., Haynes, D. W. G., Shilton, K. B. & Williams, R. (1972) Alpha-1-antitrypsin deficiency and neonatal hepatitis. *British Medical Journal,* **3,** 435.

Reubner, B. H., Bhagavan, B. S., Greenfield, A. J., Campbell, P. & Danks, D. M. (1969) Neonatal hepatic necrosis. *Paediatrics,* **43,** 693.

Sass-Kortsak, A. (1974) Management of young infants presenting with direct reacting hyperbilirubinaemia. *Paediatric clinics of North America,* **21,** 777.

Schweitzer, I. L., Wing, A., McPeak, C. & Spears, R. L. (1972) Hepatitis B antigen in mothers and infants. *Journal of the American Medical Association,* **222,** 1092.

Schweitzer, I. L., Mosley, J. W., Ashcavai, M., Edwards, V. M. & Overby, L. B. (1973) Factors influencing neonatal infection by hepatitis B virus. *Gastroenterology,* **65,** 277.

Silverman, A., Roy, C. C. & Cozzetto, F. J. (1971) In *Pediatric Clinical Gastroenterology,* p. 299. St. Louis: Moseby.

Svegar, T. (1974) Personal communication to Aagenaes, O., Fagerhol, M., Eligio, K., Munthe & Hovig, T. (1974) Pathology and pathogenesis of liver disease in alpha-1-antitrypsin deficient individuals. *Postgraduate Medical Journal,* **50,** 365.

Svegar, T. (1976) Liver disease in alpha-1-antitrypsin efficiency detected by screening of 200 000 infants. *New England Journal of Medicine*, **294**, 1316.

Talbot, I. C. & Mowat, A. P. (1975) Liver disease in infancy: histological features and relationship to alpha-1-antitrypsin phenotype. *Journal of Clinical Pathology*, **28**, 559.

Taylor, A. (1968) Autosomal trisomy and hepatitis syndromes. *Journal of Medical Genetics*, **5**, 227.

Thaler, M. M. & Gellis, S. S. (1968) Studies in neonatal hepatitis and biliary atresia: long term prognosis. *American Journal of Diseases of Childhood*, **116**, 257.

Walker, W. (1971) Haemolytic disease in the newborn. In *Recent Advances in Paediatrics*. 4th edition, p. 131, ed. Gairdner, G. & Hull, D. London: Churchill.

Watson, G. H. & Miller, V. (1973) Arteriohepatic dysplasia. Familial pulmonary artery stenosis and neonatal liver disease. *Archives of Disease in Childhood*, **48**, 459.

Wilkinson, E. J., Raab, K., Browning, C. A. & Hosty, T. A. (1974) Familial hepatic cirrhosis in infants associated with alpha-1-antitrypsin SZ phenotype. *Journal of Pediatrics*, **85**, 159.

Zeltzer, P. M., Neerhout, R. C., Fonkalsrud, E. W. & Stiehm, E. R. (1974) Differentiation between neonatal hepatitis and biliary atresia by measuring serum alpha-phetoprotein. *Lancet*, **1**, 373.

17. Infections of the liver

W. C. Marshall and A. P. Mowat

Viral infections
Parasitic infections
Bacterial infections
Reye's syndrome
Other diagnostic considerations
Acute liver failure

Viruses, bacteria, fungi, protozoa and helminths may be responsible for an infectious process involving the liver. The viral infections can be divided into those which can be termed 'hepatotrophic', that is hepatitis viruses and another group in which hepatic involvement is but part of a more widespread infection. The agents which can cause infections of the liver are listed in Table 17.1. Some infections have a worldwide distribution whilst others are acquired in more or less defined geographical areas, but with increased frequency and speed of travel, patients with these infections may be seen in unexpected circumstances. This chapter considers, in the main, infections of the liver occurring outside the neonatal period. Neonatal infections are dealt with in Chapter 16.

VIRAL INFECTIONS

Hepatitis viruses

Viral hepatitis viruses occur in all countries of the world, and at least two distinct viruses are involved. These have been distinguished in the past by different incubation periods and different routes of infection. The many terms which have been applied to these forms of hepatitis, a number of which are listed in Table 17.2, illustrate the gaps in knowledge which have existed. The terminology which is currently accepted for the two principal types of viral hepatitis is hepatitis virus type A and hepatitis virus type B.

Table 17.1 Agents responsible for infection of the liver in childhood

Hepatitis A virus	*Toxoplasma gondii*	Leptospirae
Hepatitis B virus	Toxocara	Bacteria
EB virus	Echinococcus	Brucellae
Cytomegalovirus	Leishmaniasis	Schistosomas
Yellow fever virus	Entameba Histolytica	Fasciola hepatica

Table 17.2 A selection of the nomenclature applied to the hepatitis viruses

Acute viral hepatitis	Transfusion hepatitis
Acute catarrhal jaundice	Serum hepatitis
Epidemic hepatitis	Long incubation hepatitis
Infectious hepatitis	Homologous serum jaundice
Short incubation hepatitis	MS-2 hepatitis
MS-1 hepatitis	SH hepatitis
IH hepatitis	Australia antigen hepatitis
Viral hepatitis type A	Viral hepatitis type B

Two events have been largely responsible for the clearer understanding of viral hepatitis; firstly, the studies by Krugman and his colleagues (Krugman, Giles and Hammond, 1967), and secondly, the discovery by Blumberg and his associates of an antigen in the serum of an Australian aborigine which reacted with serum from a patient with haemophilia who had received multiple transfusions. This was named Australia antigen (Blumberg, Alter and Visnich, 1965) but later became known as hepatitis-associated antigen (HAA), and serum hepatitis (SH) antigen when it was found to be closely associated with the aetiology of hepatitis B (Prince, 1968; Giles *et al.*, 1969).

Major advances have followed these discoveries and have included the successful transmission of both of the hepatitis viruses in species of non-human primates and the development of methods to measure antibody to both of the agents; but the important step of cultivation of the virus in tissue or organ cultures still eludes investigators.

Hepatitis type A

This form of hepatitis has a worldwide distribution, and in children is far commoner than hepatitis B. It is endemic in many countries and also occurs in minor and major epidemics. In the United Kingdom the majority of cases occur in the late autumn and the first half of winter.

Transmission. Transmission is generally by the faecal/oral route, but some epidemics have been caused by contamination of water and food (Mosley, 1959; Mason and McLean, 1962; Meyers *et al.*, 1975; Chaudhuri, Cassie and Silver, 1975). Close contact in a crowded environment and poor hygiene predispose to the spread of infection from person to person. In countries with inadequate sanitation, therefore, there is a greatly increased probability of infection in childhood.

Clinical features. The illness is usually mild and the incidence of asymptomatic or anicteric infection can be high, particularly in children. Jaundice is very infrequent in children under 3 years of age (Capps, Bennett and Stokes, 1952). Symptoms occur following an incubation period of 15 to 50 days, and for three to five days preceding the onset of jaundice there can be marked anorexia, nausea, vomiting, abdominal pain, mild diarrhoea and fever. In the young child the duration and severity of the preicteric symptoms are usually short and mild, and may even be absent; the first indication of the infection may be the appearance of jaundice. The liver is usually enlarged and tender, and lymphadenopathy and splenomegaly may sometimes be present.

Bile appears in the urine just before the onset of the icteric phase, which generally lasts seven to 10 days and, as with most of the other features, is generally shorter in younger children. As jaundice appears there is frequently a considerable improvement of other symptoms. Fulminant hepatitis is extremely rare in the child; when it occurs there is a rapid development of deep jaundice, widespread haemorrhagic features and rarely acute renal failure. Prompt recognition of the early signs of hepatic failure and the early institution of the treatment measures described later are of great importance.

Laboratory findings and diagnosis. In a typical case of hepatitis type A, the early stages are essentially the same as in hepatitis B infection and the pathological changes in the liver during the acute stage of the infection are indistinguishable from hepatitis B. These changes consist of hepatocellular swelling, necrosis and a mononuclear cellular infiltrate which is predominantly in the portal zones. Detailed descriptions of the histological changes are found in a review by Popper (1967) and in the *Lancet* (1971).

The biochemical and virological findings are schematically illustrated in Figure 17.1. A mild leucocytosis during the incubation period may be followed by leucopaenia and lymphopaenia, and atypical lymphocytes are not infrequently seen. The ESR may be raised in the preicteric stage but has no prognostic significance. Increase in serum transaminases is the first biochemical abnormality to be detected and precedes the appearance of jaundice; SGOT levels remain elevated for up to three weeks in most cases. A few days after the increase in transaminases, the thymol turbidity increases and remains abnormal for one to two weeks after transaminases have returned to normal. Together with the rise in thymol turbidity there is a moderate to marked increase in the levels of IgM. This immunological response can be a useful means of differentiation between the two forms of acute viral hepatitis (see Table 17.3). An increase in the prothrombin time may be an indication of extensive liver damage.

In the past the diagnosis has been based on the epidemiological and clinical features, and more recently by the exclusion of hepatitis B using tests for hepatitis B antigen and antibody, and by the exclusion of other infective causes. The discovery that the virus can be propagated in certain species of marmosets (Deinhardt *et al.,* 1966; Holmes *et al.,* 1969; Mascoli *et al.,* 1973) has led to the development of methods to measure specific antibody. A highly specific neutralising antibody test was first described, but as this required the use of marmosets it was clearly too expensive and cumbersome for routine use. Antigen prepared from liver extracts of infected marmosets has enabled techniques to detect antibody by means of complement fixation (CF) and immune adherence (IA) to be developed (Provost *et al.,* 1975a; Miller *et al.,* 1975). Both types of antibody are maintained for periods of up to nine years after infection (Krugman, Friedman and Lattmier, 1975). Complement-fixation antibody titres rapidly rise during the period of jaundice, whereas the rise of IA antibody

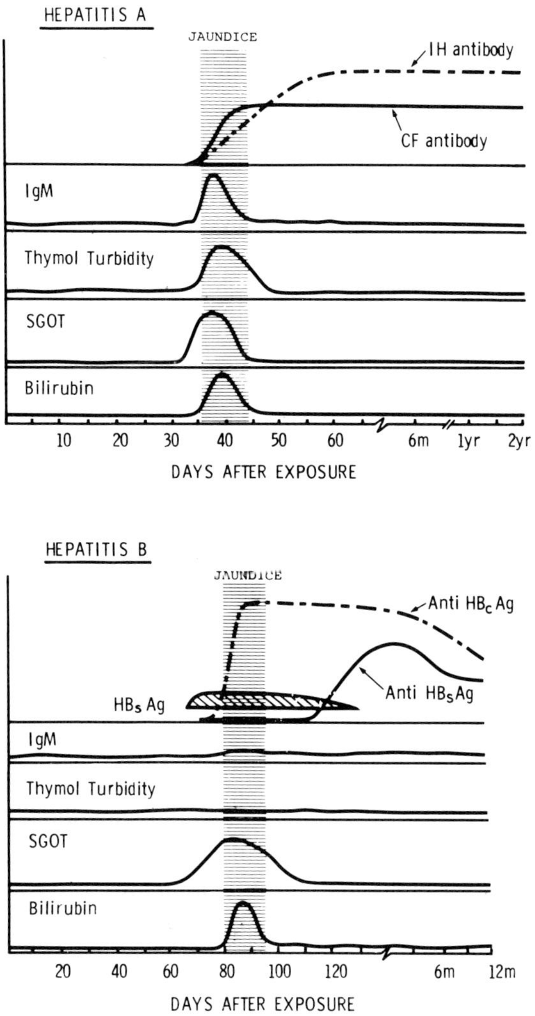

Fig. 17.1 Schematic illustration of the sequential virological, immunological and biochemical events in icteric cases of hepatitis A and B

occurs more slowly but eventually reaches higher levels than CF antibody (Fig. 17.1). Early in the infection the patient's serum may possess anticomplementary activity, which is probably due to the presence of circulating antigen-antibody complexes. These serological tests have yet to be fully utilised and will result in a greater understanding of the epidemiology of this infection. It is already clear that in countries where the disease is endemic most individuals acquire their infection at an early age and remain immune. In countries where the infection is not endemic, which may be in part due to high standards of hygiene, there exists a large pool of susceptible adults.

Using the techniques of electronmicroscopy and immune-electron microscopy, which have been so successful in the study of hepatitis B virus, particles

Table 17.3 Major differentiating features of hepatitis A and B

	Hepatitis A	Hepatitis B
Incubation period	15 to 50 days	50 to 180 days
Age distribution	Children and young adults	Rare in young children; usually adolescents and adults
Route of infection	Oral; rarely parenteral	Parenteral or oral
Epidemiology	Endemic and common source of outbreaks	History of parenteral exposure, or sporadic
Fever	Frequent in early stages	Infrequent
Severity of disease	Usually mild or subclinical in children	Frequently moderate to severe
Extrahepatic features	Very rare	Occasional
Elevated serum transaminases	Transient	More prolonged
Serum IgM	Usually high	Normal or mild elevation
Thymol turbidity	Usually elevated	Usually normal
Hepatitis B antigen in serum	Not detected	Present
Protective effect of pooled immunoglobulin	Effective	Not protective
Immunity	Homologous	Homologous

have been observed in the stools of patients with hepatitis type A (Ferris *et al.*, 1970; Feinstone, Kapikian and Purcell, 1973); the particles are 27 nm size (Fig. 17.2), are found in the acute phase of the illness and can be present five days before the rise in serum transaminases, but cannot be found at the time when serum transaminases have reached peak levels (Dienstag *et al.*, 1975). Patients are infectious during the preicteric phase and there is probably a marked decrease in infectivity at the height of the icteric phase. A chronic infective or carrier state has not been demonstrated. The hepatitis A virus is an RNA virus and is inactivated by boiling for five minutes, irradiation with ultraviolet light and by formalin.

Prevention and treatment. Although it is not yet possible to prevent infection by means of active immunisation, passive immunisation with pooled immunoglobulin is highly effective (Krugman, 1963; Reid, 1971). It is interesting that all the lots of commercial immunoglobulin which were tested by Miller *et al.* (1975) contained antibody to hepatitis A. It is of particular value to travellers to endemic areas, where a single dose of 750 mg provides protection for up to seven months. It can also be used immediately after exposure (0·05 to 0·1 ml/kg), when it may either prevent infection or result in a subclinical or a greatly modified

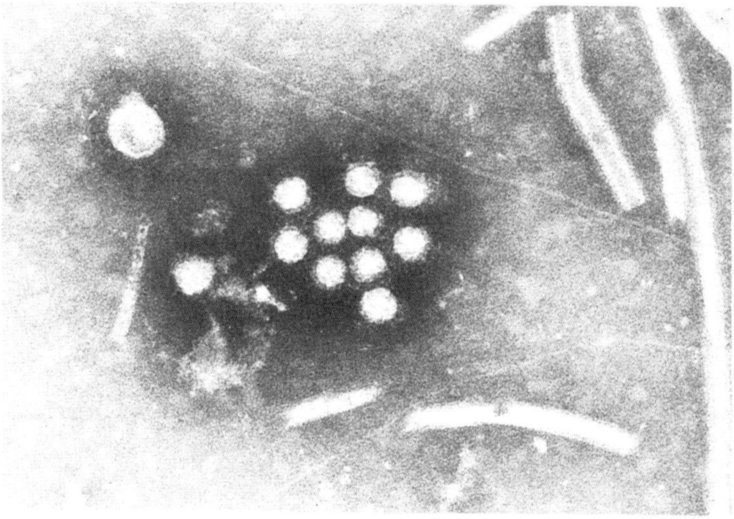

Fig. 17.2 Electronmicroscopic appearances of hepatitis A particles in a faecal suspension from an infected chimpanzee (magnification × 178 750) (Reproduced by courtesy of Dr June Almeida)

illness. It is recommended in contacts within a family, and in groups such as in schools and institutions.

There is no specific treatment. Hepatotoxic drugs must be avoided, and bed rest during the acute phase is important. The child will naturally wish to increase activity as he recovers and this should not be curtailed, but strenuous physical activity during the acute phase is dangerous (Krikler, 1971). Diet in the acute phase should include an adequate fluid and carbohydrate intake but will largely be governed by the child's own wishes.

Hepatitis type B

Although infections with hepatitis B virus are relatively uncommon problems in paediatric practice in westernised countries, there are a number of circumstances which are important. These include transplacental or perinatal infections (see Ch. 16), the prevalence of infections in institutions for the mentally handicapped, the risk of infection in children with disorders of immune function, e.g. patients with leukaemia and other malignancies, and patients with haemophilia who require multiple transfusions with blood or blood products. The introduction of routine screening of donor blood for hepatitis B antigen has greatly reduced the risk of infection from transfusions.

Transmission. The view that infection with this virus was only acquired by the parenteral route has been shown to be incorrect during the past decade, and it is now established that infection can be transmitted by the oral route (Krugman *et al.*, 1967); this study also indicated that the incubation period varied from 50 to 180 days. A very small proportion of children who acquire the infection become persistent carriers of the hepatitis B antigen, and these patients belong to

Table 17.4 Nomenclature proposed by the Committee on Viral Hepatitis set up by the U.S. National Academy of Sciences

HBV	Hepatitis B virus
HB_sAg	Hepatitis B surface antigen found on the 42 nm and 20 nm particles
HB_cAg	Hepatitis B core antigen which is found within the core of the 42 nm (Dane) particle
Dane particle	42 nm particles containing both HB_sAg and HB_cAg
Anti HB_s	Antibody to HB_sAg
Anti HB_c	Antibody to HB_cAg

certain identifiable groups. These include infants who become infected before or at birth in whom persistent antigenaemia is almost universal (Szmuness and Prince, 1971; Hollinger *et al.*, 1972), children with malignant disease such as leukaemia, children receiving immunosuppressive therapy (Sutnick *et al.*, 1971), patients requiring multiple transfusions with blood or blood products and children with Down's syndrome. There is no available method to terminate the carrier state, but it must be recognised and affected children must be clearly identified by hospital staff so that appropriate precautions can be taken for the collection and testing of blood samples. Gloves should be worn for the collection of blood and care should be taken in disposal of the used syringe and needle. All specimens sent to laboratories should be clearly labelled indicating that hepatitis B is proven or suspected.

Relationship to Australia antigen. A vast literature has accumulated in recent years confirming a relationship between Australia antigen and viral hepatitis type B. Studies of the components of the antigen and those using various methods to detect the antigen and antibody have tended to cause confusion. Currently accepted nomenclature, proposed by the committee on viral hepatitis of the U.S. National Academy of Sciences, is shown in Table 17.4.

Clinical features. The clinical features of hepatitis B are almost identical to hepatitis A. If information is available the incubation period can be helpful in differential diagnosis (see Table 17.3). Extrahepatic manifestations, such as rashes and arthritis, occur in hepatitis B and only very rarely in hepatitis A, but these are very uncommon in children so are of little help. Anicteric infection is frequent but is probably less common than in hepatitis A infections. Fever is infrequent and jaundice is generally more prolonged than in hepatitis B.

Laboratory findings and diagnosis. Laboratory tests provide the most reliable means of establishing the presence of hepatitis B infection, and these are shown in Table 17.5. These tests vary in specificity and sensitivity, and each test should

Table 17.5 Comparison of principal laboratory methods for detecting HB_sAg

Method	Sensitivity	Specificity	Time for method
Immunodiffusion	Low	High	24 hours
Counter-immunoelectrophoresis	Moderate	High	2 hours
Complement fixation	Moderate	Moderate	24 hours
Reversed passive latex agglutination	Moderate	Lowest	15 minutes
Reversed passive haemagglutination	High	Lowest	2 hours
Radioimmunoassay	Highest	Low	72 hours

be confirmed by another. Immunodiffusion is the least sensitive and, if allocated a sensitivity of 1, then other tests are of the following relative sensitivities: counter immunoelectrophoresis (1–4), complement fixation (2–10), passive haemagglutination and solid-phase radioimmunoassay (1000–10 000) and radioimmunoprecipitation (10 000–100 000) (WHO, 1975). The most recently described antibody system is related to the 20 nm particle in the core of the Dane particle which is probably the virion of hepatitis B. The level of anti HB_cAg appears to be related to the duration of infection. The time of onset and the pattern of response of the various antibodies are shown in Figure 17.1.

The immunoglobulin levels may be helpful as there is little or no elevation of IgM in hepatitis B, in contrast to high levels of IgM in the early stage of hepatitis A. There is also little or no rise in thymol turbidity (Fig. 17.1).

Visualisation of the antigen by electronmicroscopy or immunoelectronmicroscopy is also a valuable and specific method to detect HB antigen (Fig. 17.3).

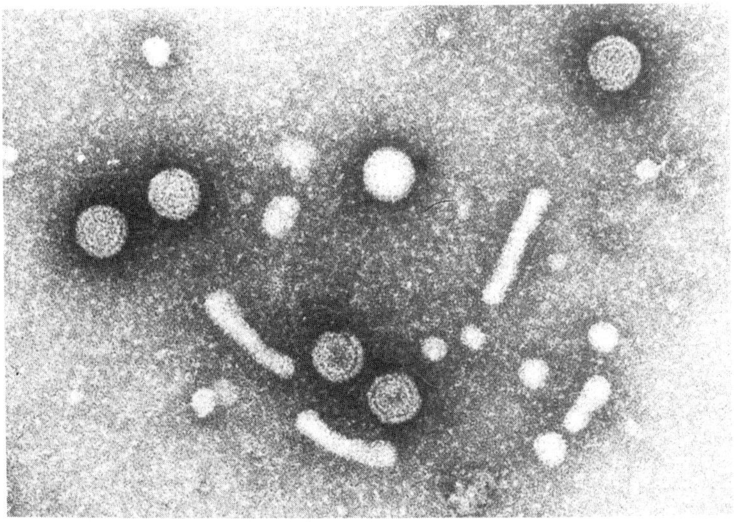

Fig. 17.3 Electronmicroscopic appearances of hepatitis B antigen showing large (42 nm) double shelled spherical particles, tubular forms and small (20 nm) spherical particles (magnification × 178 750) (Reproduced by courtesy of Dr June Almeida)

Immunodiffusion techniques have revealed antigenic differences between hepatitis B antigens (Le Bouvier, 1973), and the various subtypes have been designated adw, adr, ayw, and ayr. These subtypes have been found to breed true in infections and they have also been shown to have a geographical distribution. Their present value is mainly epidemiological and it is too early to know whether they have clinical significance. A further antigenic complex 'e' has also been described and there is now evidence that the presence of this antigen in serum of carrier mothers favours vertical transmission to her offspring (Okada *et al.*, 1976).

Treatment and prevention. No specific treatment is available and limitation of activity and a well-balanced diet is all that is necessary in the mild or moderately severe case. Special attention must be paid in the nursing of these patients because of the risk of cross-infection, and this applies particularly to those who are collecting and testing blood samples. The infection may be prevented by passive immunoprophylaxis using specific hepatitis B immunoglobulin. However, only limited supplies are available and the optimal circumstances for its use have not been clearly defined. Pooled immunoglobulin is of no value.

Other viruses

The recent development of virological and serological methods that diagnose hepatitis A and B has raised the distinct possibility of determining the existence of other hepatitis viruses, which presumably will be designated C and D, etc. (*Lancet*, 1975). This possibility has already been suggested in studies on post-transfusion hepatitis which were not due to hepatitis A or B, or to any other known viral causes of hepatitis such as EB virus and cytomegalovirus (Feinstone *et al.*, 1975). The discovery of a third or even fourth hepatitis virus would clearly be an important advance. In addition, it appears that the hepatitis A could be an enterovirus (Feinstone *et al.*, 1973; Provost *et al.*, 1975b), it is conceivable that distinct serotypes of hepatitis A virus exist as with the other enteroviruses.

EB virus (infectious mononucleosis)

Most infections with EB virus, a member of the herpesvirus group, occur in adolescents and young adults (Evans, 1972). The detailed descriptons of the symptomatology of EBV infection are beyond the scope of this chapter, but involvement of the liver is a common feature (Hoagland and McLusky, 1956; Rosalki, Gwyn-Jones and Verney, 1960; Dunnett, 1963). The frequency of hepatic involvement is such that it should not be considered a complication but rather a part of the normal infectious process with EB virus (Hoagland, 1967; Fernbach and Starling, 1972).

The clinical spectrum of liver disease extends from hepatomegaly with or without tenderness, to a picture resembling acute 'infectious' hepatitis. In the latter case there are almost always other features of the infection such as prolongation of fever, pharyngeal involvement, adenopathy, rashes and splenomegaly; differentiation from hepatitis type A is rarely a clinical problem. In the young child clinical evidence of liver disease is less frequent than in adults and the overall clinical illness is generally milder (Hsia and Gellis,

1952; Starling and Fernbach, 1968). However, severe liver involvement with prolonged jaundice may nevertheless occur and may even be fatal (Allen and Bass, 1963; Harries and Ferguson, 1968).

The haematological features, atypical lymphocytosis and a positive hetrophile antibody (Paul Bunnell) test, are usually present but the latter may be negative in the young child (Tamir *et al.*, 1974). Specific IgG and IgM antibody tests for EBV (Niederman *et al.*, 1968; Edwards and McSwiggan, 1974) are available for serological diagnosis. Cases in which there is an infectious mononucleosis-like clinical illness with negative hetrophile antibody tests should also be examined serologically for the possibility of cytomegalovirus infection, as this virus very occasionally produces a similar clinical and haematological picture (*vide infra*).

There is no specific treatment, but in severely ill patients a dramatic improvement can be achieved with corticosteroids.

Cytomegalovirus

The major clinical impact of cytomegalovirus (CMV), another of the herpesviruses, is related to intrauterine infections and the resulting multisystem disease including involvement of the liver (see Ch. 16).

Postnatal CMV infection is uncommon in childhood. Seroepidemiological studies indicate that the incidence of complement-fixing antibody in children up to 10 years of age in Europe and North America is only between 7 and 33 per cent (Krech, Jung and Jung, 1971). The vast majority of these infections are asymptomatic or are associated with a very mild febrile illness with no specific features. Very rarely, however, a mononucleosis-like disease or symptoms resembling mild acute viral hepatitis may occur (Hanshaw *et al.*, 1965; Klemola *et al.*, 1966; Krech *et al.*, 1968; Weller, 1971). Hepatic involvement is generally mild but is a frequent feature of those patients who present with a mononucleosis-like syndrome (Sterner *et al.*, 1968; Jordan *et al.*, 1973); complete recovery usually occurs. Jaundice is very mild or absent, and the principal abnormality is elevation of serum transaminases. Inflammatory cells with minimal necrosis are found in the liver (Sterner *et al.*, 1968).

Certain groups of children are at special risk from developing symptomatic CMV infection. Patients undergoing heart surgery with extracorporeal circulation may develop a 'postperfusion syndrome' three to five weeks later; this consists of a fever, atypical lymphocytosis and splenomegaly. In addition there may also be hepatomegaly, jaundice, anaemia, lymphadenopathy and abnormal liver function tests (Embil *et al.*, 1968). Another susceptible group are children with leukaemia and other forms of malignant disease, in whom the reported incidence of CMV infection is between 3 to 11 per cent (Henson *et al.*, 1972; Hughes, Feldman and Cox, 1974). In these patients, who presumably have some degree of immunodeficiency as a result of their underlying disease or the treatments they are receiving, it is not yet clear whether the infections are primary or due to reactivation of a latent CMV infection. It is likely that both occur.

The diagnosis of CMV can be readily established by isolation of the virus from urine, blood and liver, by antibody tests showing seroconversion or by the presence of CMV IgM antibody.

No specific treatment is available, but the use of antiviral agents such as cytosine or adenine arabinoside should be considered in very severe infections.

Yellow fever

Involvement of the liver by the yellow fever virus, a member of the group B arboviruses, characteristically consists of a necrosis in the midzone of the liver lobule with an absence of an inflammatory reaction, but there may also be necrosis in other areas. Symptoms follow a variable incubation period of usually between three and seven days and consist of fever, headache, muscle and epigastric pain; these symptoms are followed by a recrudescence of the fever, enlargement of the liver and the appearance of jaundice. Heavy albuminuria is a consistent feature and haemorrhagic manifestations are striking in severe cases. Hepatitis A and B must be considered in the differential diagnosis, but albuminuria is rare in viral hepatitis and prolonged fever is not a feature.

The virus is present in the blood during the first week of the disease and can be detected by intracerebral injection into the brain of infant mice. Antibody (complement-fixing and HI) tests are also available for diagnosis (WHO, 1967).

Yellow fever vaccines are effective in prevention, and circulating antibody persists for about 10 years. The history of the use of yellow fever vaccines is of special relevance to viral hepatitis. Serum hepatitis was observed in persons receiving earlier vaccines, and this was due to the incorporation of human serum into the vaccines. The most notable effect of this resulted in the massive 'epidemic' of 28 585 cases of viral hepatitis in the U.S. Army in 1942 (*Journal of American Medical Association*, 1942). There is no evidence that the currently available vaccines can cause hepatic infection; loss of 'hepatotrophism' is one of the features of attenuation of the virus.

Other viruses

Involvement of the liver may also occur in other viral infections. These include herpes simplex, Coxsackie B and Varicella–Zoster virus, but for practical purposes serious liver disease due to these agents is a feature of neonatal infections. In the older child, adenoviruses and reoviruses may rarely involve the liver.

PARASITIC INFECTIONS

Toxoplasma gondii

The majority of infections with the protozoon *Toxoplasma gondii* are either subclinical or associated with features of a non-specific febrile illness. Occasionally a glandular fever-like illness occurs, or very rarely there is a high fever, pneumonitis and a maculopapular rash. Acute hepatitis, with enlargement of the liver, mild jaundice and elevation of serum transaminase levels, may also occur, together with serological evidence of the infection (Vischer, Bernheim and Engelbrecht, 1967); general malaise and adenopathy may occur in cases with liver involvement. In the absence of serological evidence of the infection or identification of the organisms in the liver, the illness may be indistinguishable from infections with hepatitis viruses. However, the prodromal symptoms usually last several weeks, in contrast to the shorter period of symptoms in hepatitis A or B. The incidence of liver disease due to *T. gondii* in childhood, other than in congenital infections, is not known; it should be suspected when other causes of hepatitis have been excluded. Disseminated infections in which the liver is also involved occur either as a primary infection or as a reactivation of a latent infection in children with malignancies or those receiving immunosuppressive drugs. Diagnosis can be established by means of several serological tests, of which the IgM fluorescent antibody test is of particular value (Remington, Miller and Brownlee, 1968).

Sulphadiazine and pyrimethamine act synergistically to block metabolic pathways of folinic acid in the toxoplasma. Chemotherapy is used to suppress the proliferation of toxoplasma until immunity is acquired. Sulphadiazine is administered in a dose of 100 mg/kg/day and pyrimethamine in a dose of 1 mg/kg/day. Treatment should be continued until immunity is acquired, which usually takes two to four weeks; an antibody response may be used as a guide for determining the duration of treatment.

Leishmaniasis

There are a number of clinical disorders which are caused by the protozoa of the genus *Leishmania* but infection with *Leishmania donovani,* which occurs in all subtropical and tropical countries except Australia, is the cause of the visceral disease Kala-azar. Infection is spread by sandfly vectors from a canine reservoir. The onset of the illness is insidious and follows an incubation period of an extremely variable period which can range from 10 days to one or two years, or even longer.

Kala-azar is essentially a disease of the reticuloendothelial system and involvement of the liver is often a prominent feature; the presence of hepatosplenomegaly, adenopathy, anaemia and pancytopaenia may closely resemble a reticulosis or leukaemia. Fever and weight loss are common.

The diagnosis can be established by Giemsa stains of bone marrow aspirates which show the characteristic Leishman-Donovani (LD) body; LD bodies can also be seen in liver, spleen and lymph node aspirates. The parasites can also be cultured from marrow and blood. Antibody tests are available which assist in the diagnosis (Shaw and Voller, 1964).

Specific treatment with sodium stibogluconate (Pentostam) is highly effective, but supportive treatment with blood transfusions for severe anaemia may also be necessary.

Toxocariasis

The most frequent organ to be involved by the larvae of the nematode *Toxocara* is the liver (Shrand, 1964; Huntley, Costas and Lyerly, 1965) which is diffusely enlarged; histologically there are irregular foci of necrosis in the portal tracts surrounded by inflammatory cells. The larvae may sometimes be seen in biopsy specimens. Serum transaminases may be elevated but jaundice is not a feature. Although levels of serum globulins can be considerably elevated, this abnormality is more variable than a persistent eosinophilia. High titres of isohaemagglutins are also found (Huntley *et al.,* 1965). Several methods of measuring specific antibody have been described and skin test antigens are advocated, but unfortunately these are not entirely specific (Kagan, 1968).

There is no effective treatment. Diethylcarbamazine in a total daily dose of 3 mg/kg administered three times daily for a period of 21 days causes death of the larvae in the tissues and symptomatic improvement in some cases. Corticosteroids are of value in patients with marked respiratory symptoms (Beshear and Hendley, 1973), but are not indicated in patients with hepatic involvement alone or with mild pulmonary disease. Infected household animals should be dewormed at frequent intervals with piperazine in doses of 200 mg/kg.

Hydatid disease *(Echinococcus granulosus)*

The most frequent mode of presentation of hydatid disease of the liver is the finding of an epigastric mass. Less frequently there may be abdominal pain or jaundice and, very rarely, anaphylactic reactions when a cyst has ruptured into the peritoneal cavity (Joske, 1974). Very rarely the cyst may rupture into the biliary tree or become infected, when it presents clinically as an hepatic abscess (Zielinsky and Elmslie, 1969). Calcification of the cysts in the liver is not infrequent. Meyers (1960) has noted that in children hepatic cysts are less frequent than pulmonary cysts, the reverse being the case in adults.

Although the intradermal Casoni skin test has been used for many years, it is known to have certain inherent disadvantages. It is probably most reliable for detecting the prevalence of infection in a community in which other helminths are not commonly found. The complement-fixation (CF) test is valuable for diagnosis and prognosis. Cysts of the liver promote the highest levels of antibody (Bradstreet, 1969). A highly sensitive indirect haemagglutination test has also been described, which is claimed to be more sensitive than the intradermal and CF tests (Garabedian, Matossian and Djanian, 1957). Treatment of hydatid disease consists of surgical removal of the cysts. Prevention of infection in dogs is an important public health measure and consists of regular administration of antihelmintics to dogs and the destruction of infected viscera. The importation of livers and other offal for use as pet foods, and the use of meats for preparation of canned pet foods, must be under close health supervision.

Amoebiasis

Abscess formation in the liver is the commonest extraintestinal complication of infection with *Entamoeba histolytica*. The amoebae enter the liver in most instances via the portal vein, but rarely infection can be caused by direct extension from the gut. There is focal necrosis which is rapidly followed by lysis of hepatic tissue. Pleural and/or pulmonary involvement may result from direct extension of the abscesses.

All ages may be affected and abscesses have been observed in very young infants (Scragg, 1960; Larracilla, Juarez and Resendiz, 1971). An enlarged, tender liver is the main clinical finding, jaundice is rare and liver function tests may be normal; anaemia is common in fulminating disease (Lamont and Pooler, 1958). During acute amoebic dysentery, tender enlargement of the liver without demonstrable abscess formation is not infrequent. Following successful treatment of the intestinal infection, the liver returns to normal size without sequelae. This has been termed amoebic 'hepatitis' by many authors (Ramachandran *et al.*, 1973). However, it is essentially a clinical diagnosis, there being no pathological evidence of invasion of the liver by amoebae.

In addition to the demonstration of the cysts or trophozoites in stools, the fluorescent antibody test is of value in diagnosis of a recent or active infection (Jeans, 1969), but other serological tests are also available (Maddison, Kagan and Elsdon-Dew, 1968).

Specific and effective treatment with metronidazole is available (see Ch. 12). Large liver cysts require surgical aspiration.

Other parasites

Infection with other parasites such as in ascariasis and fascioliasis can, less commonly, involve the liver or biliary tree, and disease of the liver and spleen has long been recognised to result from invasion of the liver by *Schistosomata.* Careful attention to the details of the history of the illness and to where the child is residing or has resided may provide important clues to an infectious cause of liver damage.

BACTERIAL INFECTIONS

In a number of acute bacterial infections, there may be enlargement of the liver with or without jaundice, abnormalities of liver function tests such as elevation of serum transaminases or alkaline phosphatase and histological changes which have been described as 'a non-specific reactive hepatitis' (Popper and Schaffner, 1957). These changes may be seen in typhoid fever and other salmonella infections, tuberculosis, Q fever, brucellosis and septicaemias caused by a wide variety of bacteria. Similar changes may also be found in ulcerative colitis and regional enteritis.

Pyogenic abscesses of the liver

Bacteria may reach the liver via the blood system, by extension from a neighbouring septic focus, as a complication of surgical procedures, or from penetrating injuries involving the liver. In children, abscesses are usually secondary to generalised infection (Rubin, Swartz and Malt, 1974). The consequences may be solitary or multiple abscesses and, depending on the pathogenesis, may be associated with abscess formation in other organs. Hepatic enlargement, tenderness and fever may be present; abdominal pain and jaundice are infrequent. A large proportion of cases are only discovered at autopsy (Dehner and Kissane, 1960). The increasing use of radioisotope scanning of the liver should result in increased recognition. The peripheral total white cell count may be elevated but this is not invariable and the only abnormality in liver function tests is elevation of serum alkaline phosphatase; serum levels of vitamin B_{12} may be increased.

A variety of bacteria have been isolated from liver abscesses which include *Staphylococcus aureus*, haemolytic and non-haemolytic streptococci, *E. coli*,

Klebsiella/Enterobacter species, *Pseudomonas aeruginosa* and *Proteus mirabilis*. Mixed infections can occur but in a proportion of cases the abscess is sterile. Important non-bacterial infections are caused by *Candida albicans* and actinomycosis. Because of the changing biology of infections, the incidence of particular pathogens will change over periods of time as they are affected by the many known and unknown factors which modify the ecology of micro-organisms.

An increased susceptibility to hepatic abscess formation is recognised in certain groups of children. For example, abscesses are especially prevalent in chronic granulomatous disease (Johnston and Baehner, 1971) but, on the other hand, are rare in patients with other defects of neutrophil function or in isolated neutropenia. Enteric bacteria and staphylococci are the principal infecting organisms in chronic granulomatous disease. Patients with acute leukaemia are also at risk. A group which may assume increasing importance in the future are patients receiving prolonged total parenteral nutrition, as this procedure becomes used more frequently in children with chronic malnutrition due to a wide variety of gastrointestinal disorders. *Candida albicans* is the chief offender in this group.

Appropriate antibiotic treatment has to be given for a prolonged period, and surgical drainage of large abscesses may be necessary.

Leptospirosis

Leptospira icterohaemorrhagica, the causal organisms of Weil's disease, are shed in the urine of infected rodents contaminating water, moist soil and vegetation, and there is usually an abrupt onset of fever, vomiting and muscular pains. The clinical illness can vary from a severe influenza-like illness to prolonged fever with symptoms and signs due to involvement of the liver, lungs, nervous system or kidneys.

The incubation period varies from two or three days to two or three weeks and there is usually an abrupt onset of fever, vomiting and muscular pains. During the next five to 10 days jaundice and hepatomegaly may develop (Sterling, 1950) with or without haemorrhagic manifestations or signs of involvement of the lungs, nervous system or kidneys; the appearance of jaundice is a grave sign. A transient macular rash may also be present. Hepato-renal failure may occasionally occur at this stage. Usually there is a slow but complete recovery which may take several weeks.

Neutrophil leukocytosis and mild anaemia are frequent, and anaemia may be severe when there are signs of severe multisystem involvement. Blood cultures are positive during the first week of symptoms, and during the second and third weeks the organisms can be seen in the urine on dark ground microscopy. Antibodies, measured by complement-fixation using a group antigen, develop after the first week rising during the next two weeks. More specific antibody tests (Turner, 1968) are available but the CF antibody test is generally satisfactory for diagnostic purposes (Communicable Disease Report, 1972). The antibiotic of choice is penicillin and, if given in large doses during the early stages of the infection, it may be effective.

REYE'S SYNDROME

This syndrome consists of an encephalopathy and fatty degeneration of viscera and was first described by Reye and colleagues in 1963; it has been reported from most countries but is rare. Although the aetiology of this condition remains unknown, certain observations point towards an infective cause. A wide range of viruses have been implicated including influenza A and B, Varicella–Zoster, mumps, EB, para-influenza and vaccinia. The clustering of recent cases reported from the United States (Corey *et al.*, 1976) is of particular interest with respect to the possible role of influenza B infections. A 'toxic' cause cannot be excluded at the present stage and aflatoxin has been suggested to be the cause in the unusual clustering of cases in Thailand (Olson *et al.*, 1971). The studies of Crocker *et al.* (1974) suggest that a synergistic toxic effect of an insecticide and a virus could cause Reye's syndrome. Many of the biochemical abnormalities found transiently in this disorder (Brown *et al.*, 1976) are related to mitochondrial function, reflecting the changes found in this organelle on electronmicroscopy. The mechanism of injury is not yet known.

Patients with this syndrome present with a short prodromal illness, often viral or suggestive of a viral illness, which is followed within a few hours or days by vomiting, confusion, delirium, stupor and then coma. Generalised seizures may also occur but focal neurological signs are absent. There may be increasing enlargement of the liver, together with elevation of serum transaminases, hypoglycaemia, hyperammonaemia and increase in the prothrombin time; jaundice is occasionally present. The most common abnormality in the cerebrospinal fluid appears to be low levels of sugar. The hepatocytes are massively infiltrated with neutral fat, but there is an absence of an inflammatory cell reaction. Similar fatty changes may also occur in the kidneys and pancreas. The mortality of this disorder in the most recent reports is at least 40 per cent. Since the cause of the disorder and the pathogenesis of the encephalopathy remain unknown, therapy is empirical. Cerebral oedema, however, is an important factor and should be minimised. Therefore, in addition to measures aimed at correction of hypoglycaemia, electrolyte disturbances, hypoxia and acidosis, fluid intake should be reduced to between 60 to 80 per cent of normal. Increasing the serum osmolality may also minimise the effects of cerebral oedema (Lovejoy *et al.*, 1975). Mannitol infusions may be necessary when manifest features of cerebral oedema are present. Although measures to combat hepatic encephalopathy are conventionally used and appear to do no harm, there is no evidence that such measures are efficacious. Exchange transfusion may correct some of the clotting abnormalities, remove putative toxins and reduce intracranial pressure (Berman *et al.*, 1975). Peritoneal dialysis and glucose and insulin therapy are of no proven value. Intensive supportive care and monitoring are essential.

OTHER DIAGNOSTIC CONSIDERATIONS

Full haematological investigations should be carried out in all children with jaundice or other signs suggestive of infection of the liver. Various haemato-

Table 17.6 Some drugs and toxins capable of causing liver damage in children

Antimicrobials Tetracycline Chlor- and oxytetracycline Erythromycin estolate Nitrofurantoin Ampicillin Sulphonamides Lincomycin/clindamycin **Antituberculous drugs** PAS Isoniazid Rifampicin Pyrazinamide Ethambutol Ethionamide **Antimetabolites** Methotrexate 6-mercaptopurine Azathioprine	**Anaesthetics** Halothane **Anticonvulsants, sedatives and antidepressants** Phenobarbitone Diphenylhyantoin Trimethadione Phenacemide Chlordiazepoxide Tricyclic antidepressants (e.g. amitriptyline, imipramine, iprindole) Monoamine oxidase inhibitors (e.g. phenelzine, iproniazid) Phenothiazine **Anti-inflammatory and analgesic agents** Phenylbutazone Indomethacin Paracetamol	**Poisons and toxins** Carbon tetrachloride Tetrachlorethane Ferrous sulphate Senecio alkaloids Aflatoxin Radiation D.D.T. Benzine derivatives Tarmic acid Muscarine Metals (arsine, beryllium, manganese) **Other agents** Methyltestosterone Oxyphenisatin Methyl-dopa Methimazole Chlorpropramide Tolbutamide

logical disorders such as the many types of congenital and acquired haemolytic anaemias have to be considered in the evaluation of these patients.

Drugs, toxins and metabolic diseases must also be considered in the differential diagnosis, especially in the sporadic or isolated cases of 'hepatitis'. A detailed discussion of the many drugs and toxins which may cause damage or dysfunction is beyond the scope of this chapter, and these can be found in standard texts and recent reviews of the subject (Sherlock, 1975; Perez, Schafner and Popper, 1972; Maxwell and Williams, 1973). Drugs and toxins may interfere with bilirubin metabolism or have a direct toxic effect on the liver cells, and these effects are usually predictable and dose related. The adverse effects of some substances are unpredictable, occurring in only a small proportion of individuals, and are probably due to some form of hypersensitivity reaction; the incidence and severity of this type of damage is not dose related. The principal drugs which are of importance in paediatric practice are listed in Table 17.6.

It is also important to be aware of the possibility of Wilson's disease, presenting as acute liver disease which in the early stages may be clinically indistinguishable from acute viral hepatitis. Coexisting haemolysis is a clue to the diagnosis. This should be considered in patients in whom recovery is delayed or where there is no epidemiological evidence to indicate the source of the 'infection'.

ACUTE LIVER FAILURE

Hepatic failure is a complex clinical syndrome associated with severe impairment of hepatic function; it may represent the end stage of cirrhosis or other chronic liver disease or develop early during the course of an acute hepatitis complicated by massive necrosis of liver cells. The term fulminant hepatic failure is limited to those patients who develop features of liver failure within eight weeks of the onset of their illness. The syndrome is characterised by a progressive encephalopathy advancing to coma, increasing jaundice, a bleeding diathesis and complex metabolic, fluid and electrolyte abnormalities. This section concentrates on the features of acute hepatic failure, although many of these are similar to those of chronic hepatic failure and the rationale of management of acute hepatic failure has to some extent been based on observations made in chronic liver failure.

Pathogenesis of liver failure

In most instances the cause is presumed to be viral hepatitis type A; infectious mononucleosis, hepatotoxic drugs such as paracetamol, or an apparent hypersensitivity reaction with drugs such as monoamine oxidase inhibitors or halothane are occasional causes. In each instance there is massive hepatocellular necrosis with parenchymal collapse. The factors which determine the severity of the hepatic lesion or govern the ability of the liver to recover are not understood.

Clinical features

Hepatic encephalopathy has diverse clinical features reflecting the involvement of all parts of the brain. Those occurring in children are similar to adults except that in children there are more commonly acute reactions, particularly disturbed behaviour and mania. Deterioration in intellectual function, personality changes and disturbed consciousness, all of varying and fluctuating severity, are seen. The most characteristic neurological abnormality is the 'flapping tremor', i.e. rapid flexion-extension movements at the metacarpal, phalangeal and wrist joints when the arms are outstretched and fingers separated; signs of pyramidal and extrapyramidal dysfunction may also occur. These neurological abnormalities are associated with bilateral slow wave activity (two to three per second) on electroencephalography, particularly over the frontal lobes. The breath has a sweetish and slightly faecal smell, so-called 'fetor hepaticus'. Hyperventilation and hyperpyrexia may be terminal phenomena. Excessive bleeding from venepunctures, bruising at injection sites, spontaneous skin haemorrhages, and gastrointestinal bleeding reflect disturbances in coagulation; prolongation of the prothrombin time, which is resistant to vitamin K administration, confirms severe hepatic dysfunction. As the jaundice deepens the liver shrinks in size, and abdominal pain, fever and vomiting may occur. In adults the mortality is between 50 and 60 per cent, but in children it is usually between 30 and 40 per cent (Trey, Lipworth and Davidson, 1970; Marks, Mauer, and Goldman, 1969).

Laboratory investigations

Serum transaminases are often increased three to four times above normal, having previously been elevated in excess of 50 times normal. Serum albumin levels are likely to be low, hypoglycaemia is frequent and the patient may be alkalotic. The blood ammonia level is often markedly increased.

Table 17.7 Clinical grades of hepatic coma

1.	Minor disturbances of conciousness and the motor system
2.	Drowsy but responsive to simple commands
3.	Stuporose, but responsive to pain
4.	Unresponsive to painful stimuli

Table 17.8 Precipitating causes of hepatic coma

Gastrointestinal haemorrhage
Hypovolaemia
Diuretics
Potassium depletion
Sedatives and anaesthetics
High protein intake
Uraemia
Infection
Constipation

Pathogenesis of encephalopathy

The precise mechanism responsible for the cerebral changes has not yet been defined. In acute liver failure the cerebral effects are reversible and mainly metabolic, although cerebral oedema is often present. The more chronic forms of liver failure are associated with an increase in the size and number of protoplasmic astrocytes, and in the late stages there may rarely be neuronal degeneration and demyelination.

A variety of metabolic changes have been associated with hepatic failure both in man and in experimental animals (Zieve, 1975). These include increased serum concentrations of ammonia, methionine, glutamine, tryptophan, methionine metabolites, short-chain fatty acids and a variety of biogenetic amines involved in central nervous system neurotransmission. In addition, there are complex changes in cerebral blood flow, and total cerebral glucose and oxygen utilisation.

Precipitating causes of hepatic coma

The precipitating causes of hepatic coma are listed in Table 17.8. All of these aggravate the metabolic abnormalities detailed above. The importance of intensive monitoring to prevent and to detect complications at an early stage cannot be overemphasised, and an understanding of the way in which the various signs and symptoms of the syndrome develop during the course of liver disease is vital. Liver failure may develop very early in the course of acute hepatitis, and the clinician should be alerted to the possibility of impending coma by any one of the following features (Silverman, Roy and Cozzetto, 1971):

1. Persisting anorexia.
2. Deepening jaundice.
3. Relapse of initial features.
4. Reduction in liver size.
5. Ascites.

6. Prolongation of prothrombin time.
7. Depressed serum albumin concentration.
8. Marked elevation of SGOT.
9. Respiratory alkalosis.
10. Hypoglycaemia.
11. Neuropsychiatric changes.

Management of hepatic coma

The maintenance of effective respiration and an adequate circulation in the prevention of possible hypoxic damage to the brain and liver is an essential part of management and is greatly facilitated by monitoring the central venous pressure; blood pressure must be maintained. Regular monitoring of serum electrolytes, blood sugar, osmolality and pH are vital, as are measurements of fluid and electrolyte losses from the gastrointestinal tract and in the urine (Williams, 1972). Fluid intake should be carefully measured so as to avoid hypovolaemia and minimise the risk of cerebral oedema. Fluids should be given in the form of 5 or 10 per cent dextrose in a volume of approximately 75 per cent of normal requirements; this may require modification according to the urinary output and the central venous pressure findings. Potassium usually has to be given well in excess of the normal intake of 2·5 mmol (2·5 mEq)/kg/24 h, since hypokalaemia leads to alkalosis which in turn enhances renal ammonia production by the kidney as well as transfer of ammonia across the blood/brain barrier. Sodium requirements are usually low because of secondary hyperaldosteronism and renal retention of sodium.

The production and absorption of ammonia from the gastrointestinal tract must be minimised, and three methods are of established value: (1) reduction or withdrawal of dietary protein, (2) gastrointestinal cleansing with enemas and magnesium sulphate in sufficient dose to produce diarrhoea, and (3) neomycin administered orally or via a nasogastric tube.

The correction of a bleeding diathesis usually necessitates the use of fresh frozen plasma or whole blood, but intravenous vitamin K (5 to 10 mg) can be tried.

The provision of sufficient calories may pose a difficult problem; initially calories should be given in the form of carbohydrates. Vitamins are usually included in the therapeutic regimen.

As well as these general supportive measures, a careful scrutiny for any of the known precipitating causes of hepatic coma (see Table 17.8) must be maintained and these corrected if possible. Sedatives should be avoided if at all possible; if sedation is absolutely necessary a single half-normal dose of diazepam may be used. Diuretics should also be avoided. In addition, other causes of coma such as subdural haematomata, meningitis and cerebral oedema must be considered and treated. Only rarely will there be appropriate therapy for the underlying liver disease, e.g. corticosteroids for chronic active hepatitis.

In addition to these standard modes of treatment, many other experimental approaches have been advocated and used (Williams and Murray-Lyon, 1975), and these are listed in Table 17.9. None of these approaches has been shown to be any more successful than standard medical management when subjected to

Table 17.9 Experimental therapy in hepatic coma

Steroids
Exchange transfusion
Peritoneal dialysis
Haemodialysis
Charcoal column haemoperfusion
Plasmaphoresis
Heterologous
Pig liver perfusion
Cross-circulation with human volunteers
Cross-circulation with baboons
Temporary heterotopic transplantation
L-Dopa therapy
Hyperbaric oxygenation

rigorous controlled trials. Steroids have been reported to both reduce and increase mortality; they probably increase the risk of infection and in this way may precipitate coma. Exchange transfusion tends to be more enthusiastically used in paediatric patients compared with adults (Zarchy, 1973) but has not been subjected to controlled trials. The difficulties of planning and executing a controlled trial in patients with hepatic coma should not be minimised.

Prognosis

There are no good parameters presently available to assess prognosis and the degree of hepatic regeneration that may be possible in a patient who survives an episode of acute liver failure. The prognosis must be guarded since a significant proportion of patients develop postnecrotic cirrhosis, but some appear to recover completely with normal liver function, liver scan and biopsy (Karvountzis, Redeker and Peters, 1974).

References

Allen, U. R. & Bass, B. H. (1963) Fatal hepatic necrosis in glandular fever. *Journal of Clinical Pathology*, **16**, 337.

Berman, W., Pizzi, F., Schut, L., Raphaely, R. & Holtzapple, P. (1975) The effects of exchange transfusion on intracranial pressure in patients with Reye Syndrome. *Journal of Pediatrics*, **87**, 887.

Beshear, J. R. & Hendley, J. D. (1973) Severe pulmonary involvement in visceral larva migrans. *American Journal of Diseases of Children*, **125**, 599.

Blumberg, B. S., Alter, H. J. & Visnich, S. (1965) A 'new' antigen in leukaemia serum. *Journal of the American Medical Association*, **191**, 541.

Bradstreet, C. M. P. (1969) A study of two immunological tests in the diagnosis and prognosis of hydatid disease. *Journal of Medical Microbiology*, **2**, 419.

Brown, T., Hug, G., Jansky, L., Bove, K., Scheve, A., Ryana, M., Brown, H., Schubert, W. K., Partin, J. C. & Lloyd-Still, J. (1976) Transiently reduced activity of carbamyl phosphate synthetase and ornithine transcarbamylase in liver of children with Reye's syndrome. *New England Journal of Medicine*, **294**, 861.

Capps, R. B., Bennett, A. M. & Stokes, J. (1952) Epidemic hepatitis in an infants orphanage. *Archives of Internal Medicine*, **86**, 6.

Chaudhuri, A. K. R., Cassie, G. & Silver, M. (1975) Outbreak of foodborne type A hepatitis in Greater Glasgow. *Lancet*, **2**, 223.

Communicable Disease Report (1972) Public Health Laboratory Service 72/36, London.

Corey, L., Rubin, R. J., Hattwick, M. A. W., Noble, G. R. & Cassidy, E. (1976) A nationwide outbreak of Reye's syndrome: its epidemiologic relationship to influenza B. *American Journal of Medicine,* **61,** 615.

Crocker, F. S., Rozee, K. R., Ozere, R. L., Digout, S. C. & Hutzinger, O. (1974) Insecticide and viral interaction as a cause of fatty visceral changes and encephalopathy in the mouse. *Lancet,* **2,** 22.

Dehner, L. P. & Kissane, J. M. (1960) Pyogenic hepatic abscesses in infancy and childhood. *Journal of Pediatrics,* **74,** 763.

Deinhardt, F., Holmes, A. W., Capps, R. B. & Popper, H. (1966) Studies on the transmission of human viral hepatitis to marmoset monkeys. *Journal of Experimental Medicine,* **125,** 673.

Deinstag, J. L., Feinstone, S. M., Kapikian, A. Z., Purcell, R. H., Boggs, J. D. & Conrad, M. E. (1975) Faecal shedding of hepatitis A antigen. *Lancet,* **1,** 765.

Dunnett, W. H. (1963) Infectious mononucleosis. *British Medical Journal,* **1,** 1187.

Edwards, J. M. B. & McSwiggan, D. A. (1974) Studies on the diagnostic value of an immunofluorescent test for EB-virus specific IgM. *Journal of Clinical Pathology,* **27,** 647.

Embil, J. A., Folkins, D. F., Haldane, E. V. & Van Rooyen, C. E. (1968). Cytomegalovirus infection following extra-corporeal circulation in children: a prospective study. *Lancet,* **2,** 1151.

Evans, A. S. (1972) Infectious mononucleosis and other mono-like syndromes. *New England Journal of Medicine,* **286,** 836.

Feinstone, S. M., Kapikian, A. Z. & Purcell, R. H. (1973) Hepatitis A: detection by immune electronmicroscopy of a virus like antigen associated with acute illness. *Science,* **182,** 1026.

Feinstone, S. M., Kapikian, A. Z., Purcell, R. H., Alter, H. J. & Holland, P. V. (1975) Transfusion—associated hepatitis not due to viral hepatitis type A or B. *New England Journal of Medicine,* **292,** 767.

Fernbach, D. J. & Starling, K. A. (1972) Infectious mononucleosis. *Pediatric Clinics of North America,* **19,** 957.

Ferris, A. A., Kaldor, J., Gust, I. D. & Cross, G. (1970) Faecal antigen in viral hepatitis. *Lancet,* **1,** 242.

Garabedian, G. A., Matossian, R. M. & Djanian, A. Y. (1957) An indirect haemagglutination test for hydatid disease. *Journal of Immunology,* **78,** 268.

Giles, J. P., McCollum, R. M., Berndtson, L. W. & Krugman, S. (1969) Viral hepatitis: Relation of Australia SH antigen to the Willowbrook MS-2 strain. *New England Journal of Medicine,* **281,** 119.

Hanshaw, J. B., Betts, R. F., Simon, G. & Boynton, R. C. (1965) Acquired cytomegalovirus infections: association with hepatomegaly and abnormal liver function tests. *New England Journal of Medicine,* **272,** 602.

Harries, J. T. & Ferguson, A. W. (1968) Fatal infectious mononucleosis with liver failure in two sisters. *Archives of Disease in Childhood,* **43,** 480.

Henson, D., Siegel, S. E., Fuccillo, D. A., Matthew, E. & Levine, A. S. (1972) Cytomegalovirus infections during acute childhood leukaemia. *Journal of Infectious Diseases,* **126,** 469.

Hoagland, R. J. (1967) *Infectious Mononucleosis.* New York: Grune and Stratton.

Hoagland, R. J. & McClusky, R. H. (1956) Hepatitis in mononucleosis. *Annals of Internal Medicine,* **43,** 1019.

Hollinger, F. B., Goyal, R. K., Hersh, T., Powell, H. C., Schulman, R. T. & Melnick, J. L. (1972) Immune response to hepatitis virus type B in Down's syndrome and other mentally retarded patients. *American Journal of Epidemiology,* **95,** 356.

Holmes, A. W., Wolfe, L., Rosenblate, H. & Deinhardt, F. (1969) Hepatitis in Marmosets: induction of disease with coded specimens from a human volunteer study. *Science,* **165,** 816.

Hsia, D. Y-Y. & Gellis, S. S. (1952) Hepatic dysfunction in infectious mononucleosis in children. *American Journal of Diseases of Children,* **84,** 175.

Hughes, W. T., Feldman, S. & Cox, F. (1974) Infectious diseases in children with cancer. *Pediatric Clinics of North America,* **21,** 600.

Huntley, C. C., Costas, M. C. & Lyerly, A. (1965) Visceral larva migrans syndromes: clinical characteristics and immunological studies in 51 patients. *Pediatrics,* **36,** 523.

Jeans, A. L. (1969) Evaluation in clinical practice of the fluorescent amoebic antibody test. *Journal of Clinical Pathology,* **22,** 427.

Johnston, R. B. & Baehner, R. L. (1971) Chronic granulomatous disease: correlation between pathogenesis and clinical findings. *Pediatrics,* **48,** 730.

Jordan, M. C., Rousseau, W. E., Stewart, J. A., Noble, G. R. & Chin, T. D. Y. (1973) Spontaneous cytomegalovirus mononucleosis. *Annals of Internal Medicine,* **79,** 153.

Joske, R. A. (1974) The changing pattern of hydatid disease with special reference to hydatid disease of the liver. *Medical Journal of Australia,* **1,** 129.

Journal of the American Medical Association (1942) Jaundice following yellow fever vaccination. *Journal of the American Medical Association,* **119,** 1110.

Kagan, I. G. (1968) Serologic diagnosis of visceral larva migrans. *Clinical Pediatrics,* **7,** 508.

Karvountzis, G. G., Redeker, A. G. & Peters, R. L. (1974) Long-term follow-up studies of patients surviving fulminant viral hepatitis. *Gastroenterology,* **67,** 870.

Klemola, E., Salini, I., Kaariainen, L. & Koivuniemi, A. (1966) Hepatosplenomegaly after 'cytomegalovirus mononucleosis' in a child. *Annales Paediatriae Fenniae,* **12,** 39.

Krech, U. H., Jung, M. & Jung, F. (1971) *Cytomegalovirus Infections of Man,* p. 26. Basel: Karger.

Krech, U. H., Jung, M., Jung, F. & Singeisen, C. L. (1968) Virologische und klinische untersuchungen bie Konnatalen und postnatalen cytomegalien. *Schweizerische Medizinische Wochenschrift,* **98,** 1459.

Krikler, D. M. (1971) Hepatitis and activity. *Postgraduate Medical Journal,* **47,** 490.

Krugman, S. (1963) The clinical use of gamma-globulin. *New England Journal of Medicine,* **269,** 195.

Krugman, S., Friedman, H. & Lattimer, C. (1975) Viral hepatitis type A: identification by specific complement fixation and immune adherence tests. *New England Journal of Medicine,* **292,** 1141.

Krugman, S., Giles, J. P. & Hammond, J. (1967) Infectious hepatitis: evidence for two distinct clinical epidemiological types of infection. *Journal of the American Medical Association,* **200,** 365.

Lamont, N. McE. & Pooler, N. R. (1958) Hepatic amoebiasis: a study of 250 cases. *Quarterly Journal of Medicine,* **27,** 389.

Lancet (1971) Morphological criteria in viral hepatitis. Reviewed by an International Group. *Lancet,* **1,** 333.

Lancet (1975) Viral hepatitis updated. *Lancet,* **1,** 1365.

Larracilla, A. J., Juarez, F. A. & Resendiz, Z. J. (1971) Amoebiasis intestinal en los tros primeros meses de la vida. *Salud Publica de Mexico,* **13,** 79.

Le Bouvier, G. L. (1973) Subtypes of hepatitis B antigen: clinical relevance. *Annals of Internal Medicine,* **79,** 894.

Lovejoy, F. H., Smith, A. L., Bresnan, M. J., Wood, J. N., Victor, D. I. & Adams, D. C. (1975) Clinical staging in Reye syndrome. *American Journal of Diseases of Children,* **128,** 36.

Maddison, S. E., Kagan, I. G. & Elsdon-Dew, R. (1968) Comparison of intradermal and serologic tests for the diagnosis of amoebiasis. *American Journal of Tropical Medicine & Hygiene,* **17,** 540.

Marks, M. I., Mauer, S. M. & Goldman, H. (1969) Exchange transfusion in the treatment of hepatic coma. *Journal of Paediatrics,* **75,** 418.

Mascoli, C. C., Ittensohn, O. L., Villarejos, V. M., Provost, P. J. & Hilleman, M. R. (1973) Recovery of hepatitis agents in the marmoset liver from human cases occurring in Costa Rica. *Proceedings of the Society of Experimental Biology and Medicine,* **142,** 276.

Mason, J. O. & McLean, W. R. (1962) Infectious hepatitis traced to the consumption of raw oysters: an epidemiological study. *American Journal of Hygiene,* **75,** 90.

Maxwell, J. D. & Williams, R. (1973) Drug induced jaundice. *British Journal of Hospital Medicine,* **9,** 193.

Meyers, N. A. (1960) Hydatid disease in a children's hospital. *Medical Journal of Australia,* **1,** 806.

Meyers, J. D., Romm, F. J., Tihen, W. S. & Bryan, J. A. (1975) Food-borne hepatitis A in a general hospital. *Journal of the American Medical Association,* **237,** 1049.

Miller, W. J., Provost, P. J., McAleer, W. J., Ittensohn, O. L., Villarejos, V. M. & Hilleman, M. R. (1975) Specific immune adherence assay for hepatitis A antibody: application to diagnostic and epidemiologic investigation. *Proceedings of the Society for Experimental Biology and Medicine, 149,* 254.

Mosley, J. W. (1959) Water-borne infectious hepatitis. *New England Journal of Medicine,* **261,** 703.

Niederman, J. C., McCollum, R. M., Henle, G. & Henle, W. (1968) Infectious mononucleosis: clinical manifestations in relation to EB virus antibodies. *Journal of the American Medical Association,* **203,** 205.

Okada, K., Kamiyama, I., Inomata, M., Imai, M., Mikakawa, Y. & Mayumi, M. (1976) E antigen in mothers serum as an indicator of vertical transmission of HBV. *New England Journal of Medicine,* **294,** 746.

Olson, L. C., Bourgeois, C. H., Cotton, R. B., Harikul, S., Grossman, R. A. & Smith, T. J. (1971) Encephalopathy and visceral fatty degeneration syndrome and etiology. *Pediatrics,* **47,** 707.

Perez, V., Schaffner, F. & Popper, H. (1972) Hepatic drug reactions. In *Progress in Liver Diseases.* Vol. IV, p. 597, ed. Popper, H. & Schaffner, F. New York: Grune and Stratton.

Popper, H. (1967) Acute hepatic necrosis in hepatitis. In *The Liver,* p. 47, ed. Read, A. E. London: Butterworth.

Popper, H. & Schaffner, S. (1957) In *The Liver : Structure and Function,* p. 404, New York: McGraw-Hill.

Prince, A. M. (1968) An antigen detected in the blood during the incubation period of hepatitis. *Proceedings of the National Academy of Sciences,* **60,** 814.

Provost, P. J., Ittensohn, O. L., Villarejos, V. M. & Hilleman, M. R. (1975a) A specific complement fixation test for human hepatitis A employing CR-326 virus antigen: diagnosis and epidemiology. *Proceedings of the Society for Experimental Biology and Medicine,* **148,** 962.

Provost, P. J., Wolanski, B. S., Miller, W. J., Ittensohn, O. L., MacAleer, W. J. & Hilleman, M. R. (1975b) Physical, chemical, morphologic dimensions of human hepatitis A strain CR-326. *Proceedings of the Society for Experimental Biology and Medicine,* **148,** 532.

Ramachandran, S., De Saram, R., Rajapakse, C. N. A. & Sivaningham, S. (1973) Hepatic manifestations during amoebic dysentery. *Postgraduate Medical Journal,* **49,** 261.

Reid, D. (1971) Prevention of hepatitis with immunoglubulin. *Postgraduate Medical Journal,* **47,** 488.

Remington, J. S., Miller, M. J. & Brownlee, I. (1968) IgM antibodies in acute toxoplasmosis: 1. Diagnostic significance in congenital cases and a method for their rapid demonstration. *Pediatrics,* **41,** 1082.

Reye, R. D. K., Morgan, G. & Baral, J. (1963) Encephalopathy and fatty degeneration of the viscera: a disease entity in childhood. *Lancet,* **2,** 749.

Rosalki, S. B., Gwyn-Jones, T. & Verney, A. F. (1960) Transaminase and liver function studies in infectious mononucleosis. *British Medical Journal,* **1,** 929.

Rubin, R. H., Swartz, M. N. & Malt, R. (1974) Hepatic abscess: changes in clinical bacteriologic and therapeutic aspects. *American Journal of Medicine,* **57,** 601.

Samaha, F. J., Blau, E. & Bernardinelli, J. L. (1974) Reye's syndrome: clinical diagnosis and treatment with peritoneal dialysis. *Pediatrics,* **53,** 336.

Scragg, J. (1960) Amoebic liver abscess in African children. *Archives of Disease in Childhood,* **35,** 171.

Shaw, J. J. & Voller, A. (1964) The detection of circulating antibody to Kala-azar by means of immunofluorescent techniques. *Transactions of the Royal Society of Tropical Medicine and Hygiene,* **58,** 349.

Sherlock, S. (1975) *Diseases of The Liver and Biliary System,* p. 340. Oxford: Blackwell.

Shrand, H. (1964) Visceral larva migrans: Toxocara canis infection. *Lancet,* **1,** 1357.

Silverman, A., Roy, C. C., & Cozzetto, F. J. (1971) In *Paediatric Clinical Gastroenterology,* ch. 22, p. 384. St. Louis: Mosby.

Starling, K. & Fernbach, D. H. (1968) Infectious mononucleosis in the pre-school child. *Journal of the American Medical Association,* **203,** 810.

Sterling, K. (1950) Hepatic function in Weil's disease. *Gastroenterology,* **15,** 52.

Sterner, G., Agell, B. O., Wahren, B. & Espmark, K. A. (1968) Acquired cytomegalovirus in older children and adults. *Scandinavian Journal of Infectious Diseases,* **2,** 95.

Sutnick, A. L., Levine, P. H., London, W. T. & Blumberg, B. S. (1971) Frequency of Australia antigen in patients with leukaemia in different countries. *Lancet,* **1,** 1200.

Szmuness, W. & Prince, A. M. (1971) The epidemiology of serum hepatitis (SH) infections: a controlled study in two closed communities. *American Journal of Epidemiology,* **94,** 585.

Tamir, D., Benderly, A., Levy, J., Ben-Porath, E. & Vonsover, A. (1974) Infectious mononucleosis and Epstein-Barr virus in childhood. *Pediatrics,* **53,** 330.

Trey, C., Lipworth, L. & Davidson, C. S. (1970) Parameters influencing survival in the first 318 patients reported to the Fulminant Hepatic Failure Surveillance Study. *Gastroenterology,* **58,** 306.

Turner, L. H. (1968) Leprospirosis II: serology. *Transactions of the Royal Society of Tropical Medicine and Hygiene,* **62,** 880.

Vischer, T. L., Bernheim, C. & Engelbrecht, E. (1967) Two cases of hepatitis due to Toxoplasma gondii. *Lancet,* **2,** 919.

Weller, T. H. (1971) The cytomegaloviruses. Ubiquitous agents with protean manifestations. *New England Journal of Medicine,* **285,** 203 and 267.

Williams, R. (1972) Problems of fulminant hepatic failure. *British Medical Bulletin,* **28,** 114.

Williams, R. & Murray-Lyon, I. M. (1975) *Artificial Liver Support Tunbridge Wells :* Pitman.

World Health Organisation (1967) Arboviruses and human disease. Technical Report Series No. 369, Geneva.

World Health Organisation (1975) Viral hepatitis. Technical Report Series No. 570, Geneva.

Zarchy, T. (1973) Is exchange transfusion worthwhile in the treatment of children with fulminant hepatitis? *Clinical Proceedings of the Children's Hospital National Medical Centre,* **29,** 17.

Zielinsky, V. E. & Elmslie, R. G. (1969) Jaundice and hydatid disease of the liver. *Medical Journal of Australia,* **1,** 839.

Zieve, L. (1975) Metabolic abnormalities in hepatic coma and potential toxins to be removed. In *Artificial Liver Support,* ed. Williams, R. & Murray-Lyon, I. M. Tunbridge Wells: Pitman.

18. Chronic liver disease

A. P. Mowat

Chronic hepatitis
Cirrhosis
Structural anomalies
Portal hypertension
Hepatobiliary lesions in cystic fibrosis

An understanding of the clinical and biochemical effects of chronic liver disease on the child requires some knowledge of the structure and function of this organ (see Ch. 2). Any disease process affecting the liver, whether the primary pathology involves the hepatocyte generally, one of its functions, the Kupffer cell, or blood or bile flow, will have to a greater or lesser extent some influence on the many functions of the liver and may have important secondary effects on bile and blood flow. It should be stressed, however, that the liver has a considerable reserve capacity and many of its functions can be maintained in the face of marked pathological changes; for example, the relative well-being of patients with extrahepatic biliary atresia during the early months of their lives. This hepatic reserve may not always be in the patient's best interests; it may lull the physician into a false sense of security with regard to the management of both medical and surgical conditions which are amenable to treatment. The assessment of the severity and the differential diagnosis of chronic liver disease is often difficult on clinical grounds. Routine liver function tests are sometimes unhelpful, and other investigations such as hepatic scanning, barium studies, selective coeliac axis arteriography and splenic venography may be necessary. In many instances, the most important single investigation is percutaneous liver biopsy.

CHRONIC HEPATITIS

Definition of chronic hepatitis requires consideration of both the clinical course of an on-going hepatic inflammation and the pathological features as seen on liver biopsy. Clinically it may be defined as on-going hepatitis persisting beyond the usual duration of acute hepatitis, namely two to three months. Even after years of continuous or relapsing biochemical abnormality, the biopsy appearances may be those of acute hepatitis. Conversely, pathological features indicating chronicity may be evident after an illness lasting apparently only three to four weeks. A raised gamma globulin, positive antinuclear factor and prolonged prothrombin time, strongly suggest chronic liver disease. Chronic persistent hepatitis is a benign lesion requiring no treatment. Where 'bridging' lesions occur (see below), however, prognosis must be guarded and careful follow-up is necessary (Boyer and Klatskin, 1970). A guarded prognosis is also required in persistent hepatitis B antigenaemia. Chronic agressive hepatitis has a bad prognosis, unless the patient responds to treatment.

Importance of liver biopsy

Liver biopsy is mandatory in assessing the need for treatment of chronic hepatitis, unless coagulation abnormalities contraindicate the investigation. The major pathological categories of chronic hepatitis are chronic persistent hepatitis and chronic aggressive hepatitis. The essential features of chronic persistent hepatitis are that the inflammatory infiltrate is virtually confined to the widened portal tracts and that the limiting plate of the hepatic lobule is intact; the lobular architecture is preserved and there is little or no increase in fibrous tissue. Chronic aggressive hepatitis is characterised by the presence of a perilobular hepatitis which leads to piecemeal erosion of the parenchyma adjacent to the portal tracts and interlobular septa. The liver cells are swollen and may assume pseudoductular arrangements. Plasma cells and lymphocytes predominate in the inflammatory response, and there is marked proliferation of fibroblasts. These changes disturb the lobular architecture, but true cirrhosis (i.e. fibrous connective tissue with nodular regeneration) is by definition absent. The presence of so-called 'bridging' lesions, in which proliferating fibroblasts and inflammatory cell aggregates link the portal tracts to each other or to hepatic veins, is a further pathological feature indicating chronicity.

It is important to appreciate that these pathological findings do not represent a distinct disease entity but rather a process which may have many causes. Further, the histological findings in the liver may vary from lobule to lobule and from time to time.

Chronic active hepatitis

This term is applied to a chronic progressive liver disorder associated with the histological appearances of chronic aggressive hepatitis (Fig. 18.1). Its pseudonyms include active juvenile cirrhosis, lupoid hepatitis, subacute hepatitis, plasma cell hepatitis, active chronic hepatitis and liver disease in young women with hypergammaglobulinaemia. The liver lesion has a marked propensity to progress to cirrhosis, and cirrhosis is already present in as many as 30 per cent of cases at the time of diagnosis. Repeated episodes of necrosis, stromal collapse and increasing fibrosis lead inevitably to cirrhosis (Sherlock, 1974).

Clinical features

Chronic active hepatitis often presents as an acute hepatitis with anorexia, nausea, fever and jaundice, but a history of contact with known cases of hepatitis is infrequent. In some patients the acute illness resolves and relapse of the jaundice may be the first clinical indication of the severity of the liver disease. In the remainder the onset is insidious with symptoms such as arthralgia, arthritis, fever, erythema nodosum or colitis; acne and livid cutaneous striae may be early features. Secondary amenorrhoea and thyroiditis may occur, and

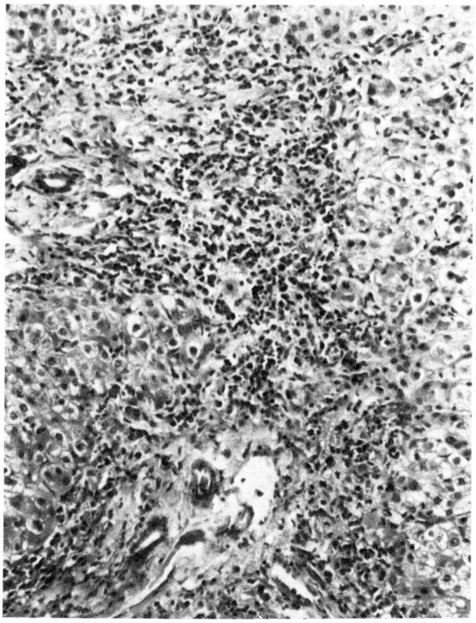

Fig. 18.1 Histological features of chronic aggressive hepatitis. The liver cells are large and swollen. There is intense mononuclear cell infiltration in the portal tracts and typical irregularities of the junctions between the hepatic parenchyma and the portal tracts; isolated swollen hepatocytes are surrounded by inflammatory cells extending out from the portal tract, the appearances of so-called 'piecemeal' necrosis.

some patients present with epistaxis and/or bruising following minor trauma. Occasionally, lethargy and anorexia may be the only symptoms (Dubois and Silverman, 1974). In all age groups approximately 70 per cent of patients are female. Affected patients are often well grown and look healthy but have hepatosplenomegaly; less commonly the other features referred to above are present. Spider naevi, digital clubbing and palmar erythema may also be evident.

Laboratory investigations and differential diagnosis

Serum bilirubin and transaminase levels are increased to a varying degree, and anaemia, thrombocytopenia and leucopenia may occur early in the course of the disease; the prothrombin time may be slightly prolonged. The total serum gamma globulin concentration is greater than 30 g/l with a marked elevation of the immunoglobulins. Antinuclear factor is positive in a high percentage of patients, some of whom show LE cell phenomena; up to 70 per cent of patients have smooth muscle antibodies, and a smaller proportion have anti-mitochondrial antibodies; abnormalities of cell-mediated immunity may also occur. The condition is rarely associated with hepatitis B antigenaemia. Percutaneous liver biopsy shows the classical features of chronic aggressive hepatitis; it may be impossible, however, to exclude cirrhosis on the basis of the biopsy findings.

Table 18.1 Causes of biliary cirrhosis

Extrahepatic biliary atresia
Intrahepatic biliary hypoplasia
Choledochal cyst
Ascending cholangitis
Cystic fibrosis
Ulcerative colitis
Byler's disease
Familial intrahepatic cholestasis

In the paediatric age group the main alternative diagnoses which should be considered are acute or chronic persistent hepatitis, Wilson's disease, liver disease associated with alpha-1-antitrypsin deficiency, cystic fibrosis and drug-induced hepatitis. In particular clinical circumstances consideration should be given to the causes of cirrhosis listed in Tables 18.1, 18.2 and 18.3.

Treatment and prognosis

Corticosteroids are the mainstay of treatment. In a controlled trial in adult patients steroids produced such a favourable response in the treated group that continuation of the trial became unjustifiable (Cook, Mulligan and Sherlock, 1971). Although no controlled trials have been reported in children, the available information suggests that the prognosis in children treated with steroids is even better than that for adults (Dubois and Silverman, 1974).

Prednisolone in a dose of 1 to 1·5 mg/kg/day should be given at the time of diagnosis, even before the histological diagnosis is confirmed if a prolonged prothrombin time precludes biopsy. The aim of treatment is to induce a complete biochemical control of the hepatitis while avoiding serious side-effects from the steroids. Full doses are usually required for the first four weeks of treatment, but thereafter it may be possible to reduce the dose gradually over

Table 18.2 Causes of postnecrotic cirrhosis

Posthepatic	Neonatal hepatitis Acute viral hepatitis Chronic active hepatitis Drugs, toxins or poisons Irradiation
Passive venous congestion	Constrictive percarditis Ebstein's anomaly Budd–Chiari syndrome Chronic congestive cardiac failure
Veno-occlusive disease (Jamaican)	
Indian childhood cirrhosis	
Ulcerative colitis	

Table 18.3 Genetic causes of cirrhosis

Wilson's disease
Galactosaemia
Fructosaemia
Glycogen storage disease type IV
Tyrosinosis
Alpha-1-antitrypsin deficiency
Cystic fibrosis
Niemann–Pick disease
Cystinosis
Cholesterol ester storage disease
Gaucher's disease
Hurler's syndrome
Byler's disease
Hepatic porphyria
Sickle-cell disease
Thalassaemia
Hereditary haemorrhagic telangiectasia
Haemochromatosis
Zellweger's syndrome
Defective cholic acid synthesis

the course of three to four months to an alternate day regimen. Excessive weight gain in the first weeks of treatment occurs almost inevitably, but serious side-effects can often be avoided. Clinical and biochemical remission is likely to occur within one to three months of starting treatment. In a minority of patients complete biochemical remission cannot be achieved without producing significant side-effects from the steroids. In these circumstances reduction of the steroid dose and addition of azathioprine (1 mg/kg/day) often results in biochemical control of the hepatitis. The patient should remain on treatment until biochemical remission has been present for at least one year; liver biopsy should be repeated at this stage, and if evidence of histological activity persists further therapy is indicated. Careful follow-up is required after therapy has been discontinued.

CIRRHOSIS

Cirrhosis defines a histological abnormality of the liver, in which the normal hepatic lobular architecture is destroyed and replaced by nodular regeneration of hepatocytes, surrounded by variable amounts of fibrous tissue. Hepatocellular necrosis promotes increased collagen deposition, which further impairs the local circulation causing further liver cell damage, and a vicious circle is established. Impaired liver function due to the loss of hepatocytes and the vascular effects of the fibrous tissue account for the main pathophysiological effects of cirrhosis. The pathological classification of cirrhosis into micronodular, macronodular and imcomplete septal cirrhosis may be applied to paediatric patients, but it is often more helpful, both from the aetiological and clinical standpoint, to consider two main groups: biliary, in which the lesion is primarily in the duct system, and postnecrotic indicating hepatocellular necrosis from whatever cause.

Clinical features and laboratory investigations

The clinical features of cirrhosis vary according to the underlying cause, but certain manifestations are common to all. These include those associated with portal hypertension (i.e. oesophageal varices, ascites, splenomegaly and hypersplenism), and anaemia, finger clubbing, and haemodynamic changes such as spider angiomata, liver palms, a rapid pulse with wide pulse pressure and warm skin, and pulmonary arteriovenous fistulae; in some instances, steatorrhoea, fatigue and anorexia are prominent. Advanced cirrhosis may be present, however, before there are significant clinical manifestations.

In patients with biliary cirrhosis jaundice is common, and pruritus, cutaneous xanthomata and malabsorption are frequently seen.

Abnormal laboratory investigations include bromsulphalein retention, low serum albumin and raised serum gamma globulin concentrations; a mild anaemia, leucopaenia and thrombocytopenia are common findings in the presence of splenomegaly; the prothrombin time may be prolonged, and a respiratory alkalosis and features of hyperaldosteronism may be present. The serum levels of alkaline phosphatase and cholesterol are often markedly raised in biliary cirrhosis.

Specific investigations are necessary for the causes of cirrhosis as listed in Tables 18.1, 18.2 and 18.3. It cannot be stressed too strongly that in all cases of chronic liver disease Wilson's disease must be excluded.

Management

The aetiology of the cirrhosis must be defined whenever possible so that specific therapy can be instituted and genetic advice offered. For the majority of patients, however, treatment is directed at the prevention of complications. In paediatric practice it is most important to minimise the effects of malabsorption. Medium-chain triglycerides decrease steatorrhoea and may improve the nutritional status. Cholestyramine is the drug of choice for relieving pruritus, and in the absence of complete biliary atresia it may also help to improve liver function. Fat-soluble vitamins must be given either as large oral supplements or intramuscularly.

Ascites should be initially treated with oral hydrochlorothiazide and spironolactone on alternate days with daily potassium supplements; life-threatening respiratory distress may result from massive ascites when intravenous frusamide or etharynic acid can be used. Frusamide may be substituted for hydrochlorothiazide if the patient becomes refractory to this drug. Most children find a restricted salt diet so unpalatable that the nutritional losses outweigh the advantages of this approach to management. In rare instances, abdominal paracentesis may be necessary. The volume of fluid removed should be limited to that which is necessary to improve the patient's discomfort; unfortunately any removed fluid rapidly reaccumulates. In adult practice, paracentesis with intravenous reinfusion of the protein-rich concentrated ascitic fluid produces satisfactory remission of refractory ascites for periods of up to eight weeks, but this approach has not been reported in children.

Iron deficiency anaemia should be corrected and therapy controlled by means of sequential serum iron levels.

Rapid deterioration in the patient's condition should suggest alimentary bleeding, septicaemia or the development of hepatoma.

STRUCTURAL ANOMALIES

Choledochal cyst, intrahepatic bile duct dilatation, polycystic disease of the liver and congenital hepatic fibrosis may occur singly or in combination. The aetiology of these lesions is not fully understood, but they are usually considered as congenital disorders; they are often associated with renal disease (Lieberman *et al.*, 1971).

Choledochal cyst

Choledochal cysts result from dilatations of the common bile duct. The cyst may take the form of a localised distention with a narrow hypoplastic terminal common bile duct, a diverticulum type cyst from one side of the common bile duct or a fusiform distention which is found particularly in older children. A congenital weakness of the bile duct wall has been suggested to be aetiologically important; the cysts vary in volume from 0·01 to 8 litres. Eighty per cent occur in girls (Saito and Ishida, 1974), 20 per cent present during the first year of life, and 30 to 50 per cent in the first 10 years. In the newborn, the clinical features may be very similar to those of extrahepatic biliary atresia or biliary ascites. In older children the classical triad of intermittent jaundice with conjugated hyperbilirubinaemia, colicky right-sided abdominal pain and a cystic tumour of varing size is found in only one-third of patients.

Diagnosis may be suspected on the basis of the clinical findings. A disproportionately high serum alkaline phosphatase concentration compared with serum transaminase levels is particularly suggestive. Other helpful investigations include barium meal, showing displacement of the duodenum if the cyst is large, ultrasonic scanning of the biliary tree, and cholangiography; cholangiography may be achieved intravenously, but more commonly transhepatic or operative techniques are required.

Treatment is surgical, and the cyst should be removed if at all possible. In many instances, it is necessary to perform a cholodochojejunostomy with a Roux-en-Y loop.

Polycystic disease of the liver and kidney

This is a poorly characterised group of conditions manifesting with cyst formation in many organs, particularly the kidneys, liver and pancreas (Lieberman *et al.*, 1971).

The 'adult' form is inherited as an autosomal dominant with high penetrance, and the predominant features are renal enlargement and renal failure. The severity of the disease is very variable and the condition can present in infancy or be found incidentally in old age. Hepatomegaly and, rarely, portal hypertension may be found.

In the 'infantile' form the features are similar, but bile duct abnormalities are conspicuous and increasing hepatic fibrosis occurs with age. Blythe and Ockenden (1971), on the basis of family studies and the clinicopathological findings, have suggested that this form can be classified into four subgroups, each of which is inherited in an autosomal recessive fashion. Group 1: presentation in the perinatal period with massive kidneys and early death from renal failure and minimal hepatic involvement; group 2: presentation in the neonatal period with progressive renal failure; group 3: presentation in infancy when portal hypertension tends to be superadded to the chronic renal failure; group 4: presentation in the first five years of life when portal hypertension and gross hepatic fibrosis are the main features.

The diagnosis should be suspected on the basis of the clinical findings and the appearances of the nephrogram on intravenous pyelography. In the 'adult' form radiology shows large kidneys with wide separation of calyses. In the 'infantile' form there is typically a delayed appearance of the dye with a streaky appearance, and also delayed clearance of the radio-opaque material. The scintiscan findings of multiple filling defects in the liver and peritoneoscopy are also helpful investigations. The diagnosis is confirmed histologically by liver biopsy. Treatment is directed at minimising the effects of the renal dysfunction, but if portal hypertension supervenes surgery may be necessary.

Congenital hepatic fibrosis

This disorder occurs sporadically or in familial form. It is characterised by marked portal fibrosis, bizarre bile duct proliferation and normal hepatic lobules. Portal hypertension commonly supervenes (Nathan and Batsakis, 1969) and there may be associated cystic abnormalities of the kidneys. These pathological changes are not accompanied by significant impairment of hepatocellular or renal function. The condition presents in the first or second decade with asymptomatic splenomegaly or with haematemesis and abdominal pain. Liver function tests are usually normal, but the serum alkaline phosphatase level may be high. Histological examination of the liver is essential for confirmation of the diagnosis. Alimentary bleeding may be an indication for portal vein diversion.

Congenital dilatation of the intrahepatic bile ducts

This very rare anomaly may occur as an isolated finding, or be found in association with dilatation of extrahepatic ducts or with congenital hepatic fibrosis (Caroli and Corcos, 1964). It is frequently complicated by severe cholangitis and septicaemia, which should be managed conservatively with antibiotic therapy. Surgery and cholangiography should not be performed unless there is evidence of complete biliary obstruction due to calculus formation (Murray-Lyon *et al.*, 1972).

PORTAL HYPERTENSION

The causes of portal hypertension may be classified according to whether the hypertension is extrahepatic, intrahepatic or postsinusoidal (see Table 18.4). The clinical features, pathophysiological changes and complications of portal

Table 18.4 Causes of portal hypertension

Extrahepatic	
Obstruction of portal or splenic vein	
	Idiopathic
	Congenital lesions
	Oomphalitis
	Umbilical vein catheterisation
	Portal pyelophlebitis
	Intra-abdominal sepsis
	Trauma
	Duodenal ulcer
	Pancreatitis
	Malignant disease
	Lymph gland enlargement
Increased blood flow	
	Arteriovenous fistulae
	Tropical splenomegaly
Intrahepatic	
	Cirrhosis
	Congenital hepatic fibrosis
	Portal zone infiltrations
	Schistosomiasis
	Acute hepatitis
	Chronic active hepatitis
	Hereditary telangiectasia (Rendu–Weber–Osler disease)
Postsinusoidal	
	Budd–Chiari syndrome
	Inferior vena caval obstruction
	Veno-occlusive disease
	Constrictive pericarditis

hypertension are similar for children and adults. Since there is a marked difference in the frequency of the various causes of portal hypertension and also in the modes of presentation, diagnostic considerations and schemes of investigation must be modified. A knowledge of the natural history of the condition as it complicates the different causes, the deleterious effects of splenectomy in many circumstances, particularly in the young child, and the technical difficulties in constructing portosystemic anastomosis between the small intra-abdominal vessels of a young child are all important considerations in planning management. Portal hypertension in childhood still carries a significant morbidity and mortality, and iatrogenic factors are contributory. Portal hypertension usually results from impeded blood flow in the portal venous system due to obstruction of the portal vein or its tributaries, a variety of lesions within the liver or obstruction to venous outflow from the liver. Rarely it results from increased blood flow to the liver usually due to arteriovenous malformations; on occasions, it may affect only part of the portal system.

The importance of detailed assessment

The importance of detailed investigation (see Table 18.5) of the cause of the portal hypertension must be stressed. Specific therapy may be available for some of the causes, and failure to identify the cause due to incomplete investigation

Table 18.5 The investigation of portal hypertension

Complete peripheral blood count
Platelet count
Liver function tests
Paul–Bunnell test
Barium meal
Liver and spleen scan
Sweat electrolytes
Caeruloplasmin
Alpha-1-antitrypsin
Urinary amino acids
Galactose-1-phosphate uridyl transferase
Chest X-ray
Electrocardiogram
Liver biopsy
Endoscopic examination
Selective venous phase angiography from superior mesenteric and coeliac arteries
Splenoportography and measurement of splenic pulp pressure
Wedged-hepatic vein pressure
Inferior venacavogram
Cardiac catheterisation

can lead to inappropriate management with sometimes grave consequences. Certain liver diseases, for example chronic active hepatitis and Wilson's disease, are capable of causing portal hypertension but respond to specific treatment if diagnosed early. Irreversible surgical procedures must be postponed if at all possible until investigations are complete (Fonkalsrud, Myers and Robinson, 1974).

Extrahepatic portal hypertension

Obstruction of the portal vein

This may occur anywhere between the portahepatis and the hilum of the spleen. The portal vein may be replaced by a fibrous remnant, contain an organised blood clot, be compressed from outside, be obstructed by a web or diaphragm or be replaced by a sheath of small channels usually described as cavernous transformation (Mikkelson, 1966). Omphalitis, peritonitis and umbilical vein catheterisation have been incriminated as possible causes, but these rarely account for more than 30 per cent of cases in most series (Voorhees *et al.*, 1965). In older children abdominal trauma, duodenal ulcer, pancreatitis, parasitic infection and localised lymph gland enlargement have sometimes been found to be the cause of portal hypertension.

Clinical features

The usual presenting features are asymptomatic splenic enlargement, or haematemesis and/or melaena from bleeding oesophageal varices; less commonly patients may present with abdominal enlargement and ascites. The onset may be at any time from six months to 15 years. Often the only abnormal physical finding is splenomegaly, but even this may be absent in the hypotensive patient following bleeding; similarly, varices may not be demonstrated on oesophagography at this time. Bleeding may follow upper respiratory tract infections and frequently stops spontaneously. Relapses occur at irregular intervals and become much less frequent as the patient reaches his late teens. Encephalopathy rarely complicates alimentary bleeding.

Intrahepatic portal hypertension

The intrahepatic vasculature is markedly disturbed by the fibrosis, the cellular regeneration and the scarring and collapse of hepatic parenchyma which characterises cirrhosis. This results in an increase in the vascular resistance within the liver, and any of the many varieties of cirrhosis may be responsible. In general portal hypertension is a late manifestation of liver disease; Wilson's disease, hereditary telangiectasia, type IV glycogen storage disease, and anicteric hepatitis, however, may result in portal hypertension without the patient appearing ill. The manifestations of the portal hypertension are similar to those of extrahepatic obstruction, but hypersplenism is commoner; gastrointestinal bleeding, however, is poorly tolerated and hepatic coma is common (Scott and Foster, 1967). The clinical features of portal hypertension secondary to congenital hepatic fibrosis are very similar to those seen in patients with extrahepatic portal hypertension; in this condition encephalopathy rarely complicates gastrointestinal bleeding.

In hereditary telangiectasia (Rendu–Weber–Osler disease) portal hypertension results from the many arteriovenous shunts within the liver; portal blood flow increases and the intrahepatic vascular resistance increases.

Postsinusoidal portal hypertension

Budd–Chiari syndrome

In this syndrome there is obliteration of the major hepatic veins or the intrahepatic portion of the inferior vena cava; it complicates conditions such as neoplasms, particularly hepatomas, hypernephroma, leukaemia, sickle-cell disease, polycythaemia and allergic vasculitis; hepatic vein thrombosis may occur in patients on oral contraceptives and should be considered in adolescents. The condition is characterised by abdominal distention of short duration, abdominal pain, hepatomegaly and ascites; jaundice and splenomegaly occur in about 25 per cent of patients, but oesophageal varices tend to be a late complication. The diagnosis should be suspected on the basis of the clinical history and the results of scintillation scanning of the liver using technetium 99; typically the caudate lobe shows good isotope uptake, while uptake in the remainder of the liver is poor due to the fact that the hepatic veins draining the caudate lobe empty directly to the inferior vena cava (Tavill *et al.*, 1975). Confirmation of the diagnosis requires angiographic and catheterisation procedures (Kibel and Marsden, 1956).

Obstruction of the inferior vena cava

The clinical features seen in children with obstruction of the extrahepatic portion of the inferior vena cava are similar to those seen in the Budd–Chiari syndrome. The majority are secondary to tumours and thrombosis, and a small proportion result from web or membrane obstruction of the vein. Vena cavae obstruction must be distinguished from the Budd–Chiari syndrome since the former is amenable to surgery; the presence of collateral veins, however, presents considerable technical difficulties. Inferior vena caval angiography and hepatic vein catheterisation are necessary for diagnosis. The nature of these membranous obstructions is unknown; some are thought to be congenital, and others acquired (Datta *et al.*, 1972; Volpe, Bergin and Overholt, 1970).

Veno-occlusive disease

In this condition the medium and smaller hepatic veins are occluded, and it is an important cause of postsinusoidal portal hypertension in children living in areas where 'bush teas', derived from plants containing senacio alkaloids, are drunk. It affects predominantly children under the age of 6 years and is fatal in about 20 per cent of patients; the disease may be subacute or chronic, and be complicated by portal hypertension. Early in the course of the disease centrilobular congestion, hepatocellular necrosis, subintimal swelling and occlusion of hepatic veins are typical findings, but these features may be absent by the time cirrhosis has developed (Stuart, 1970).

Management of portal hypertension

In patients with extrahepatic portal hypertension the frequency of gastrointestinal bleeding often decreases with age, and bleeding is rarely fatal particularly in the initial episode. Decompression of the portal system by portocaval shunting can relieve disturbing and even incapacitating symptoms in infants with intrahepatic portal hypertension, but these procedures rarely influence long-term survival. Early surgical intervention before full diagnostic appraisal should therefore be discouraged (Voorhees and Price, 1974; Fonkalsrud *et al.*, 1974).

Laboratory investigations

The investigations required for the full evaluation of portal hypertension are outlined in Table 18.5. Simple procedures should be carried out initially, and the results of these will provide guidance as to which of the further tests are likely to be necessary. An upper gastrointestinal series is mandatory; visualisation of the stomach and duodenum is important, not only because varices may be found at these sites, but also because both cirrhosis and portal hypertension predispose the patient to peptic ulceration. Selective angiography of the splenic and mesenteric arteries, with films taken during the venous phase, will often clearly outline the anatomy of the portal venous system particularly with a preinfusion of Priscoline; the risk of complications associated with this procedure is small providing the femoral arteries are sufficiently wide to catheterise easily. Resolution may be inferior compared to that obtained with splenoportography; even in experienced hands, however, the latter procedure may be complicated by intraperitoneal haemorrhage from the spleen, which can be so severe that splenectomy becomes necessary. Splenoportography should therefore not be performed unless it is planned to proceed to splenectomy, preferably in conjunction with some shunt procedure. Under the age of 10 years splenectomy predisposes the patient to infection;

also, shunts are likely to thrombose in this age group. In addition, by removing the spleen benign portosystemic anastomosis by-passing the coronary-oesophageal drainage system are removed.

Acute bleeding episodes

The management of acute bleeding episodes involves close monitoring of vital signs and appropriate transfusion of preferably fresh whole blood. The insertion of a central venous pressure line is important in avoiding the risks of over-transfusion which, as a result of distention of varices, may perpetuate bleeding. Pitressin intravenously or via a superior mesenteric artery is safe and effective. Intravenous therapy is generally administered for only 20 to 40 minutes, but a constant arterial infusion is possible for as long as four to five days. If these measures fail to arrest the bleeding a paediatric Sangstaken–Blakemore tube can be inserted, but experience is required for its successful use. If the patient has known liver disease or clinical features suggestive of chronic liver disease, measures to combat hepatic encephalopathy should be undertaken.

Surgery

It is important to bear in mind that any surgical procedure which decompresses portal pressure by diverting blood into channels which by-pass the liver, may cause a deterioration in liver function and hepatic encephalopathy; this is particularly the case in the presence of liver disease, but this can also occur in the non-cirrhotic patient (Voorhees and Price, 1973). Even when portal hypertension is known to be present, bleeding may have other causes and endoscopy is essential in planning surgery.

In children with extrahepatic portal hypertension the portal vein is usually not available for surgery. Most other measures such as splenorenal and mesocaval shunts are likely to be followed by thrombosis unless a shunt with a diameter of greater than 1 cm can be guaranteed. At present a mesocaval shunt, with or without a graft from the superior mesenteric vein to the inferior vena cava, is the procedure of choice (Lambert, Tank and Turcotte, 1974). Even in experienced centres surgery is often followed by complications unrelated to the portal hypertension, and surgery should be avoided if at all possible (Fonkalsrud *et al.*, 1974). In patients with portal hypertension due to congenital hepatic fibrosis portacaval shunting is effective in controlling the hypertension and should certainly be considered when bleeding is significant. When cirrhosis is established any shunting procedure will result in a deterioration of liver function and carries the risk of hepatic encephalopathy. For these poor risk patients more conservative measures, such as injection of oesophageal varices by sclerosing material or mesocaval anastomosis, should be considered.

HEPATOBILIARY LESIONS IN CYSTIC FIBROSIS

Hepatobiliary lesions occur in the majority of patients with cystic fibrosis (see Table 18.6) and, since up to 80 per cent of children with cystic fibrosis are expected to reach the age of 20, physicians caring for such children and adolescents must be prepared to deal with the problems resulting from liver disease.

Table 18.6 Incidence of hepatobiliary lesions in cystic fibrosis

Criteria	Percentage abnormal		Reference
Liver enlargement	0·5		Crozier, 1974
	62		Feigelson *et al.*, 1972
Abnormal scan	80		Feigelson *et al.*, 1972
Serum alkaline phosphatase			
<4 years	0		
<16 years	47		Boat *et al.*, 1974
Liver biopsy	50	}	
Gammaglutamyl transpeptidase	30–60	} 90	Isenberg *et al.*, 1974
Cholecystogram	40	}	

Pathogenesis

The pathogenesis of the liver disease in cystic fibrosis is considered to be similar to the pathogenesis of the other organ abnormalities. The mucus-producing glands along the bile ducts are affected and result in the secretion of hyperviscid bile which obstructs the bile ductular radicals. This results in focal biliary obstruction with eosinophilic concretions within the bile ducts, bile duct reduplication, destruction of liver cells, inflammatory cell infiltrate and an increase in fibrous tissue; this process may begin in fetal life and proceed without symptoms until many areas of the liver are affected, with destruction of hepatocytes and their replacement by fibrous tissue. As the fibrous tissue contracts and the remaining liver cells grow in a disorganised fashion, the normal architecture of the liver becomes disturbed, resulting in cirrhosis.

A variety of factors may contribute to the hepatobiliary lesions which occur in cystic fibrosis, and these are listed in Table 18.7.

Prolonged neonatal conjugated hyperbilirubinaemia occurs in a small proportion of cases; of these, 50 per cent will have had meconium ileus. The pathological changes vary from established biliary cirrhosis to mild cholestasis (Valman, France and Wallis, 1971). Management includes supportive treatment, flushing the extrahepatic bile ducts at laparotomy and the administration of steroids. Complete biochemical and histological recovery may occur, even when jaundice has persisted for as long as six months.

Abnormalities of the gall bladder and biliary tree are common (Rousing and Sloth, 1973), and between 30 and 50 per cent of patients have small gall bladders or gall bladders which do not fill on cholecystography; gall-stones and cholangitis without associated cirrhosis occur not infrequently.

Fatty metamorphosis is common, haemosiderosis may be associated with increased iron absorption in patients who are not receiving full doses of pancreatic supplements and vitamin E deficiency may add to the pigment deposition within hepatocytes.

Clinical features

The majority of patients with liver involvement are asymptomatic, and splenomegaly may be the first indication of liver disease. The liver may be easily palpable as a result of downward displacement due to lung disease; liver scanning will confirm true liver enlargement and is the most sensitive indicator

Table 18.7 Hepatobiliary lesions in cystic fibrosis

Focal biliary fibrosis progressing to cirrhosis
Prolonged neonatal intrahepatic cholestasis
Small gall bladder (35 to 50 per cent of cases)
Gall-stones
Cholangitis
Cardiac cirrhosis
Drug-induced hepatitis
Fatty metamorphosis
Haemosiderosis
Viral hepatitis A and B
Cytomegalovirus

of hepatic involvement (Feigelson, Pecau and Perez, 1972). Occasionally massive haematemesis or ascites may be the first clinical indication of liver disease.

Management

As in other forms of cirrhosis the place of portal decompression in the management of bleeding varices is unresolved. Moreover, portacaval shunting may be technically difficult because of retroperitoneal oedema and fibrosis, and the operation of choice is probably a mesocaval shunt. Severe pulmonary disease is a contraindication to surgery. In carefully selected patients, however, effective surgery may be of benefit (Tyson, Schuster and Shwachman, 1968).

References

Boat, T. F., Doershuk, C. F., Stern, R. C. & Matthews, L. W. (1974) Serum alkaline phosphatase in cystic fibrosis. *Clinical Pediatrics,* **13,** 505.

Boyer, J. L. & Klatskin, G. (1970) Pattern of necrosis in acute viral hepatitis. *New England Journal of Medicine,* **283,** 1063.

Blythe, H. & Ockenden, B. G. (1971) Polycystic of the kidneys and liver presenting in childhood. *Journal of Medical Genetics,* **8,** 257.

Caroli, J. & Corcos, V. (1964) La dilatation congenital des voies biliares intrahepatique. *Revue Medicale Surgical du Mal du Foie,* **39,** 1.

Cook, G. C., Mulligan, R. & Sherlock, S. (1971) Controlled prospective trial of corticosteroid therapy in active chronic hepatitis. *Quarterly Journal of Medicine,* **40,** 159.

Crozier, N. D. (1974) Cystic fibrosis—a not-so-fatal disease. *Pediatric Clinics of North America,* **21,** 935.

Datta, D. V., Saha, S., Singh, S. A. K., Gupta, D. B., Aikat, B. K., Chugh, K. S. & Chhuttani, P. N. (1972) Chronic Budd–Chiari syndrome due to obstruction of the intrahepatic portion of the inferior vena cava. *Gut,* **13,** 372.

Dubois, R. A. & Silverman, A. (1974) Treatment of chronic active hepatitis in children. *Postgraduate Medical Journal,* **50,** 386.

Feigelson, J., Pecau, Y. & Perez, R. (1972) Liver scanning and function in cystic fibrosis. *Acta Paediatrica Scandinavica,* **61,** 337.

Fonkalsrud, E. W., Myers, N. A. & Robinson, M. J. (1974) Management of extrahepatic portal hypertension in children. *Annals of Surgery,* **180,** 487.

Isenberg, J. N., L'Heureux, P., Warwick, W. J. & Sharp, H. (1974) Detection of cirrhosis in cystic fibrosis: lack of correlation with gamma-glutamyltranspeptidase and biliary tract roentgenogram. *Gastroenterology,* **66,** 887.

Kibel, M. A. & Marsden, M. B. (1956) Inferior venacaval and hepatic vein thrombosis; the Chiari syndrome in childhood. *Archives of Disease in Childhood,* **31,** 225.

Lambert, M. J., Tank, E. S. & Turcotte, J. G. (1974) Late sequelae of mesocaval shunt in children. *American Journal of Surgery,* **125,** 19.

Lieberman, E., Salinas Madrigal, L., Gwinn, J. L., Brennen, L. P., Fine, R. N. & Landing, B. H. (1971) Infantile polycystic disease of kidneys and liver; clinical, pathological and radiological correlations and comparisons with congenital hepatic fibrosis. *Medicine,* Baltimore, **50,** 277.

Mikkelson, W. P. (1966) Extrahepatic portal hypertension in children. *Annals of Surgery,* **111,** 333.

Murray-Lyon, I. M., Shilkin, K. B., Laws, D. W., Illing, R. C. & Williams, R. (1972) Non-obstructive dilatation of the intrahepatic biliary tree with cholangitis. *Quarterly Journal of Medicine,* **41,** 477.

Nathan, M. & Batsakis, J. G. (1969) Congenital hepatic fibrosis. *Surgery, Gynaecology and Obstetrics,* **128,** 1033.

Rousing, H. & Sloth, K. (1973) Microgallbladder and biliary calculi in mucoviscidosis. In *Acta Radiologica (Diagnostica),* Stockholm, **14,** 585.

Saito, S. & Ishida, M. (1974). Congenital choledochal cyst (Cystic dilatation of the common bile duct). In *Progress in Paediatric Surgery,* **6,** 63.

Scott, H. W. & Foster, J. H. (1967) Surgical experience in the management of cirrhosis of the liver in children. *American Journal of Surgery,* **113,** 102.

Sherlock, S. (1974) Progress report. Chronic Hepatitis. *Gut,* **15,** 581.

Stuart, K. L. (1970) Veno-occlusive disease. In *Diseases of Children in the Sub-tropics and Tropics.* 2nd edition, ed. Jelliff, D. B., p. 185. London: Arnold.

Tavill, A. S., Wood, E. J., Kreel, L., Jones, E. A., Gregory, M. & Sherlock, S. (1975) The Budd–Chiari syndrome: correlation between the hepatic scintography and the clinical, radiological and pathological findings in 19 cases of hepatic venous outflow obstruction. *Gastroenterology,* **68,** 509.

Tyson, K. R. T., Schuster, S. R. & Shwachman, H. (1968) Portal hypertension in cystic fibrosis. *Journal of Pediatric Surgery,* **3,** 271.

Valman, H. B., France, N. E. & Wallis, P. G. (1971) Prolonged neonatal jaundice in cystic fibrosis. *Archives of Disease in Childhood,* **46,** 805.

Volpe, J. A., Bergin, J. J. & Overholt, E. L. (1970) Budd–Chiari syndrome caused by a web as a result of visceral thrombophlebitis migrans. *American Journal of Digestive Diseases,* **15,** 469.

Voorhees, A. B. J., Harris, R. C., Britten, R. C., Price, J. B. & Santulli, G. V. (1965) Portal hypertension in children. *Surgery,* **58,** 540.

Voorhees, A. B. J. & Price, J. B. (1973) Portal-systemic encephalopathy in the non-cirrhotic patient. *Surgery,* **107,** 659.

Voorhees, A. B. J. & Price, J. B. (1974) Extrahepatic portal hypertension. *Archives of Surgery,* **108,** 338.

19. Tumours of the liver

Jean W. Keeling

Hamartoma
Hepatoblastoma
Hepatocellular carcinoma
Rhabdomyosarcoma
Metastatic and other tumours

Table 19.1 Comparative frequency of different primary tumours of the liver in childhood (Keeling, 1971)

Hamartoma	7
Hepatoblastoma	32
Hepatocellular carcinoma	4
Rhabdomyosarcoma	3

Primary tumours of the liver occurring during childhood are much less common than metastatic ones and account for less than 6 per cent of all tumours seen in children's hospitals throughout the world. Despite their rarity, however, they must be considered in the differential diagnosis of hepatomegaly since early and radical surgery offers the best chance of cure. Four types of primary liver tumours occur in childhood: benign localised hamartoma and three malignant neoplasms, hepatoblastoma, hepatocellular carcinoma and embryonic rhabdomyosarcoma of the bile ducts (Table 19.1). The first two types usually present under the age of 3 years and may even be present at birth, whilst the latter two are seen in older children.

HAMARTOMA

Clinical features and diagnosis

Liver hamartomata usually present in the first two years of life and many are found on routine examination of the infant either shortly after birth or during the ensuing months. There may be no symptoms other than a painless or slightly tender abdominal swelling. Occasionally large tumours may cause difficulties during delivery, or death from haemorrhage due to intrapartum trauma; angiomatous hamartoma of the liver is a rare cause of neonatal jaundice (Claireaux, 1960). A rapid increase in abdominal girth due to filling of cystic

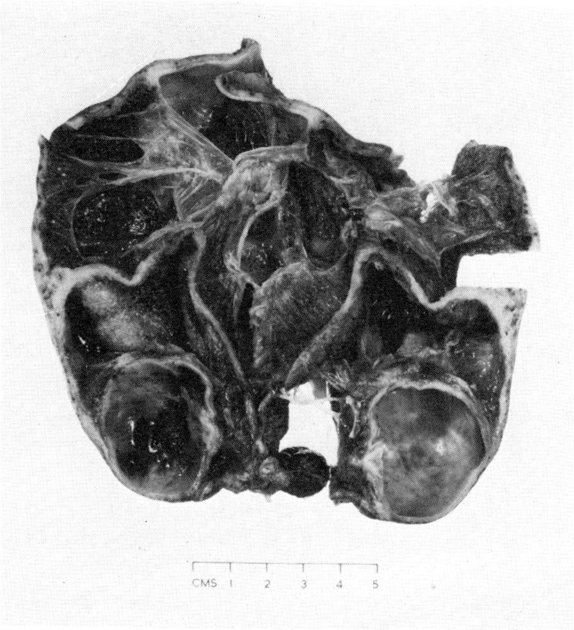

Fig. 19.1 Bisected hamartoma showing several epithelial-lined cysts and haemorrhages

components with fluid or to haemorrhage into the tissue mass may occur and suggest a malignant tumour. Those with a large angiomatous component may cause high output cardiac failure due to arteriovenous shunting.

Pathology

The hamartoma is encapsulated and may measure up to 15 cm in diameter. Pedunculated tumours are covered by liver capsule, and those with a large angiomatous component have a red-purplish cut surface; dilated, blood-filled channels are seen and haemorrhages are common (Fig. 19.1).

Histologically, they are composed of endothelial-lined spaces, usually filled with blood, lying in a loose connective tissue stroma; other hamartomata are composed of a mixture of solid tissue and cystic areas, the solid parts often having a yellowish appearance which consist of bands of liver cells, often with marked bile retention, separated by fibrous bands. Groups of bile ducts are scattered throughout the mass and it is the distention of these ducts which results in cyst formation, the smaller ones being lined by bile duct epithelium, whereas in the larger ones the epithelium is entirely flattened.

Treatment

Early laparotomy is essential in the management of hamartomata. Some of the tumours are attached to the liver by a pedicle and are easily removed, but in most, partial hepatectomy is necessary. In the newborn it may be preferable to delay hemihepatectomy in view of the associated high mortality of such extensive surgery at this time (Keeling, 1971).

HEPATOBLASTOMA

Clinical features and diagnosis

Hepatoblastoma is by far the commonest of the primary liver tumours in childhood and usually presents before the age of 3 years, although exceptionally it may occur in the older child. It can also present at birth or the neonatal period, indicating development *in utero*. The presenting symptoms include abdominal distention, vomiting and anorexia, and signs of precocious puberty may be present; both *in vivo* and *in vitro* production of chorionic gonadotrophin by hepatoblastoma have been demonstrated (Braunstein *et al.*, 1972). A straight abdominal X-ray confirms hepatic enlargement and may show adrenal and tumour calcification. An intravenous pyelogram should be performed to exclude Wilms' tumour, since secondary liver deposits are commoner than primary liver tumours and both neuroblastoma and nephroblastoma commonly occur in this age group. Liver scintillation scanning, inferior venacavography or hepatic arteriography will help to locate the tumour within the liver and may distinguish between a solitary tumour and multiple tumour deposits.

Arteriography may be of considerable assistance to the surgeon in anticipating possible planes of resection and may help to avoid extensive infarction of the liver, which can be fatal following apparently complete resection of the tumour. Serum alpha-fetoprotein estimation may be useful since elevated levels occur in hepatoblastoma as well as in hepatocellular carcinoma, whereas levels are normal in tumours metastasising to the liver; production of this protein by hepatoblastoma in tissue culture has been demonstrated. Biopsy is the only sure method of diagnosis. Open biopsy is preferred to needle biopsy since tumour samples may be confidently obtained, and also because of the danger of haemorrhage from such a vascular tumour.

No generalised liver disorder has been reported in infants developing hepatoblastoma nor has malignant change been found in a pre-existing hamartomatous malformation. There is no increased incidence of congenital malformations in infants who develop hepatoblastoma and no concurrence of a particular defect as found in the Wilms' aniridia syndrome. Hepatoblastoma has, however, been reported in a family (Fraumeni *et al.*, 1969) where two infant sisters developed the tumour. Several authors report a slight male preponderance from 3:2 to 5:2.

Pathology

Hepatoblastoma is an embryonic tumour of the infant liver comparable with nephroblastoma in its wide range of histological appearances. The tumour is a firm, encapsulated brownish-tan mass, and fibrous bands can be seen running across the cut surface. It occurs five times more commonly in the right lobe of the liver compared with the left (Keeling, 1971). The tumour tissue itself is yellowish-tan, and areas of haemorrhage several centimeters in diameter and of cystic degeneration are common (Fig. 19.2).

The histological appearances of this tumour are very variable. Some tumours consist predominantly of tissue resembling fetal liver, whilst others contain a large proportion of other types of tissue. The tumours which resemble fetal liver are composed of small cells with oval nuclei and a narrow ring of deep

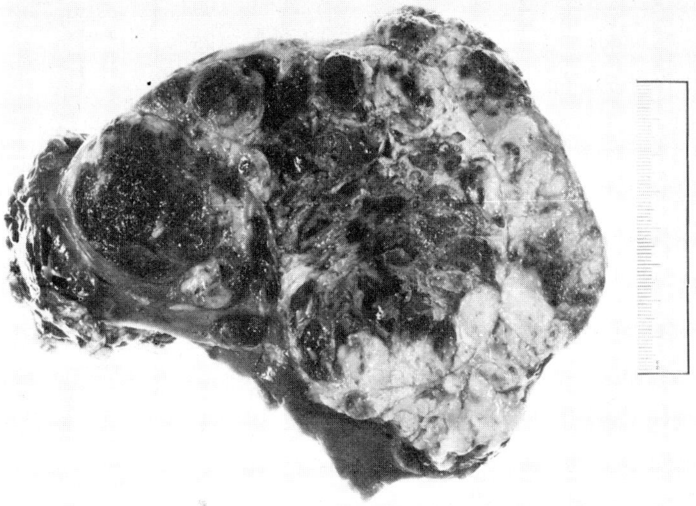

Fig. 19.2 Massive lobulated hepatoblastoma with multiple areas of haemorrhage (Keeling, 1971, by courtesy of the Editor of the *Journal of Pathology*)

eosinophilic cytoplasm, and sometimes organisation into cords and trabeculae is seen (Fig. 19.3), whilst in other cases cells may be arranged in solid sheets. The appearances of the immature liver cells compare with those of the fetal liver at different stages of development, both between different tumours and in different areas within the same tumour, the cells becoming larger and having relatively more cytoplasm as development proceeds. Other hepatoblastomas may be composed of immature liver tissue with a variable admixture of areas of smaller, darker-staining cells with inconspicuous cytoplasm within which developing

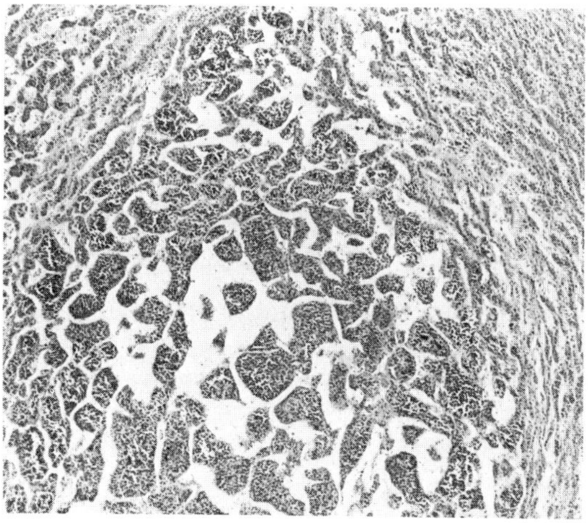

Fig. 19.3 Hepatoblastoma containing immature hepatocytes arranged in trabeculae (magnification × 31)

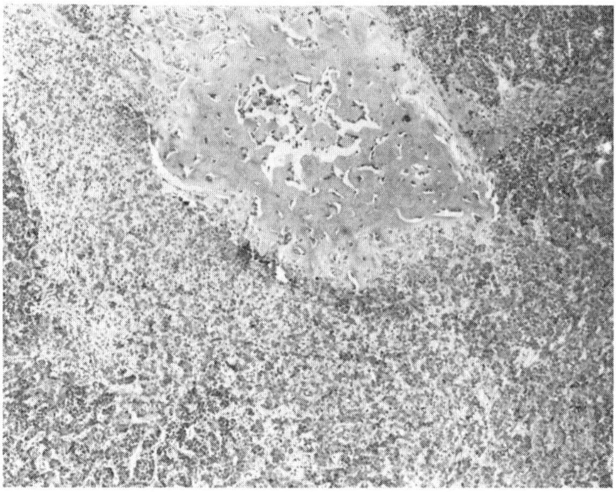

Fig. 19.4 Islands of osteoid arising from metaplasia of bile duct-like epithelium in hepatoblastoma (magnification × 31)

bile ducts may be found. These small dark cells are also capable of metaplasia to squamous cells, and keratin pearls may be found. Islands of osteoid may also be seen arising from the metaplastic bile duct cells (Fig. 19.4). Sometimes, mineralisation of the osteoid to bone may occur, and occasionally this may be demonstrated radiologically. Embryonic mesenchymal tissue can be found in all hepatoblastomas if a careful search is made. Thus, hepatoblastomas are all mixed tumours and probably best considered as a single group rather than subdividing them according to their histological components, since there is no difference in behaviour between them. Differences by light and electron microscopy are demonstrable between the liver cells in hepatoblastomas and the hepatocellular carcinoma of older children, and it is incorrect to group the predominantly liver cell hepatoblastoma with hepatocellular carcinoma, as the former are more likely to be cured by resection.

Hepatoblastoma spreads locally to lymph nodes in the porta hepatis and around the coeliac axis, and to the diaphragm; spread via the bloodstream occurs to the lungs and thence frequently to the bones and brain.

Treatment

The efficacy of treatment is difficult to assess since rapid advances in recent years in the quality of supportive treatment, radiotherapy and chemotherapy effectively mean that no two cases are treated in the same way. If the tumour is solitary and lies within one lobe, hemihepatectomy offers the best chance of success. Operative mortality, however, is high, with reported figures varying from 24 to 31 per cent, haemorrhage from the raw surface of the liver being a particular hazard. The only satisfactory way of assessing radiotherapy and different chemotherapeutic regimes will be by means of a carefully planned multicentre trial.

HEPATOCELLULAR CARCINOMA

Clinical features and diagnosis

Carcinoma of the liver, indistinguishable from the tumour found in adults, usually occurs in children over the age of 6 years. Presenting symptoms include abdominal pain, vomiting, loss of weight and abdominal distention. Jaundice is uncommon in the early stages, but often occurs terminally. Liver function tests are frequently normal, but serum alpha-fetoprotein levels may be increased. Plain abdominal X-ray will confirm liver enlargement and inferior venography, hepatic arteriography or liver scintillation scanning will localise the tumour. This is particularly useful if surgery is contemplated. The tumour may arise in a previously healthy liver or complicate other liver diseases and metabolic disorders involving the liver. Carcinoma has been found in livers with pre-existing cirrhosis, extrahepatic biliary atresia and intrahepatic biliary atresia. It has been recorded in a child in whom giant cell hepatitis in infancy progressed to cirrhosis. Metabolic disorders which have been complicated by liver carcinoma include glycogen storage disease, Neimann–Pick disease and hereditary tubular dysplasia (de Toni-Fanconi). In this last disorder, its occurrence has been recorded both during childhood and in adult life. To date, no cases of cirrhosis or hepatic fibrosis occurring in children with alpha-antitrypsin deficiency have been complicated by hepatocellular carcinoma, although tumours have been found in adults with liver disease occurring in the absence of this enzyme (Borg and Eriksson, 1972).

Complications of hepatocellular carcinoma in childhood include severe generalised osteoporosis and disturbances in lipid metabolism. The osteoporosis is thought to be a protein-sparing mechanism and may be accompanied by growth retardation; a return to radiological normality has been observed following hemihepatectomy. Elevated serum levels of cholesterol, cholesterol esters and total lipids may occur; the hypercholesterolaemia may be secondary to the low serum protein levels, and the raised total lipid levels may reflect some degree of hepatic insufficiency (Teng *et al.*, 1961).

Pathology

Hepatocellular carcinoma may occur as a single mass occupying most of a liver lobe, potentially suitable for resection, or as multiple tumour nodules present throughout the whole of the organ. The tumours are lobulated, encapsulated, yellow in colour and frequently have small scattered haemorrhages.

Histologically, the tumour is composed of large cells with palely staining reticular nuclei with prominent nucleoli, and large amounts of pale eosinophilic cytoplasm, resembling hepatocytes; often there is little nuclear or cellular pleomorphism. The tumour cells are frequently arranged in irregularly sized trabeculae and bile ducts are absent. Intracellular bile retention is common, giving rise to the yellow colour of the tumour.

The tumours metastasise widely and early to local lymph nodes and via the bloodstream to the lungs.

Treatment

Treatment is less satisfactory than that of hepatoblastoma, and consists of hemi-hepatectomy, either alone or with radiotherapy, or radiotherapy and chemotherapy. Treatment may prolong survival by months when compared with the natural course of the disease, but no long-term survivals have been achieved.

RHABDOMYOSARCOMA

Clinical features and diagnosis

Rhabdomyosarcomata of the bile ducts occur in older children, usually over the age of 6 years. Symptoms include jaundice, abdominal pain, anorexia and abdominal swelling; these symptoms may be accompanied by severe jaundice of the obstructive type.

Pathology

The tumours are cream-coloured and firm in texture. Yellowish areas of cystic degeneration are frequently found, but no liver-like tissue is present within the tumour. Translucent botryoid nodules of tumour may protrude singly or in groups into dilated bile ducts, resembling the appearance of this type of tumour in the infant bladder or vagina (Fig. 19.5). The tumour may be solitary, but frequently multiple tumours are found, which may be widely separated and surround bile ducts with healthy ducts between them. When a main bile duct is affected, the proximity of the other main duct, hepatic artery and portal vein makes resection impossible.

Histologically, these tumours are composed of large, elongated, mesenchymal cells having large nuclei which exhibit marked pleomorphism, and cytoplasm often has a foamy appearance. Tubules lined by cuboidal cells are scattered through the tumour and are frequently surrounded by a palisaded halo of mesenchymal cells. Cytoplasmic striations can be demonstrated by phosphotungstic acid—haematoxylin staining in strap-like and 'tadpole' cells, but are not as frequently seen as in rhabdomyosarcomata of the urogenital sinus. Areas of cystic degeneration are common, particularly in large tumours.

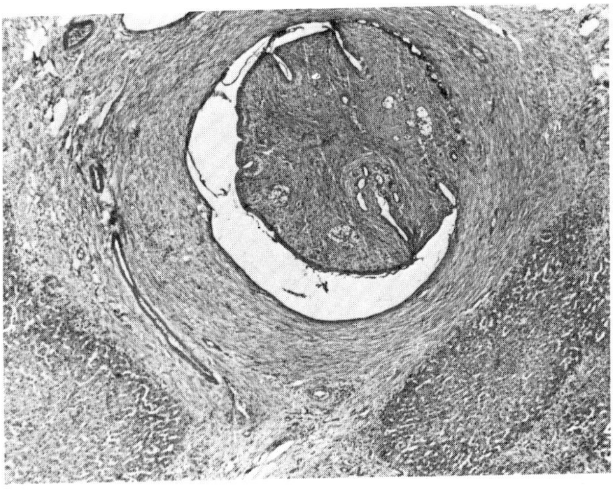

Fig. 19.5 Small rhabdomyosarcoma arising from smooth muscle in a bile duct and protruding into the lumen (magnification × 31)

Metastatic tumour deposits may be found in lymph nodes in the porta hepatis, and blood-borne spread to the lung may occur early.

Treatment

Attempts have been made at surgical excision, but neither this nor any chemotherapeutic regimes has been successful.

METASTATIC AND OTHER TUMOURS

Metastatic tumours of the liver are much commoner than primary ones in childhood. It is difficult to assess their true incidence since some may be so small as not to give rise to signs or symptoms. It is when they cause marked liver enlargement that confusion may arise, particularly in the presence of an unobtrusive primary tumour. Many of these can be distinguished from primary liver tumours by radiological, biochemical and haematological investigations, but in some cases it is necessary to resort to laparotomy for diagnosis. Experience at The Hospital for Sick Children over a 20-year period indicates that the number of metastatic tumours requiring open biopsy to distinguish them from primary tumours was approximately equal to the number of primary tumours seen during that time.

Neuroblastoma is the commonest tumour to metastasise to the liver in childhood, and multiple deposits are frequently present (Fig. 19.6). The primary site

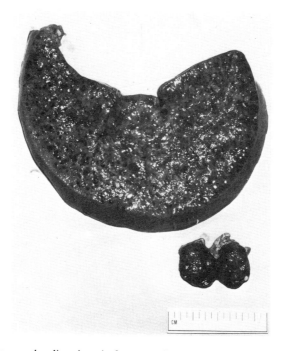

Fig. 19.6 Multiple secondary liver deposits from a small primary adrenal neuroblastoma

is usually abdominal, either in the adrenal or the sympathetic chain. Nephroblastoma and teratoma may also be responsible for large secondary deposits in the liver.

The liver may be diffusely infiltrated by tumours of the reticuloendothelial system, such as lymphosarcoma or histiocytosis X, and the liver enlargement may be so prominent as to overshadow lymph node and splenic involvement. Bone marrow aspiration will often distinguish a lymphosarcoma from a primary liver tumour, but liver biopsy may sometimes be necessary for diagnosis.

Very rarely, a true teratoma of the liver may occur (Yarborough and Evashnick, 1956; Misugi and Reiner, 1965). These can contain entirely mature tissues, when resection offers a good chance of a complete cure, or alternatively contain a mixture of mature, embryonic and frankly carcinomatous tissue, when widespread metastatic tumours may already be present when the child is first seen.

References

Borg, N. O. & Eriksson, S. (1972) Liver disease in adults with $alpha_1$ antitrypsin deficiency. *New England Journal of Medicine,* **287,** 1264.

Braunstein, G. D., Bridson, W. E., Glass, A., Hull, E. W. & McIntire, K. R. (1972) In vivo and in vitro production of chorionic gonadotrophin and alpha fetoprotein by a virilising hepatoblastoma. *Journal of Clinical Endocrinology & Metabolism,* **35,** 857.

Claireaux, A. E. (1960) Neonatal hyperbilirubinaemia. *British Medical Journal,* **1,** 1528.

Fraumeni, J. F. Jr., Rosen, J. P., Hull, E. W., Barth, R. F., Shapiro, S. R. & O'Connor, J. F. (1969) Hepatoblastoma in infant sisters. *Cancer,* **24,** 1086.

Keeling, J. W., (1971) Liver tumours in infancy and childhood. *Journal of Pathology,* **103,** 69–85.

Misugi, K. & Reiner, C. B. (1965) A malignant true teratoma of liver in childhood. *Archives of Pathology,* **80,** 409.

Teng, C. T., Daeschner, C. W., Singleton, E. B., Rosenberg, H. S., Cole, V. W., Hills, L. L. & Brennan, J. C. (1961) Liver disease and osteoporosis in children. 1. Clinical observations. *Journal of Pediatrics,* **59,** 684–702.

Yarborough, S. M. & Evashnick, G. (1956) Case of teratoma of the liver with 14 years post-operative survival. *Cancer,* **9,** 848.

20. Disorders of the pancreas

J. P. K. McCollum and J. T. Harries

Cystic fibrosis
Congenital pancreatic hypoplasia (Shwachman's syndrome)
Embryological malformations
Pancreatitis
Pancreatic cysts
Malnutrition

Table 20.1 Disorders of the pancreas in childhood

Congenital
Cystic fibrosis
Congenital pancreatic hypoplasia (Shwachman's syndrome)
Embryological malformations
Ectopic pancreas
Annular pancreas
Congenital lipase deficiency
Trypsinogen deficiency
Acquired
Pancreatitis
Acute
Chronic
Cysts
Tumours
Malnutrition

In childhood disorders of the pancreas are relatively uncommon but, with the development and application of new investigatory techniques, they may become increasingly recognised in the future. Table 20.1 lists the established congenital and acquired disorders of the pancreas which are encountered in childhood. Of these the commonest and most important is cystic fibrosis.

This chapter concentrates on disorders of the exocrine pancreas, but tumours of the endocrine pancreas, however, may rarely result in disease in childhood as a result of hypersecretion of a variety of polypeptide hormones. For example, gastrin-producing tumours can lead to severe and recurrent peptic ulceration, the so-called Zollinger–Ellison syndrome (see Isenberg, Walsh and Grossman, 1973). Hypersecretion of insulin or glucagon results in hypoglycaemia and insulin-resistant diabetes, respectively. Severe watery diarrhoea, hypokalaemia and hypochlorhydria (Verner–Morrison syndrome) may be associated with endocrine tumours which produce vasoactive intestinal peptide hormone (see Isenberg *et al.*, 1973).

Congenital lipase and trypsinogen deficiency are extremely rare and have already been considered in Chapter 11.

CYSTIC FIBROSIS

Cystic fibrosis is a multiorgan disease characterised by chronic lung disease, pancreatic insufficiency, liver dysfunction and increased concentrations of electrolytes in sweat. All these manifestations can probably be accounted for by a primary disorder of the exocrine and mucus-secreting glands. The condition was first reported by Fanconi, Uehlinger and Knauer in 1936, and the defect in sweat electrolytes was first described in 1953 (di Sant'Agnese *et al.*, 1953).

Cystic fibrosis is predominantly a Caucasian disease with an incidence of about one in 2000 live births (Danks, Olan and Anderson, 1965) with a carrier frequency of 5 per cent, and is transmitted as an autosomal recessive trait. One in 20 of the population will be heterozygotes, and the likelihood of two heterozygotes mating can be estimated to be about one in 400.

Pathogenesis

The nature of the primary metabolic defect in cystic fibrosis remains unknown, and no single hypothesis has yet been shown to account for the varied manifestations of the disease. It seems clear, however, that the clinical and pathological features of cystic fibrosis are a direct consequence of obstruction of small ducts by mucus.

Composition of secretions

Compared with other organic substances the fucose content of glycoproteins obtained from duodenal juice, sweat, urine, submaxillary saliva, bronchial and rectal mucus is increased compared with that found in similar secretions in normal subjects. The calcium concentration of submaxillary saliva is also often increased. The sodium and chloride concentrations in sweat are consistently increased and potassium content is also sometimes elevated; the increased content of sodium and chloride is due to defective ductular reabsorption of these two ions. Sodium and chloride are also increased in submaxillary and mixed saliva, but are normal or only slightly increased in parotid secretions; they are normal in tears and duodenal fluid. In those patients with normal function of the acinar cells of the pancreas, both the volume and bicarbonate content of pancreatic secretion is reduced indicating defective tubular function.

Circulating factors

Up to 90 per cent of patients with cystic fibrosis, a large proportion of heterozygotes and 5 to 10 per cent of normal subjects possess serum 'factors' which induce asymmetrical ciliary beats in rabbit trachea and oyster gills. Similar factors have been found in sweat, and submaxillary and parotid saliva of affected patients, and have been shown to inhibit sodium reabsorption in the human sweat gland. Patient sera also inhibits erythrocyte (Na^+-K^+)-ATPase, and glucose-stimulated short-circuit current in the rat jejunum *in vitro* (Cole and Sella, 1975; Araki, Field and Shwachman, 1975). Whether these factors are one of the same and represent a primary abnormality remains to be determined.

Essential fatty acid deficiency

Biochemical evidence of essential fatty acid (i.e. linoleic and arachidonic acid) deficiency is commonly found in cystic fibrosis, and it has been suggested that this, together with secondary abnormalities of prostaglandin metabolism, may represent a primary abnormality (see Chase 1976). Elliott (1976), in an uncontrolled study, reported some improvement in patients following essential fatty acid supplementation. Further controlled studies are required to confirm these preliminary observations.

Cell culture studies

Leucocyte and fibroblast culture techniques have demonstrated a number of abnormalities in patients and heterozygotes—for example, abnormal metachromatic staining, increased activity of the lysosomal enzyme α-glucosidase and increased concentrations of acid mucopolysaccharides (Krauss *et al.*, 1971).

Clinical and laboratory features

The diagnosis of cystic fibrosis should be suspected in any child with chronic recurrent upper or lower respiratory tract infections, particularly if such symptoms are associated with failure to thrive and pale, oily, bulky, foul-smelling stools; in contrast to patients with coeliac disease the appetite is often increased and may be ravenous. The patient's appearance may vary from a severely malnourished child to a healthy one. Nasal polyps are common. Ten to 15 per cent of patients present in the first few days of life with meconium ileus, and the diagnosis and management of this serious complication is considered in Chapter 4. Occasionally rectal prolapse may be the presenting feature; this disappears with dietary treatment and surgery is rarely necessary. Rarely infants with cystic fibrosis can present with intracranial or cutaneous bleeding due to vitamin K deficiency. Occasionally the presenting features may be those of cirrhosis and portal hypertension with hypersplenism. Because of excessive losses of sodium chloride in sweat, increased sweating during hot weather can lead to hypovolaemia, dehydration and shock. Prolonged neonatal jaundice should alert the physician to a possible diagnosis of cystic fibrosis.

The spectrum of the onset and severity of the clinical features of cystic fibrosis varies widely. For example, 15 to 20 per cent of patients present with pulmonary symptoms having no symptoms or signs of pancreatic insufficiency; similarly the reverse situation may hold true. Any child exhibiting any of the above general clinical features should be suspected of having cystic fibrosis until proven otherwise by means of sweat tests.

Pulmonary features

The vast majority of patients develop respiratory symptoms during childhood, and in 60 to 70 per cent these develop during the first year of life. Initial symptoms may be acute and severe, or mild and recurrent. Cough may be paroxysmal and accompanied by vomiting, suggesting a diagnosis of pertussis; wheezing may be a predominant feature. Approximately 75 per cent of patients have developed the pulmonary symptoms described above by the age of 2 years. Untreated, the respiratory symptoms progress with the production of purulent sputum. Radiologically there is evidence of hyperinflated lungs, areas of segmental or lobar collapse, and later a thickened bronchial wall pattern develops; a diagnosis of cystic fibrosis can be strongly suspected from these radiological appearances. The natural history of the pulmonary manifestations is progression to bronchiectasis, emphysema, recurrent focal or lobular atelectasis and sometimes pneumothorax; cor pulmonale, haemoptysis and right-sided heart failure may be terminal events in the progressive and irreversible lung damage that can occur. The most important pathophysiological factor in the genesis of the lung disease is obstruction of the bronchial tree by viscid secretions with distal collapse and/or infection. Generally speaking chronic obstructive airway disease with secondary infection dominates the clinical picture and usually determines the morbidity and life expectancy.

Respiratory tests usually reveal a reduced pO_2 and prolongation of the expiratory flow rate early in the course of the disease. The vital capacity may be decreased, and residual volume and airway resistance increased.

Gastrointestinal manifestations

In a small proportion of patients the gastrointestinal manifestations of cystic fibrosis may precede those of pulmonary involvement by several months or years. These include failure to thrive and abdominal distention in a child with a ravenous appetite and foul-smelling, bulky stools, intestinal obstruction due to meconium ileus within the first few days of life, rectal prolapse and intestinal obstruction in the older child or young adult due to faecal impaction. Approximately 80 per cent of patients have severe pancreatic dysfunction which may be progressive. Pancreatic dysfunction results from obstruction of small ducts by viscid secretions with destruction of acinar tissue; these events are reflected by the histopathological changes shown in Figure 20.1. These changes progress with age, as illustrated in Figures 20.1 and 20.2, and are in marked contrast to those seen in Shwachman's syndrome (see Fig. 20.3).

Malabsorption of protein and fat-soluble vitamins can result in hypoalbuminaemia and vitamin deficiency states. Osteomalacia, hypoprothrombinaemia and bleeding due to vitamin K deficiency, vitamin A deficiency with xerophthalmia and raised intracranial pressure, and vitamin E deficiency with ceroid deposition in smooth muscles have all been reported (see Kopel, 1972). Faecal losses of fat and nitrogen are considerable in untreated cystic fibrosis.

Recurrent abdominal pain of varying severity and location is not an uncommon symptom. Faecal impaction, flatulence and pancreatitis should be considered in the differential diagnosis. Peptic ulceration is only rarely seen in cystic fibrosis.

It is probable that the intestinal malabsorption cannot be entirely explained on the basis of pancreatic insufficiency, and defective small intestinal mucosal

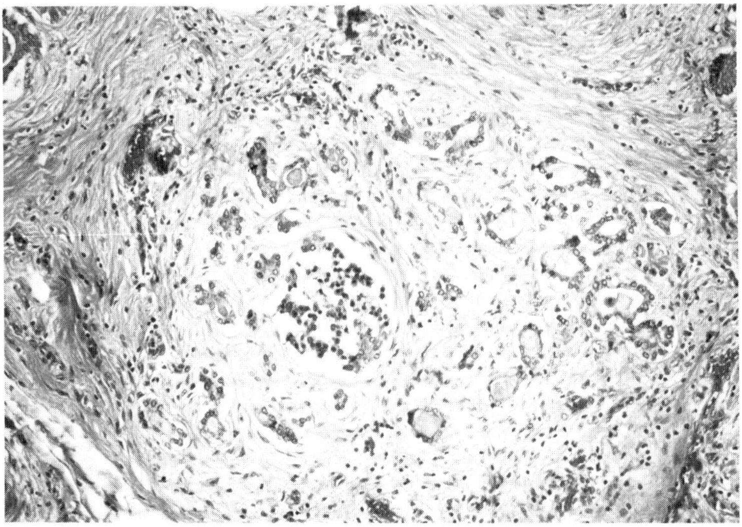

Fig. 20.1 Pancreas from a patient aged 6 years with cystic fibrosis. There is an increase in fibrous tissue infiltrated by lymphocytes, both within and between the pancreatic lobules. Acinar tissue is depleted, and the small ductules are distended by lamellar eosinophilic concentrations. The islets of Langerhans appear normal (magnification × 130). (Reproduced by kind permission of Dr J. R. Pincott)

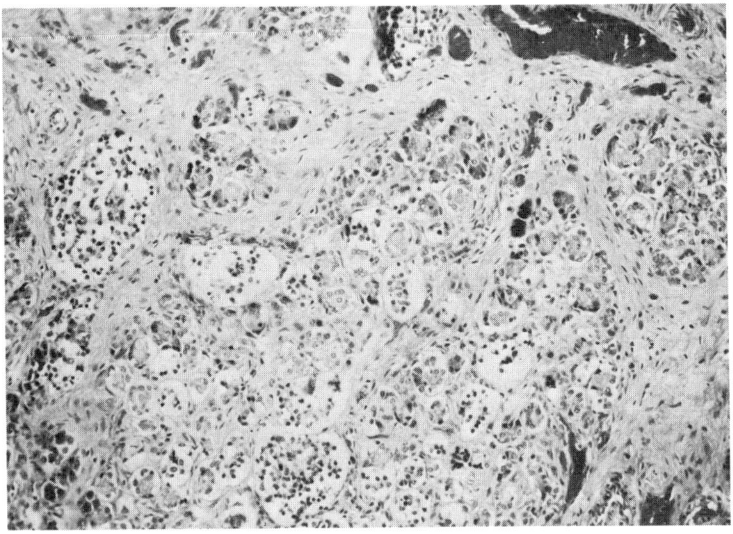

Fig. 20.2 Pancreas from a patient aged 5 months with cystic fibrosis. The histopathological changes are much less striking than in the older child; nevertheless, intra- and interlobular fibrosis and eosinophilic ductular concentrations are present (magnification × 130). (Reproduced by kind permission of Dr J. R. Pincott)

function and disturbances of bile salt metabolism may contribute in some patients.

Small intestinal mucosal function. There is no good evidence that the structure of the small intestine is abnormal in cystic fibrosis. A few patients have been reported to also have coeliac disease, but this is probably a chance association. Mucosal function has not been extensively studied in cystic fibrosis, but a few observations suggest that mucosal dysfunction may contribute to the malabsorption.

Light and electronmicroscopic studies of small intestinal biopsies have shown the normal microvilli of the enterocytes to be covered by a coarse fibrillar substance, probably mucus (Freye *et al.,* 1964). This substance was closely adherent to the normally found 'glycocalyx', and was absent from normal biopsies and from one patient without steatorrhoea. Disacchariduria (Gibbons, 1969) and reduced mucosal lactase and L-alanyl-L-phenylalanine hydrolase activities have also been reported in cystic fibrosis (Antonowicz *et al.,* 1968; Morin *et al.,* 1976). Phenylalanine is absorbed by a separate transport system to lysine, and *in vitro* mucosal uptake of phenylalanine has been shown to be impaired, whereas lysine uptake was normal. (Morin *et al.,* 1976).

These observations should add impetus to future studies concerned with the mucosal phase of small intestinal absorption in cystic fibrosis.

Disturbances of bile salt metabolism. The enterohepatic circulation of bile salts is broken in cystic fibrosis due to defective ileal absorption of bile salts. Consequently the faecal output of bile salts is increased to a degree similar to that seen following ileal resections (Weber *et al.,* 1973). These abnormalities are improved by the administration of pancreatic supplements or by reducing the intake of dietary fat. The concentration of total bile salts in duodenal fluid is reduced with a marked increase in the ratio of glycine to taurine conjugated bile salts (McCollum *et al.,* 1976). Coupled with the low pH of duodenal fluid, these abnormalities can be anticipated to interfere with formation of bile salt micelles and to impair solubilisation of dietary fat and fat-soluble vitamins. In addition bile salts are activators of pancreatic esterase which is necessary for the hydrolysis of esters of vitamin E and other substances (Muller *et al.,* 1976). The markedly reduced activity of pancreatic esterase which occurs in cystic fibrosis (McCollum *et al.,* 1976) may be a contributory factor to the established vitamin E deficiency which occurs in such patients (Harries and Muller, 1971). Free bile acids are known to enhance the colonic absorption of dietary oxalate, and this may explain the hyperoxaluria which occurs in cystic fibrosis (Ogilvie *et al.,* 1976); with increasing survival patients may be at risk of developing renal oxalate stones in later life.

Hepatobiliary lesions. The hepatobiliary lesions and their management are considered in detail in Chapter 18. With the increasing survival of patients hepatobiliary lesions will become commoner. Any adolescent or adult with unexplained portal hypertension should have a sweat test (Stern *et al.,* 1976).

Table 20.2 Differential diagnosis of cystic fibrosis

Asthma and recurrent chest infections
Nasal polyps
Bronchiectasis
Histoplasmosis
Tuberculosis
Shwachman's syndrome
Congenital lipase deficiency
Enterokinase deficiency
Trypsinogen deficiency
Coeliac disease
Cows' milk protein intolerance
Other diarrhoeal states
Meconium plug syndrome
Rectal prolapse
Persistent neonatal jaundice
Cirrhosis
Portal hypertension
Intussusception after the age of 3 years

Dysfunction of the endocrine pancreas

The number of patients who develop diabetes mellitus which requires treatment is increasing. Glucose intolerance may be present for several years prior to the development of clinical diabetes and, in contrast to other diabetics, ketosis is rarely seen in cystic fibrosis. It is assumed that the diabetes is secondary to islet cell destruction.

Infertility

Adult males with cystic fibrosis are sterile (Kaplan *et al.*, 1968). The ejaculum is reduced in volume, contains no spermatozoa, has a reduced concentration of fructose and increased concentrations of citric acid and acid phosphatase activity. The testes are normal or slightly reduced in size, the epididymides are poorly developed and the body and tail are often absent, and the vas deferens is usually absent. These abnormalities develop *in utero* and have been found in patients shortly after birth. Testicular hormonal function and sexual activity may not be impaired.

The incidence of inguinal hernia, hydrocoeles and undescended testes is markedly increased in affected males.

Diagnosis

The conditions which should be considered in the differential diagnosis of cystic fibrosis are listed in Table 20.2. The implications of a diagnosis of cystic fibrosis to the patient and family are profound, and a high degree of clinical suspicion is essential.

The commonest cause of pancreatic dysfunction in childhood is cystic fibrosis, Shwachman's syndrome probably being the second commonest cause. The main features which differentiate these two conditions are listed in Table 20.3.

Table 20.3 Main differentiating features between Shwachman's syndrome and cystic fibrosis

	Cystic fibrosis	Shwachman's syndrome
Localisation of primary pancreatic defect	Ductular	Acinar
Infections	Pulmonary	Random
Sweat test	Positive	Negative
Haematological and skeletal abnormalities	Absent	Present
Growth	May be normal	Severely impaired

Sweat test

The sweat test is the single most reliable technique for establishing a diagnosis of cystic fibrosis. The concentrations of sodium and chloride are determined in sweat collected by pilocarpine iontophoresis (Gibson and Cooke, 1959; Shwachman and Mahmoodian, 1967). The finding of a sweat sodium concentration of greater than 70 mmol/l on at least two separate collections of more than 100 mg of sweat is consistent with the diagnosis of cystic fibrosis. The test should be performed by a laboratory which has experience of the technique. The diagnosis is confirmed by accompanying evidence of pancreatic insufficiency and/or pulmonary involvement.

A few children suspected of having cystic fibrosis have equivocal sweat tests with sodium and chloride concentration varying from 50 to 70 mmol/l. These children require repeated sweat tests, careful assessment of pulmonary and pancreatic function and long-term follow-up. A variety of factors should be considered in interpreting the results of a sweat test. Sweat electrolytes are normally increased during the first few days of life, and sodium and chloride concentrations may be as high as 70 to 80 mmol/l in the stimulated sweat of some infants. Sodium and chloride concentrations increase after the age of 17 years to mean values of 47 and 30 mmol/l, respectively. Generally speaking the larger the volume of sweat collected, the more accurate will be the determination, and electrolyte values in amounts of sweat of less than 100 mg should be interpreted with great caution. Elevated sweat electrolytes may occasionally be found in other conditions such as adrenal insufficiency, malnutrition, diabetes insipidus, ectoadrenal dysplasia, allergic diseases and type I glycogen storage disease. Salt loading may increase sweat electrolytes, and repeated stimulation of the same area of skin can result in a reduced volume of sweat and increased electrolyte concentrations.

Pancreatic function

Pancreatic function can be assessed following stimulation with intravenous cholecystokinin-pancreozymin and secretin, or following a test meal (see Ch. 3).

Eighty per cent of patients have evidence of pancreatic insufficiency. The volume, pH and bicarbonate concentration of the pancreatic juice are reduced, and the activities of the pancreatic enzymes are markedly impaired or absent. Occasionally, enzyme activities may be normal or increased in the face of reduced volume and bicarbonate outputs; this finding provides supportive evidence to the concept that the primary pancreatic defect is a functional tubular one, and that exocrine dysfunction develops secondary to ductular obstruction.

The stool trypsin test is an unreliable method of assessing pancreatic function and its routine use should be discouraged.

Screening tests

The determination of albumin (Prosser *et al.,* 1974), enzymes (Robinson and Elliott, 1976) and serum proteins (Ryley *et al.,* 1976) in faecal material, the quantification of sodium and potassium in nail clippings (Antonelli, Ballati and Annibaldi 1969) and the chloride plate and filter paper technique have all been reported as useful screening procedures for detecting children with cystic fibrosis. All of these tests, however, have their limitations, and at present there is no simple good test which can justify its application to massive newborn screening programmes.

Treatment

There is no specific treatment since the basic abnormality has not been defined and, since the clinical manifestations vary depending on the degree of involvement of different organs, management will vary from patient to patient according to their needs. The primary aims of management are the prevention and treatment of pulmonary obstruction and infection, and to maintain the patient in a satisfactory nutritional state. It should be emphasised that the major cause of morbidity and mortality in cystic fibrosis is a direct result of the pulmonary manifestations; accumulation of viscid secretions causes bronchial and bronchiolar obstruction, and infection.

Tubular obstruction

A variety of methods have been advocated to remove viscid secretions. These include mucolytic agents (e.g. n-acetylcysteine), bronchodilators, expectorants, mist-tent therapy and physiotherapy. The single most important therapy is regular physiotherapy which involves postural drainage and breathing exercises. The parents are taught the technique so that the child receives regular physiotherapy in the home; in mild disease the child receives therapy once daily, whereas in more severely affected patients therapy is administered three or four times daily.

Infection

The commonest infecting agent is *Staphylococcus aureus.* Other organisms which can be recovered from the sputum include *Pseudomonas aeruginosa, Klebsiella pneumoniae* and *Haemophilus influenzae.* The choice of antibiotic, the duration of treatment and the prevention of infection by prophylactic antibiotics are controversial issues, and policies vary among individual physicians (see Mearns, 1974). For example Lawson (1969) advocates continuous antibiotic therapy from the time of diagnosis, whereas this is not the view of others (Mearns, 1974).

We agree with most of the therapeutic scheme proposed by Mearns (1974) and refer the reader to this excellent review for further details. Generally speaking, acute exacerbations are treated with antibiotics which the cultured organisms are sensitive to. Tetracycline and oxytetracycline should be avoided in children under the age of 7 years because of their effects on teeth. Antibiotics are continued for one to two months following resolution of the acute infection. Intensive physiotherapy is necessary during acute exacerbations of respiratory disease.

The indications for prophylactic antibiotic therapy have not been completely clarified, particularly when applied to the first year of life. The value of continuous antibiotics during the first year of life has not been proven. Because of their side-effects and the possible emergence of antibiotic-resistant strains of bacteria, it is our view that prophylactic antibiotics throughout the first year of life are not indicated. Patients with minimal pulmonary involvement during upper respiratory tract infections should receive antibiotics for seven to 10 days. Some patients with irreversible lung damage benefit from continuous antibiotics.

Aerosol treatment (with neomycin, gentamicin, paromomycin or cloxacillin) may be useful in infants and older children with minimal lung involvement, but the value of this form of treatment in patients with severe disease is questionable.

Other approaches to pulmonary disease

In selected patients surgical resection of chronic areas of atelectasis and sepsis or bronchiectatic areas may be beneficial. Tracheostomy and bronchial lavage may be a life-saving procedure in severely ill patients, but the effects of lavage are usually only transient. Patients who develop cor pulmonale require digitalis and, if necessary, restriction of fluid and salt, and diuretics.

Nutrition

The maintenance of adequate nutrition depends on the control of both the pulmonary disease and the malabsorption. In a recent study of adolescents and young adults with cystic fibrosis, Lapey *et al.* (1974) found that growth failure and state of nutrition correlated more closely with pulmonary disease than with the degree of pancreatic insufficiency. The management and long-term effects of large intestinal resections for meconium ileus deserve special attention and are considered in detail in Chapter 7.

A diet containing adequate calories (e.g. up to 840 kJ per kg per day in young infants) and a low fat and high protein content forms the basis of dietetic management (see Francis, 1975). A variety of pancreatic enzyme preparations are available for replacement therapy, and the treatment of pancreatic insufficiency with pancreatic extracts has recently been reviewed by Saunders and Wormsley (1975). Children require continuous and adequate amounts of pancreatic extracts. Dietary restrictions and pancreatic extracts, however, may not be necessary in older children and young adults (Lapey *et al.*, 1974). A powder preparation (e.g. 0·5 g Pancrex V Forte powder for infants, increasing to 2 g by the age of 2 years) mixed with water or fruit juice and given immediately before meals is usually adequate for infants and young children. In older children six to 10 tablets of the same brand of pancreatic extract are required with each meal. Cotazym or nutrizym preparations can be given in equivalent amounts. The degree of steatorrhoea and azotorrhoea and the response to replacement therapy varies widely from patient to patient, but generally speaking pancreatic extracts only partially correct the increased faecal excretion of fat and nitrogen. This may be related to instability of the administered enzymes in the acidic environment of the stomach and duodenum, as well as to impaired micellar solubilisation of the products of lipolysis (McCollum *et al.*, 1976). It is probably for these reasons that some patients benefit from oral supplements of sodium bicarbonate. Adequate amounts of vitamin supplements should be given to all patients. There is no good evidence that the inclusion of medium-chain triglycerides in the diet or the use of elemental diets are superior to the above described measures. In the group of patients with normal pancreatic function neither dietary restriction, pancreatic extracts nor vitamin supplements is necessary.

General

Salt supplements may be advisable if excessive sweating occurs in association with hot weather or fever.

The patients should be seen at intervals of one to two months so that respiratory problems can be detected and treated promptly. Routine sputum or cough swabs should be performed and the sensitivity of pathogens to antibiotics determined.

The emotional and social implications of an incurable disease may be profound to the child and family. Constant support and sometimes psychiatric help are important aspects of all-round management.

Prognosis

The prognosis has improved considerably over the past 25 to 30 years. In the United States the survival rate at 10 years was 1 per cent prior to 1939, whereas for the years 1966 to 1968 25 per cent of patients were alive at 20 years (Warwick and Pogue, 1969). Longitudinal life tables have been constructed for patients attending the Queen Elizabeth Hospital for Children, London from 1966 to 1972 (Mearns, 1974); 72 per cent were alive at 12 years and 45 per cent at 20 years. The quality of life of survivors is at least equally important to the duration of survival, and the findings of Mearns (1974) suggest that the prognosis is not necessarily worse in patients who present with early and severe symptoms compared with those who present later. Cystic fibrosis is no longer a disease of childhood, and the reasons for increased survival are probably multifactorial as they are controversial.

CONGENITAL PANCREATIC HYPOPLASIA (Shwachman's syndrome)

Although this condition is commonly referred to as Shwachman's syndrome (Shwachman *et al.*, 1964), it was in fact first described by Nezelof and Watchi in 1961. It is a rare disorder, the most important differential diagnosis being cystic fibrosis (McCollum, Muller and Harries, 1975), and the main features which differentiate these two diseases are shown in Table 20.3. As with cystic fibrosis it is a multisystem disease characterised by pancreatic insufficiency, skeletal and haematological abnormalities, sometimes overwhelming infections and normal sweat electrolyte concentrations. A familial incidence is common and an autosomal recessive mode of inheritance is probable.

Pathogenesis

The pathogenesis of Shwachman's syndrome is not understood. Embryological development of pancreatic and acinar cells and myeloid tissue occurs at about the same time, and it has been suggested that intrauterine infection at this time may play a role in pathogenesis (Hruban *et al.*, 1963); this seems unlikely, however, since the condition may occur in siblings of successive pregnancies, and in one family both the father and daughter had neutropenia (Burke *et al.*, 1967).

Clinical and laboratory features

Shwachman's syndrome usually presents in infancy with steatorrhoea and failure to thrive and is almost always associated with haematological abnormalities, most commonly neutropenia (Nezelof and Watchi, 1961; Shwachman *et al.*, 1964); anaemia, thrombocytopenia and marrow hypocellularity are also not uncommon. The patients have an increased susceptibility to infection, particularly of the respiratory tract and skin, and up to 20 per cent die from overwhelming infections. Reduced levels of serum immunoglobulins have been reported (Doe, 1973). Metaphyseal chondrodysplasia occurs in at least 20 per cent of cases, and bony changes are most pronounced in the femoral necks and may lead to coxa vara deformities in later life (Stanley and Sutcliffe, 1973). Thoracic dystrophy contributes to the increased susceptibility to respiratory tract infections in some patients (Danks *et al.*, 1976). Muscular hypotonia and

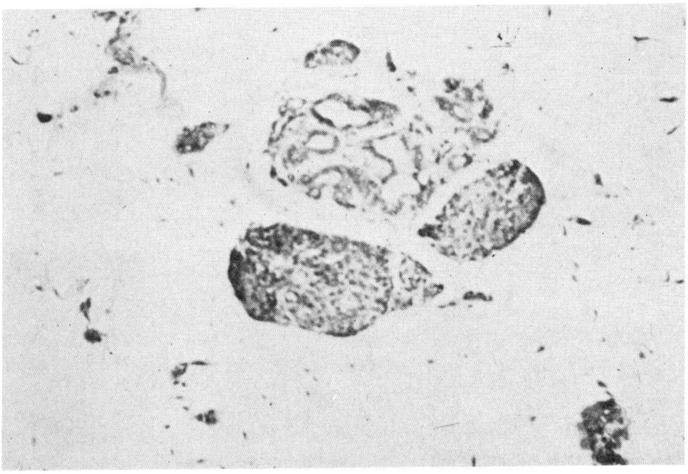

Fig. 20.3 Histological appearances of the pancreas in Shwachman's syndrome. Acinar tissue is very sparse with preservation of the islets of Langerhans and the ducts. The acinar cells are almost completely replaced by fat, and there is an absence of fibrosis and inflammatory cells.

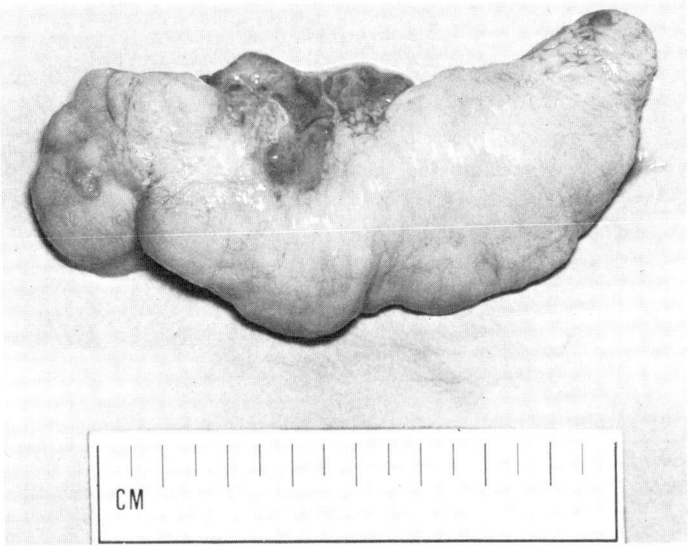

Fig. 20.4 Macroscopic appearances of the pancreas in Shwachman's syndrome. The gland appears as a lobulated, fat-laden structure

hypopigmentation of the retina may also be associated features. Diabetes mellitus is a rare complication (Shmerling *et al.*, 1969).

In contrast to cystic fibrosis the acinar component of pancreatic function is predominantly affected, ductular function being relatively normal. The secretory volume of the pancreas is normal, but bicarbonate output may be slightly reduced in some patients. Enzyme activities are markedly reduced or absent, lipase being most severely affected (McCollum *et al.*, 1975). Histologically, acinar tissue is extremely sparse or absent with preservation of the islets of Langerhans in a gland entirely replaced by fat. The ducts and lining epithelial cells are normal, and there is an absence of fibrosis and inflammatory cells (see Fig. 20.3). Macroscopically the gland resembles a piece of lobulated fat, as shown in Figure 20.4.

The proximal small intestinal mucosa is morphologically normal (Shmerling *et al.*, 1969) and the steatorrhoea is due to pancreatic insufficiency.

Treatment

Treatment with pancreatic extracts and/or a low fat diet which can be supplemented with medium-chain triglycerides usually improves the steatorrhoea with weight gain; vitamin supplements should be administered. The characteristically short stature of these patients, however, does not respond to treatment and cannot be attributed to malabsorption; the pathogenesis of the dwarfism is not clear but may be related to the skeletal defects. Treatment with pancreatic extracts has no affect on the skeletal and haematological abnormalities or on the susceptibility of the patients to infections. Surgery may be necessary for coxa vara deformities later in childhood.

EMBRYOLOGICAL MALFORMATIONS

Annular pancreas

An annular pancreas describes pancreatic tissue which encircles the descending part of the duodenum, and results from a defect in the embryological development of the pancreas from the primitive duodenum (see Ch. 1). Symptoms of upper intestinal obstruction may develop soon after birth. Plain films of the abdomen typically show a dilated proximal duodenum and the 'double-bubble' sign (i.e. fluid levels in the stomach and duodenum), with the more distal regions of the small intestine devoid of gas. Pregnancy is frequently complicated by hydramnios, and other congenital anomalies such as malrotation, imperforate anus, Down's syndrome and cleft palate are often associated.

Ectopic pancreas

Ectopic pancreatic tissue may be located in the stomach or in any part of the small intestine. It may lead to bleeding, obstruction or intussusception.

PANCREATITIS

Table 20.4 lists the causes of pancreatitis in childhood, and these can be divided into acute and chronic recurrent pancreatitis.

Acute pancreatitis

Viruses

Mumps is the commonest cause of acute pancreatitis in childhood. It should be emphasised, however, that clinical pancreatitis is a relatively rare complication of mumps. A few days following the parotid swelling severe epigastric pain, vomiting and diarrhoea develop, and these symptoms together with fever and bradycardia persist for about a week. The serum amylase is elevated even in the

Table 20.4 Causes of pancreatitis in childhood

Acute
Viruses, particularly mumps
Acute haemorrhagic pancreatitis
Trauma
Pancreatic duct obstructions
Following organ transplantation
Tumours
Idiopathic
Chronic recurrent
Hereditary
Familial lipaemia
Hyperparathyroidism
Cystic fibrosis
Following organ transplantation
Lipodystrophy
Idiopathic

absence of symptoms, and rarely the disease may be accompanied by transient diabetes. The vast majority of patients make a complete recovery. Other viral infections such as measles, congenital rubella and coxsackie B and influenza A viral infections have also been implicated as rare causes of acute pancreatitis in childhood.

Acute haemorrhagic pancreatitis

The diagnosis should be borne in mind in any patient receiving corticosteroids (Riemenschneider, Wilson and Vernier, 1968). The onset of symptoms is sudden and may be accompanied by shock, ascites and renal failure, and subsequently hypoglycaemia. The serum amylase is increased, and there may be hyperglycaemia, glucosuria, leucocytosis and proteinuria. Some patients develop fat necrosis of the long bones. The mortality of this type of pancreatitis can be as high as 75 per cent.

Trauma

Acute pancreatitis may follow blunt abdominal trauma and has recently been described in child abuse (Pena and Medovy, 1973). After the acute symptoms have subsided a pseudocyst may develop as a result of fluid entering the lesser sac of omentum; this may be accompanied by abdominal distention and a palpable mass and, as a result of gastric displacement and pressure, lead to symptoms and signs of subacute obstruction. The cysts should be surgically drained as soon as possible. The prognosis is generally good.

Pancreatic duct obstruction

Obstruction of the pancreatic duct due to congenital malformations may occasionally cause acute pancreatitis. Pancreatitis secondary to obstruction of the duct by *Ascaris lumbricoides* (Dobbs, 1935) appears to be less common than in the past.

Following organ transplantation

Acute pancreatitis was reported in 5 per cent of adults following renal transplantations (Corrodi *et al.*, 1975), and may rarely complicate organ transplantation in children. The pancreatitis can be haemorrhagic in some patients. Possible contributing causes are therapy with immunosuppressive drugs, early hypercalcaemia following transplantation, surgery and infections.

Tumours

Primary or metastatic tumours of the pancreas may initiate an episode of acute pancreatitis severe enough to produce pseudocyst formation and ascites (Niccolini, Graham and Banks, 1976).

Idiopathic

Acute pancreatitis may develop in the absence of any of the above described predisposing factors.

Chronic recurrent pancreatitis

Hereditary pancreatitis

Recurrent attacks of abdominal pain begin in childhood and may be accompanied by lysinuria and cystinuria (Gross, Ulrich and Maher, 1961); most families, however, do not have aminoaciduria (McElroy and Christiansen, 1972; Sibert, 1973). The condition is inherited in an autosomal dominant fashion. In the careful study of Gross, Gambill and Ulrich (1962), the mean age of onset was 11·8 years, and hereditary pancreatitis made up 13 per cent of all cases of pancreatitis. The aetiology of familial pancreatitis is controversial. Dilatation of the pancreatic ducts secondary to a presumed obstructive element and hypertrophy of the sphincter of Oddi (Robechek, 1967) have been reported in patients subjected to laparotomy. Sphincterectomy relieved symptoms in two of the three patients described by Robechek (1967). Adham, Dyce and Haverback (1968) reported an increase in serum trypsin binding activity in some of their patients and suggested that their finding could have aetiological significance.

Upper gastrointestinal bleeding and pancreatic pseudocysts may develop as the disease progresses. Similarly, pancreatic calcification, diabetes and insufficiency of the exocrine pancreas may also develop.

Other causes of chronic recurrent pancreatitis

Chronic recurrent pancreatitis may also occur in patients with familial lipaemia (Kennedy and Collett, 1949; Poulsen, 1950), hyperparathyroidism (Carey and Fitzgerald, 1968), cystic fibrosis (Shwachman, Lebenthal and Khan, 1973), following organ transplantation (Corrodi *et al.*, 1975), lipodystrophy (Smith *et al.*, 1975) and also in children with none of the above predisposing causes.

PANCREATIC CYSTS

Pancreatic cysts may be classified as pseudocysts, retention cysts, congenital and neoplastic cysts. By far the commonest type of cyst encountered in childhood is a pseudocyst, and the causes are listed in Table 20.5.

These pseudocysts vary in size, are lined by non-epithelial tissue and contain pancreatic secretions, plasma, blood and inflammatory exudate. They arise as a result of pancreatic duct obstruction in a pancreas which is still capable of secreting juice. The clinical manifestations are variable and the onset may be acute or insidious. Symptoms include pain, anorexia, vomiting and weight loss. Physical findings include abdominal tenderness and a mass, and jaundice. They are variable in size and may fill the entire abdominal cavity or be so small as to

Table 20.5 Causes of pancreatic pseudocysts in childhood

Acute (haemorrhagic) pancreatitis
Hereditary pancreatitis
Trauma
Primary or secondary tumours of the pancreas
Idiopathic

be impalpable. Complications include infection, perforation, haemorrhage due to rupture into the gastrointestinal tract or erosion into a major artery, jaundice due to common bile duct obstruction, intestinal obstruction, and pleural effusions. Pseudocysts have a tendency to adhere to the stomach and displace it anteriorly, and oedema of the gastric mucosa is not an uncommon finding.

The treatment of choice is surgical drainage and generally speaking the prognosis is good. Only rarely is excision of the cyst necessary.

MALNUTRITION

Morphological abnormalities of the pancreas such as vacuolisation of the acinar cytoplasm, fibrosis, epithelial metaplasia and cystic dilatation of the ducts are well recognised in malnourished children. These changes reflect atrophy of the pancreas.

Barbezat and Hansen (1968) studied pancreatic secretion following stimulation with cholecystokinin-pancreozymin and secretin in children with kwashiorkor and marasmus who had a mean age of approximately 2 years. Pancreatic amylase, lipase, trypsin and chymotrypsin activities were markedly reduced, and improved with treatment. Low serum albumin concentrations were associated with low pancreatic enzyme activities and vice versa. In contrast, the volume and pH response to secretin was not impaired.

Treatment must be primarily directed towards improving nutritional status, and the use of pancreatic supplements should be discouraged since this approach avoids the fundamental nutritional problem which faces the children.

References

Adham, N. F., Dyce, B. & Haverback, B. J. (1968) Elevated serum trypsin binding activity in patients with hereditary pancreatitis. *American Journal of Digestive Diseases,* **13,** 8.

Antonelli, M., Ballati, G. & Annibaldi, L. (1969) Simplified nail clipping test for diagnosis of cystic fibrosis. *Archives of Disease in Childhood,* **44,** 218.

Antonowicz, I., Reddy, V., Khaw, K. T. & Shwachman, H. (1968) Lactase deficiency in patients with cystic fibrosis. *Pediatrics,* **42,** 492.

Araki, H., Field, M. & Shwachman, H. (1975) A new assay for cystic fibrosis factor: effects of sera from patients with cystic fibrosis in the in vitro electrical properties of rat jejunum. *Pediatric Research,* **9,** 932.

Barbezat, G. O. & Hansen, J. D. L. (1968) The exocrine pancreas and protein calorie malnutrition. *Pediatrics,* **42,** 77.

Burke, V., Colebatch, J. H., Anderson, C. M. & Simons, M. J. (1967) Association of pancreatic insufficiency and chronic neutropenia in childhood. *Archives of Disease in Childhood,* **42,** 147.

Carey, M. C. & Fitzgerald, O. (1968) Hyperparathyroidism associated with chronic pancreatitis in a family. *Gut,* **9,** 700.

Chase, H. P. (1976) Fatty acids, prostaglandins, and cystic fibrosis. *Pediatrics,* **57,** 441.

Cole, C. H. & Sella, G. (1975) Inhibition of ouabain-sensitive ATPase by the saliva of patients with cystic fibrosis of the pancreas. *Pediatric Research,* **9,** 763.

Corrodi, P., Knoblauch, M., Binswanger, U., Scholzel, E. & Largiader, F. (1975) Pancreatitis after renal transplantation. *Gut,* **16,** 285.

Danks, D. M., Olan, J. & Anderson, D. M. (1965) Genetic study of fibrocystic disease of the pancreas. *Annals of Human Genetics,* **28,** 323.

Danks, D. M., Haslam, R., Mayne, V., Kaufmann, H. J. & Holtzapple, P. G. (1976) Metaphyseal chondrodysplasia, neutropenia, and pancreatic insufficiency presenting with respiratory distress in the neonatal period. *Archives of Disease in Childhood,* **51,** 697.

di Sant'Agnese, P. A., Darling, R. C., Perera, G. A. & Shea, E. (1953) Abnormal electrolyte composition of sweat in cystic fibrosis of the pancreas. *Pediatrics,* **12,** 549.

Dobbs, R. H. (1935) Acute pancreatitis in childhood. *Lancet,* **2,** 989.

Doe, W. F. (1973) Two brothers with congenital pancreatic exocrine insufficiency, neutropenia and dysgammaglobulinaemia. *Proceedings of the Royal Society of Medicine,* **66,** 1125.

Elliott, R. B. (1976) A therapeutic trial of fatty acid supplementation in cystic fibrosis. *Pediatrics,* **57,** 474.

Fanconi, G., Uehlinger, E. & Knauer, C. (1936) *Wiener medizinische Wochenschrift,* **86,** 753.

Francis, D. E. M. (1975) *Diets for Sick Children.* 3rd edition. Oxford: Blackwell.

Freye, H. B., Kurtz, S. M., Spock, A. & Capp, P. (1964) Light and electron microscopic examination of the small bowel of children with cystic fibrosis. *Journal of Pediatrics,* **64,** 575.

Gibbons, I. S. E. (1969) Disaccharides and cystic fibrosis of the pancreas. *Archives of Disease in Childhood,* **44,** 63.

Gibson, L. E. & Cooke, R. E. (1959) A test for concentration of electrolytes in sweat in cystic fibrosis of the pancreas utilizing pilocarpine by iontophoresis. *Pediatrics,* **23,** 545.

Gross, J. B., Gambill, E. E. & Ulrich, J. A. (1962) Hereditary pancreatitis. *American Journal of Medicine,* **33,** 358.

Gross, J. B., Ulrich, J. A. & Maher, F. T. (1961) Further observations on the hereditary form of pancreatitis. The Exocrine Pancreas. *Ciba Foundation Symposium,* p. 278, ed. de Reuck, A. V. S. & Cameron, M. P. Boston: Little, Brown.

Harries, J. T. & Muller, D. P. R. (1971) Absorption of different doses of fat soluble and water miscible preparations of vitamin E in children with cystic fibrosis. *Archives of Disease in Childhood,* **46,** 341.

Hruban, Z., Oda, Y., Warner, N. E. & Wright, F. H. (1963) Pancreatic fibrosis with intracellular inclusions. *Archives of Pathology,* **76,** 122.

Isenberg, J. I., Walsh, J. H. & Grossman, M. I. (1973) Zollinger-Ellison syndrome. *Gastroenterology,* **65,** 140.

Kaplan, E., Shwachman, H., Perlmutter, A. D., Rule, A., Khaw, K. T. & Holsdaw, D. S. (1968) Reproductive failure in males with cystic fibrosis. *New England Journal of Medicine,* **279,** 65.

Kennedy, R. L. J. & Collett, R. W. (1949) Chronic relapsing pancreatitis and hyperlipaemia. *American Journal of Diseases of Children,* **78,** 80.

Kopel, F. B. (1972) Gastrointestinal manifestations of cystic fibrosis. *Gastroenterology,* **62,** 483.

Krauss, I., Antonowicz, I., Shah, H., Lazarus, H. & Shwachman, H. (1971) Metachromasia and assay for lysosomal enzymes in skin fibroblasts cultured from patients with cystic fibrosis and controls. *Pediatrics,* **47,** 1010.

Lapey, A., Kattwinkel, J., di Sant'Agnese, P. A. & Laster, L. (1974) Steatorrhea and azotorrhea and their relation to growth and nutrition in adolescents and young adults with cystic fibrosis. *Journal of Pediatrics,* **84,** 328.

Lawson, D. N. (1969) Panel discussion on microbiology and chemotherapy of the respiratory tract in cystic fibrosis, p. 225. *Proceedings of the Fifth International Cystic Fibrosis Conference, Cambridge,* ed. Lawson, D., London: Cystic Fibrosis Research Trust.

McCollum, J. P. K., Muller, D. P. R. & Harries, J. T. (1975) Congenital pancreatic hypoplasia with neutropenia and skeletal abnormalities. *Proceedings of the Royal Society of Medicine,* **68,** 304.

McCollum, J. P. K., Mathias, P. M., Sciberras, D., Muller, D. P. R., Newman, C., Harries, J. T. & Norman, A. P. (1977) Factors influencing the serum concentrations of vitamin E and essential fatty acids in cystic fibrosis. *Proceedings of the 7th International Congress for Cystic Fibrosis, Paris.* In press.

McElroy, R. & Christiansen, P. A. (1972) Hereditary pancreatitis in a kinship associated with portal vein thrombosis. *American Journal of Medicine,* **52,** 228.

Mearns, M. (1974) Cystic fibrosis. *British Journal of Hospital Medicine,* **4,** 497.

Morin, C. L., Roy, C. C., Bonin, A. & Lasalle, R. (1976) Small bowel mucosal dysfunction in patients with cystic fibrosis. *Proceedings of the 7th International Congress for Cystic Fibrosis, Paris.* In press.

Muller, D. P. R., Manning, J. A., Mathias, P. M. & Harries, J. T. (1976) Studies on the intestinal hydrolysis of tocopheryl esters. *International Journal for Vitamin and Nutrition Research,* **2,** 207.

Nezelof, C. & Watchi, M. (1961) L'hypoplasie congenitale lipomateuse du pancreas exocrine chez l'enfant. *Archives Francaises de Pediatrie,* **18,** 1135.

Niccolini, D. G., Graham, J. H. & Banks, P. A. (1976) Tumor-induced acute pancreatitis. *Gastroenterology,* **71,** 142.

Ogilvie, D., McCollum, J. P. K., Packer, S., Manning, J., Oyesiku, J., Muller, D. P. R. & Harries, J. T. (1976) Urinary outputs of oxalate, calcium and magnesium in children with intestinal disorders: a potential cause of renal calculi. *Archives of Disease in Childhood,* **51,** 790.

Pena, S. D. J. & Medovy, H. (1973) Child abuse and traumatic pseudocyst of the pancreas. *Journal of Pediatrics,* **83,** 1026.

Poulsen, H. M. (1950) Familial lipaemia. *Acta Medica Scandinavica,* **138,** 413.
Prosser, R., Owen, H., Bull, F., Parry, B., Smerkinich, J., Goodwin, H. A. & Dathan, J. (1974) Screening for cystic fibrosis by examination of meconium. *Archives of Disease in Childhood,* **49,** 597.
Riemenschneider, T., Wilson, J. F. & Vernier, R. L. (1968) Glucocorticoid-induced pancreatitis in children. *Pediatrics,* **41,** 428.
Robechek, P. J. (1967) Hereditary chronic relapsing pancreatitis: a clue to pancreatitis in general? *American Journal of Surgery,* **113,** 819.
Robinson, P. G. & Elliott, R. B. (1976) Cystic fibrosis screening in the newborn. *Archives of Disease in Childhood,* **51,** 301.
Ryley, H. C., Neale, L. M., Prosser, R. & Dodge, J. (1976) Screening for cystic fibrosis by analysis of serum protein in faeces. *Archives of Disease in Childhood,* **51,** 641.
Saunders, J. H. B. & Wormsley, K. G. (1975) Pancreatic extracts in the treatment of pancreatic exocrine insufficiency. *Gut,* **16,** 157.
Shmerling, D. H., Prader, A., Hitzig, W. H. & Giedion, A. (1969) The syndrome of exocrine pancreatic insufficiency, neutropenia, metaphyseal dysostosis and dwarfism. *Helvetica Paediatrica Acta,* **24,** 547.
Shwachman, H., Diamond, L. K., Oski, F. A. & Khaw, K. T. (1964) The syndrome of pancreatic insufficiency and bone marrow dysfunction. *Journal of Pediatrics,* **65,** 645.
Shwachman, H., Lebenthal, E. & Khan, K. T. (1973) Acute attacks of pancreatitis in patients with cystic fibrosis. *Fourth Annual Meeting of the European Working Group for Cystic Fibrosis,* p. 24. Warsaw: Polish Paediatric Association.
Shwachman, H. & Mahmoodian, H. (1967) Pilocarpine iontophoresis sweat testing. Results of seven years' experience. Fourth International Conference on Cystic Fibrosis of the Pancreas, 1966, Part I. Berne, Grindelwald. *Modern Problems in Pediatrics,* **10,** 158.
Sibert, J. R. (1973) Hereditary pancreatitis in a Newcastle family. *Archives of Disease in Childhood,* **48,** 618.
Smith, P. M., Morgans, M. E., Clark, C. G. & Lennard-Jones, J. E., and Gunnlaugsson, O. & Jonasson, T. A. (1975) Lipodystrophy, pancreatitis, and eosinophilia. *Gut,* **16,** 230.
Stanley, P. & Sutcliffe, J. (1973) Metaphyseal chondrodysplasia with dwarfism, pancreatic insufficiency and neutropenia. *Pediatric Radiology,* **1,** 119.
Stern, R. C., Stevens, D. P., Boat, T. F., Doershuk, C. F., Izant, R. J. & Matthews, L. W. (1976) Symptomatic hepatic disease in cystic fibrosis: incidence, course, and outcome of portal systemic shunting. *Gastroenterology,* **70,** 645.
Warwick, W. J. & Pogue, R. E. (1969) Computer studies in cystic fibrosis. p. 320, *Proceedings of the Fifth International Cystic Fibrosis Conference,* Ed. Lawson, D. Cambridge. London: Cystic Fibrosis Research Trust.
Weber, A. M., Roy, C. C., Morin, C. L. & Lasalle, R. (1973) Malabsorption of bile acids in children with cystic fibrosis. *New England Journal of Medicine,* **289,** 1001.

Index

Abdominal trauma, 103, 348, 349
Abetalipoproteinaemia, 27, 132, 204
Achalasia, 4, 96
Achlorhydria
  intrinsic factor in, 19
  predisposing factor in gastroenteritis, 166
Acrodermatitis enteropathica, 159
Active chronic hepatitis; *see* Chronic active hepatitis
Active juvenile cirrhosis; *see* Chronic active hepatitis
Acute terminal ileitis
  Anisalis, 117
  relationship to Crohn's disease, 117
  Yersinia enterocolitica, 117
Adenosine triphosphatase
  cellular location, 26
  effect of cystic fibrosis serum on, 336
  function, 26
  inhibition by bile acids, 187
Adenyl cyclase
  activation
    E. coli toxin, 11, 27, 170–171
    V. cholera toxin, 11, 27, 170–171
    S. typhimurium, 171
    prostaglandins, 27
    vasoactive inhibitory peptide, 27
  cellular location, 26
  function, 26
  prenatal development, 11
Adrenal glands
  aldosterone and colonic function, 28
  calcification
    in hepatoblastoma, 328
    in Wolman's disease, 256
  hyperaldosteronism, 315
  insufficiency
    fat malabsorption in, 27
    sweat electrolytes in, 342
Aflatoxin
  cause of liver disease, 135
  in Reye's syndrome, 301
Aganglionosis; *see* Hirschsprung's disease
Agenesis of anus, 78–80
Agenesis of rectum, 78–80
Alpha-fetoprotein
  extrahepatic biliary atresia and, 281
  hepatic carcinoma and, 328, 331
  hepatic metastasis and, 328
  hepatoblastoma and, 59, 328
  teratoblastoma and, 59
Alpha-l-antitrypsin deficiency, 151, 275–276
Ammonia; *see* Hyperammonaemia
Amoebiasis, 219–221, 298–299
Amylase
  activation, 31
  function, 29, 202
  normal values, 54, 55
  pancreatitis and, 349
  postnatal development, 13–14, 34
  prenatal development, 13
  protein-energy deficiency and, 137, 351
Anaerobic bacteria; *see also* Stagnant loop syndrome
  in hypogammaglobulinaemia, 167
  metabolism of bile salts, 187
  in stagnant loop syndrome, 126
Anal fissure, 99
Ankylostomiasis, 213–214
Annular pancreas
  cleft palate and, 348
  Down's syndrome and, 348
  duodenal obstruction and, 68
  imperforate anus and, 348
  malrotation and, 348
  pathogenesis, 7
Anorectal anomalies
  associated anomalies, 80
  clinical features, 79
  diagnosis and management, 79–80
  prognosis, 80
Anovulvular fistula, 78–80
Appendicitis
  aetiology and pathology, 90
  in ascariasis, 212
  clinical features and diagnosis, 90–91
  differential diagnosis, 90–91
  management, complications and prognosis, 91
Apple peel anomaly, 70
APUD cells, 23, 30
Ascariasis, 211–212, 299
Atresia
  duodenum, 68
  ileum, 69–71, 92
  jejunum, 69–71, 92
  oesophagus, 64–65
  pathogenesis, 8
  pylorus, 66
  rectum, 78–80
Australia antigen, 287, 292

Bacterial contamination; *see* Stagnant loop syndrome
Bacterial hepatitis
pyogenic abscess, 299–300
leptospirosis, 300
Bacterial overgrowth; *see* Stagnant loop syndrome
Bacterial toxins
E. coli, 11, 27, 169–171
S. dysenteriae, 170
V. cholera, 11, 27, 169–171
Bacteroides, 166
Barium enema
indications, 40, 41
in management of intussusception, 93
Barium meal and follow through, 40
Barium swallow, 39–40
Beckwith's syndrome, 82
Beri-beri, 131
Beta-lactoglobulin, 153
Bifidobacteria, 167
Bile; *see also* Bile salts
composition, 31
control of secretion, 32
function, 31
Bile salts
absorption of, 23, 121–122
activation of pancreatic enzymes and, 31, 340
bile flow and, 32
cystic fibrosis and, 340
defective synthesis, 282–283
enterohepatic circulation of, 121–122
extrahepatic biliary atresia, diagnosis of, 281
hyperoxaluria and, 126–127
intestinal resection and, 72, 120, 122–124, 126
investigation of, 54–55
lipid absorption and, 31, 121
micelles and, 122
normal values, 55
postnatal development of, 34
protein-energy deficiency and, 136
protracted diarrhoea and, 187
stagnant loop syndrome and, 124, 126, 167
Biliary atresia
extrahepatic, 278–282
intrahepatic, 282–283
Biliary cirrhosis; *see* Cirrhosis
Bilirubin; *see also* Hyperbilirubinaemia
biochemistry, 260, 266–268
Biopsy
liver, 44–46
rectal, 46–47
small intestine, 42–44
Bleeding from gastrointestinal tract, causes of; *see also* Cirrhosis. Peptic ulcer. Portal hypertension
ankylostomiasis, 131, 214
cows' milk intolerance, 154
Crohn's disease, 112–117
duplications, 80–81
endoscopy as cause, 48
endoscopy in diagnosis, 48
Bleeding from gastrointestinal tract, causes of; (*continued*)
familial polyposis coli, 98
fascioliasis, 223
generalised juvenile polyposis, 98–99
hereditary pancreatitis, 350
hereditary tyrosinaemia, 253
hiatus hernia, 95
intussusception, 92
juvenile polyps, 99
Meckel's diverticulum, 42, 94
pancreatic pseudocysts, 350, 351
Peutz-Jeghers syndrome, 98
rectal biopsy, 47
schistosomiasis, 224
small intestinal biopsy, 44, 148
strongyloides, 213
trichuriasis, 215
ulcerative colitis, 105–111
Blue diaper syndrome, 201
Breast feeding
acrodermatitis enteropathica and, 159
antiviral properties of, 167
effect on stool flora, 166, 167
gastroenteritis and, 167
hyperbilirubinaemia and, 267–269
immunoglobulin content of, 10, 34, 167
lactoferrin in, 167
pH of, 167
Budd-Chiari syndrome, 320
Bush tea
cause of liver disease, 135, 321

Caecum, undescended, 4
Calcification; *see also* Adrenal glands
causes, 39
in hepatoblastoma, 328
in hereditary pancreatitis, 350
in hydatid disease, 298
in meconium peritonitis, 84
in schistosomiasis, 224
Calcitonin, 19
Capillaria philippinensis, 212
Carcinoid syndrome, 92
Cellular immunity
in chronic active hepatitis, 312
in coeliac disease, 144
in cows' milk intolerance, 153
in intestinal lymphangiectasia, 232
Cholangitis, 281, 317
Cholecystokinin-pancreozymin
bile secretion and, 32
gallbladder contraction and, 32–33
investigation of pancreatic function, 54
pancreatic secretion and, 30
secreting cells, 18, 30
Choledochal cyst, 6, 273, 279, 316
Cholestyramine
bile secretion and, 32
extrahepatic biliary atresia, diagnosis of, 281
ileal resection and, 72, 124, 127
liver disease and, 278, 282, 315
protracted diarrhoea and, 187

Chronic active hepatitis
clinical features, 311–312
extrahepatic manifestations, 311–312
histology of, 311, 312
laboratory investigations and differential diagnosis, 312–313
pseudonyms, 311
treatment and prognosis, 313–314
Chronic hepatitis, 310–325
Cirrhosis; *see also* Hepatitis syndrome of infancy. Chronic hepatitis. Hyperbilirubinaemia. Liver failure
abetalipoproteinaemia and, 204
alpha-l-antitrypsin deficiency and, 275–276
carcinoma in, 331
causes, 313, 314
chronic active hepatitis and, 311
classification, 314
clinical features and investigations, 315
definition, 314
galactosaemia and, 258
glycogen storage disease and, 257
haemochromatosis and, 263
hereditary tyrosinaemia and, 253
histology, 314
management, 315–316
Wilson's disease and, 262
Clostridium perfringes, 170
Coeliac disease
aetiology, 142–144
associated diseases, 151
clinical features, 147–148
complications, 150–151
cystic fibrosis and, 340
definition, 142
diagnostic criteria, 149–150
genetic and environmental factors, 144–145
incidence, 144
intestinal loss of protein, 228
investigations, 148–149
management, 151–152
pathology, 145–147
Colitis; *see also* Ulcerative colitis. Ulcerative enteritis
cows' milk intolerance and, 154
Congenital chloridorrhoea, 206–208
Congenital dilatation of intrahepatic bile ducts, 317
Congenital folate malabsorption, 206
Congenital glucose-galactose malabsorption, 204
Congenital hepatic fibrosis, 316, 317
Congenital lipase deficiency, 205
Congenital pancreatic hypoplasia; *see* Shwachman's syndrome
Congenital sucrase-isomaltase deficiency, 204
Constipation; *see* Megacolon
Copper
in protein-energy deficiency, 137
in Wilson's disease, 262
Cows' milk protein intolerance
clinical features, 153–154
coeliac disease and, 150–151
diagnostic criteria, 154
Cows' milk protein intolerance (*continued*)
eosinophilic gastroenteropathy and, 160
management, 154
pathogenesis, 153
pathology, 153
protracted diarrhoea and, 186
Coxsackie B virus; *see* Hepatitis syndrome of infancy
Crigler-Najjar syndrome, 261, 269
Crohn's disease
aetiology, 112
cause of hepatitis, 299
clinical features, 113–115
complications, 116–117
diagnosis, 115
epidemiology, 112
extraintestinal manifestations, 117
management, 115–116
pathology, 113
Curling's ulcer, 96
Cushing's ulcer, 96
Cyclic AMP
small intestinal secretion and, 26–27, 170–171
synthesis, 26, 170
Cyclic GMP, 33
Cystic fibrosis
basic defect in, 336–337
bile salt metabolism and, 340
clinical and laboratory features, 337–341
coeliac disease and, 151
differential diagnosis, 341, 342
dysfunction of endocrine pancreas, 341
faecal impaction in, 338
gastointestinal manifestations, 338–341
hepatobiliary lesions in, 323–324, 340
histology of pancreas, 338–339
incidence, 336
infertility, 341
intestinal loss of protein in, 228
neonatal jaundice and, 276
pancreatic function, 342–343
prognosis, 345
pulmonary features, 337–338
screening of newborn, 343
small intestinal mucosal function, 340
sweat test, 342
treatment, 343–345
tyrosine metabolism and, 252
Cystinuria, 201, 350
Cytomegalovirus; *see also* Hepatitis syndrome of infancy. Infections of the liver
cause of diarrhoea, 171
cause of hepatitis, 295–296
extrahepatic biliary atresia and, 279

Dehydration
hypernatraemic, 175–176
hyponatraemic, 176
management, 178–182
normonatraemic, 173–175
Dermatitis herpetiformis, 151
Diaphragm of duodenum, 68
Diaphragmatic hernia, 81

Diets; *see also* Medium-chain triglycerides
cirrhosis and, 315
coeliac disease and, 151–152
cows' milk intolerance and, 154
Crohn's disease and, 115
cystic fibrosis and, 344–345
galactosaemia and, 259
glycogen storage diseases and, 258
hepatic coma and, 305
hepatitis syndrome of infancy and, 278
hereditary fructose intolerance and, 260
protein-losing enteropathies and, 232–233
protracted diarrhoea and, 188–190, 191, 194–195
Shwachman's syndrome and, 347
small intestinal resection and, 127
tyrosinaemia and, 254
ulcerative colitis and, 108
urea cycle disorders and, 255
Wolman's disease and, 256
Diphyllobothrium latum, 219
Disaccharide intolerance, 184–186
Dubin-Johnson syndrome, 261
Duovirus; *see* Rotavirus
Duplications, 80–81

EB virus; *see* Infectious mononucleosis
Ecology of gut flora, 166, 268
Ectopic anus, 79
Ectopic gastric mucosa
in duplications, 80–81
in Meckel's diverticulum, 94
Ectopic pancreas, 94, 348
Egg protein intolerance, 152
Encopresis, 242–245
Endoscopy; *see* Investigatory techniques, 38–60
Enterobiasis, 215–216
Enterocolitis; *see* Necrotising enterocolitis
Enterogastrone, 18
Enteroglucagon, 125
Enterokinase
deficiency, 201
function, 29, 200
prenatal development, 13
Enteropathies of small intestine
acrodermatitis enteropathica, 159
ankylostomiasis, 214
bacterial and viral enteritis, 155–156
causes, 142
coeliac disease, 145–147
cows' milk protein intolerance, 153
dermatitis herpetiformis, 151
drugs, 160
eosinophilic gastroenteropathy, 160
folate deficiency, 132
giardiasis, 158
histiocytosis X, 160
iron-deficiency, 131, 132, 160
lymphoma, 160
necrotising enterocolitis, 83, 160
pellagra, 132
protein-energy deficiency, 132
radiation, 160

Enteropathies of small intestine (*continued*)
soy protein intolerance, 154
stagnant loop syndrome, 126
strongyloides, 213
transient gluten intolerance, 154–155
tropical sprue, 158–159
Eosinophilic gastroenteropathy, 160
Epigastric hernia, 102
Erythroblastosis, 276
Escherichia coli
colicines and, 166
heat-stable toxin, 11, 27, 170
heat-labile toxin, adenyl cyclase and, 11, 27, 170–171
K88 antigen and, 167, 169
plasmids and, 169
role in gastroenteritis, 169–171
spread of infection, 173
Esterase
activation by bile salts, 30, 340
in cystic fibrosis, 340
normal values, 55
pancreatic, 30
in Wolman's disease, 255
Exomphalos
associated anomalies, 82
gastroschisis, 82
omphalocoele, 82
pathogenesis, 4
Extrahepatic bile ducts
abnormalities in cystic fibrosis, 323
atresia, 278–282
dilatation, 316, 317
invasion in ascariasis, 299
invasion in fascioliasis, 299
perforation, 277
rupture of hydatid cyst into, 298
Extrahepatic biliary atresia
aetiology, 278–279
carcinoma in, 331
clinical and laboratory features, 279
diagnosis, 279–281
extrahepatic manifestations, 279
histology, 278, 280
surgical management, 281–282

Faecal soiling; *see* Encopresis
Familial disorders of bilirubin metabolism
biochemistry, 260
Crigler-Najjar syndrome, 261
Dubin-Johnson syndrome, 261
Gilbert's syndrome, 260
Rotor syndrome, 261
Familial hypomagnasaemia, 208
Familial hypophosphataemic rickets, 208
Fascioliasis, 223, 299
Fasciolopsiasis, 223–224
Fat
absorption, 19, 26, 27, 28, 30, 31, 121–122
effect on gastric emptying, 18
malabsorption
in abetalipoproteinaemia, 27, 204
in Addison's disease, 27

Fat
  malabsorption (*continued*)
    causing watery diarrhoea, 124
    in cirrhosis, 315
    in coeliac disease, 148
    in congenital lipase deficiency, 205
    following intestinal resection, 121–122
    in glycogen storage diseases, 257
    investigation of, 51–52
    in newborn, 34
    in protein-energy deficiency, 136
    in Shwachman's syndrome, 346
    in stagnant loop syndrome, 126
    in strongyloides, 213
Femoral hernia, 102
Fistula *in ano*, 100
Flagyl
  in amoebiasis, 221, 299
  in appendicitis, 91
  in giardiasis, 223
Flukes
  fascioliasis, 223
  fasciolopsiasis, 223–224
  schistosomiasis, 224–225
Foreign bodies
  endoscopy in management, 48
  oesophageal, 84
  radiological investigation, 39
  trichobezar, 102–103
Fructosaemia; *see* Hereditary fructose intolerance
Fructose
  hereditary intolerance, 259, 275
  in ejaculum of cystic fibrosis, 341
  secondary malabsorption, 186
Functional faecal elimination disorders; *see also* Psychological disturbances
  aetiological factors and classification, 240, 242–243
  diarrhoea, 241–242
  encopresis, 242–245
  incontinence, 241
  soiling, 241
  treatment, 237, 239, 241–242, 244–245
Functional intestinal obstruction, 86

Galactosaemia, 258–259, 267, 275
Gallbladder; *see also* Gallstones
  absent, 6
  control of contraction, 33
  in cystic fibrosis, 323
  cyclic GMP in contraction of, 33
  development, 5
  double, 6
  function, 32–33
  puncture during liver biopsy, 46
  structure, 32
  torsion, 6
Gallstones
  cause of hyperbilirubinaemia, 273
  following intestinal resection, 122
  intra-abdominal calcification and, 39
  investigation, 40
Gammaglobulin; *see also* Immunoglobulins
  in colostrum, 34
  placental transfer, 35
Gastric acid
  antibacterial properties of, 18, 166
  effect on gastrin secretion, 19
  in fetus, 10
  following small intestinal resection, 49, 125
  investigation of, 49
  in Menetrier's disease, 49
  in newborn, 34
  in pernicious anaemia, 49
  in peptic ulcer, 49
  in Verner-Morrison syndrome, 49
  in Zollinger-Ellison syndrome, 49
Gastric emptying, 18
Gastric inhibitory peptide hormone, 19, 125
Gastrin
  effect on bile secretion, 32
  effect on pancreatic secretion, 30
  following small intestinal resection, 49, 125
  function, 19
  prenatal development, 10
  regulation of secretion, 19
  secreting cells, 18, 19
  in Zollinger-Ellison syndrome, 335
Gastroenteritis; *see* Infective diarrhoea and vomiting
Gastrografin
  in treatment of meconium ileus, 40, 73
Gastro-oesophageal reflux, 94–95; *see also* Hiatus hernia
Gastroschisis, 82
Giant cell hepatitis; *see* Hepatitis syndrome of infancy
Giant hypertrophy of gastric mucosa, 228–229
Giardiasis, 158, 221–223
  association with hypogammaglobulinaemia, 158, 222
  enteropathy of small intestine and, 158, 222
Gilbert's syndrome, 260, 267
Gliadins, 142, 143
Glucagon, 125, 335
Glucose
  absorption, 26
  absorption in fetus, 10
  congenital malabsorption, 204
  investigations of malabsorption, 50–51
  secondary malabsorption, 186, 187
Gluten intolerance; *see* Coeliac disease
  permanent, 141–152
  transient, 154–155, 186
Glycocalyx
  composition, 25
  in cystic fibrosis, 340
  function, 25–26
Glycogen storage diseases
  biochemistry, 256
  carcinoma in, 331
  clinical features, 257
  diagnosis, 258
  laboratory findings, 257

Glycogen storage diseases (*continued*)
sweat electrolytes in, 342
treatment, 258
Granular proctitis, 111–112
Growth hormone, 150

Haemochromatosis, 262–263
Haemorrhoids, 100
Hamartoma of liver, 326–327
Hartnup disease, 201
Hawaii agent, 172
Henoch-Schonlein syndrome, 92
Hepatic abscess
in amoebiasis, 298
in ascariasis, 211
in hyatid disease, 218–219, 298
pyogenic, 299–300
Hepatic coma; *see* Hepatic failure
Hepatic failure
clinical features, 303
laboratory investigations, 303
management, 305, 306
pathogenesis, 303
pathogenesis of encephalopathy, 304
precipitating causes of coma, 304–305
prognosis, 306
Hepatic infections
bacteria, 299–301
non-bacterial causes, 300
parasites, 296–299; *see also* Parasitic infections
viruses, 286–296; *see also* Hepatitis syndrome of infancy. Hepatitis A virus. Hepatitis B virus. Hepatitis viruses
Hepatic necrosis
acute neonatal, 277
in alpha-1-antitrypsin deficiency, 276
in amoebiasis, 298
in cirrhosis, 314
in erythroblastosis, 276
in hepatic failure, 303
in hepatitis syndrome of infancy, 272
in protein-energy deficiency, 134
in toxocariasis, 297
in yellow fever, 296
Hepatic tumours
carcinoma, 331–332
cause of Budd-Chiari syndrome, 320
hamartoma, 326–327
hepatoblastoma, 328–330
metastatic, 333
rhabdomyosarcoma, 332–333
Hepatitis A virus
clinical features, 287–288
differentiation from hepatitis B, 289, 290
histology, 288
laboratory findings and diagnosis, 288–290
prevention and treatment, 290–291
transmission, 287
Hepatitis B virus
clinical features, 292
chronic active hepatitis and, 312
chronic hepatitis and, 311
differentiation from hepatitis A, 287, 290
Hepatitis B virus (*continued*)
extrahepatic biliary atresia and, 279
hepatitis syndrome of infancy and, 274
laboratory findings and diagnosis, 292–294
nomenclature, 292
relationship to Australia antigen, 287, 292
transmission, 291–292
treatment and prevention, 294
Hepatitis syndrome of infancy
acute hepatic necrosis and, 277
alpha-1-antitrypsin deficiency and, 275–276
association of pulmonary stenosis, 276
choledochal cyst and, 277
course and prognosis, 277
erythroblastosis and, 276
extrahepatic biliary atresia and, 278–282
extrahepatic manifestations, 274
familial, 276
fructosaemia and, 275
galactosaemia and, 275
gallstones and, 277
hepatitis A virus and, 275
histology, 272, 280
idiopathic, 277
infecting agents, 273, 274
intrahepatic biliary hypoplasia and, 282–283
intrahepatic cholestasis and, 277
management, 278
microcystic disease and, 277
Rotor syndrome and, 277
tyrosinosis and, 275
Hepatitis viruses; *see also* Hepatitis syndrome of infancy
adenoviruses, 296
Coxsackie B, 296
cytomegalovirus, 295–296
hepatitis A virus, 287–291
hepatitis B virus, 291–294
herpes simplex, 296
infectious mononucleosis, 294–295
nomenclature, 287
reoviruses, 296
Varicella-Zoster, 296
yellow fever, 296
Hepatoblastoma, 328–330
alpha-fetoprotein in, 59
Hepatocellular carcinoma
clinical features and diagnosis, 331
pathology, 331
treatment, 331–332
Hereditary fructose intolerance
biochemistry, 259
cause of hyperbilirubinaemia, 275
clinical features, 259–260
diagnosis, 260
treatment, 260
Hereditary telangiectasia, 320
Hernia
diaphragmatic, 81
epigastric, 102
femoral, 102
hiatus, 94–95
inguinal, 101

Hernia (*continued*)
supraumbilical, 102
umbilical, 102
Herpes simplex virus, 296
Hiatus hernia, 94–95; *see also* Gastro-oesophageal reflux
Hirschsprung's disease
clinical features and diagnosis, 74–75
complications, 76
differentiation from functional megacolon, 243–244
late onset Hirschsprung's disease, 76–77
management and prognosis, 75–76
necrotising enterocolitis in, 83
pathogenesis, 9
protracted diarrhoea and, 188
ultra-short segment disease, 77–78
very-short segment disease, 77–78
Histiocytosis X
hepatic involvement in, 334
rectal biopsy in, 47
small intestinal enteropathy in, 160
HL-A8 antigen
in coeliac disease, 144
in cows' milk intolerance, 153
Hookworm; *see* Ankylostomiasis
Hydatid disease, 218–219, 298
Hydramnios
in annular pancreas, 348
in congenital chloridorrhoea, 207
in jejunal and ileal atresia, 70
in small intestinal atresia, 10, 69
in tracheo-oesophageal fistula, 64
Hymenolepiasis, 219
Hyperammonaemia
management, 255, 305
in Reye's syndrome, 301
normal levels ammonia, 58
secondary to liver disease, 254, 303, 304
in urea cycle disorders, 254–255
Hyperbilirubinaemia; *see also* Cirrhosis. Hepatitis syndrome of infancy. Jaundice. Hepatic failure. Hepatic infections. Hepatic tumours
Hyperbilirubinaemia, conjugated
Budd-Chiari syndrome and, 320
causes, 273–277
chronic active hepatitis and, 311–314
chromosomal abnormalities and, 276
cirrhosis and, 314–316
course and prognosis, 277
cystic fibrosis and, 276, 337
extrahepatic biliary atresia and, 278–282
hamartoma and, 326
hepatic carcinoma and, 331
intrahepatic biliary hypoplasia and, 282–283
management, 278
Niemann-Pick disease and, 276
pancreatic pseudocysts and, 351
rhabdomyosarcoma and, 332
Hyperbilirubinaemia, unconjugated
breast feeding and, 268
classification, 267
Hyperbilirubinaemia, unconjugated (*continued*)
Crigler-Najjar syndrome and, 261, 269
Dubin-Johnson syndrome and, 261
galactosaemia and, 258, 267
Gilbert's syndrome and, 260
hypothyroidism and, 269
infections and, 268, 275
kernicterus and, 269–270
management, 270–272
physiological, 267–268
Rotor syndrome and, 261
transient familial, 269
tyrosinaemia and, 253
Hyperoxaluria
cause of renal calculi, 126
in cystic fibrosis, 340
following ileal resection, 126–127
pathophysiology, 127, 340
Hypertrophic pyloric stenosis
associated anomalies, 67
cause of hyperbilirubinaemia, 267
clinical features, 67
management and prognosis, 67–68
Hypoganglionosis; *see* Pseudo-Hirschsprung's disease
Hypoglycin, 135
Hypoproteinaemia; *see also* Protein. Protein-energy deficiency. Protein-losing enteropathies
in ankylostomiasis, 214
in cirrhosis, 315
in coeliac disease, 150
in cystic fibrosis, 338
in giant hypertrophy of gastric mucosa, 229
in intestinal lymphangiectasia, 229
in Menetrier's disease, 229
in protein-energy deficiency, 351
risk of kernicterus in, 270

Iminoglycinuria, 201
Immunity; *see also* Immunoglobulins
prenatal development, 10, 11
Immunoglobulins
in chronic active hepatitis, 312
in coeliac disease, 141–152
in cows' milk, 153
in giardiasis, 158, 222
in human milk, 153
in Shwachman's syndrome, 346
IgA
in coeliac disease, 143
in cows' milk, 153
in cows' milk intolerance, 153
in fetus, 11
in human milk, 153, 167
in intestinal lymphangiectasia, 232
isolated deficiency of, 151, 167
in protracted diarrhoea, 158
secreting cells, 22
secretory IgA, 22, 167
IgE
in coeliac disease, 143
in cows' milk intolerance, 153

Immunoglobulins (*continued*)
IgG
in coeliac disease, 143
in intestinal lymphangiectasia, 232
placental transfer of, 11
secreting cells, 22
IgM
in coeliac disease, 143
in cows' milk intolerance, 153
in cytomegalovirus hepatitis, 295
in fetus, 11
in hepatitis A virus, 288, 290
in hepatitis B virus, 293
in intestinal lymphangiectasia, 232
in protracted diarrhoea, 158
secreting cells, 22
in toxoplasmosis, 297
Imperforate anus; *see* Anorectal anomalies
Infectious mononucleosis, 294–295
Infective diarrhoea and vomiting
clinical features, 173–176
dehydration in, 173–176
differential diagnosis, 176–177
early complications, 182–183
infecting agents, 169–173
management, 177–182
pathophysiology, 170–171
predisposing factors, 165–169
prognosis, 191–192
protracted diarrhoea
differential diagnosis, 187–188
management, 188–191
pathophysiology, 184–187
Inguinal hernia, 101, 341
Intestinal lymphangiectasia
causes, 228
primary, 229–233
secondary, 233
Intrahepatic biliary hypoplasia, 282–283
Intravenous feeding, 190
Intrinsic factor
in achlorhydria, 19
in B_{12} absorption, 18–19
biologically inert, 206
congenital deficiency, 205
secreting cells, 17
Intussusception, 92–93
caused by polyps, 98–99
caused by vitello-intestinal duct remnants, 94
Investigatory techniques
absorption of haematinics, 53
anorectal manometry, 75
carbohydrate absorption, 49–51
endoscopy, 47–48
fat absorption, 51–52
fluid and electrolyte absorption, 52–53
gastric acid secretion, 49
liver biopsy, 44–46
liver function, 55–59
pancreatic function, 53–55
peroral small intestinal biopsy, 42–44
protein absorption, 52
radioisotopic scanning, 41–42
Investigatory techniques (*continued*)
radiology, 38–41
rectal biopsy, 46–47
Iron
absorption, 19
in ankylostomiasis, 214
in coeliac disease, 148
in cows' milk intolerance, 53
in Crohn's disease, 112–117
in cystic fibrosis, 323
in haemochromatosis, 262
in intestinal resection, 123
investigation of absorption, 53
in protein-energy deficiency, 131
in protein-losing enteropathies, 228, 230
Irritable bowel syndrome; *see* Psychological disturbances

Jaundice; *see also* Bilirubin. Hyperbilirubinaemia
physiological, 267–268

Kala-azar: *see* Leishmaniasis
K cells, 144
Kernicterus
in breast feeding, 269
in Crigler-Najjar syndrome, 261
definition, 269
risk factors, 269
unconjugated hyperbilirubinaemia and, 266–272
Klebsiella, 83
Kwashiorkor; *see also* Protein-energy deficiency
bile salt metabolism in, 135–136
carbohydrate absorption in, 137
fat absorption in, 136
intestinal loss of protein in, 228
protein absorption in, 136

Lactase
congenital deficiency, 203
in cystic fibrosis, 340
function, 203
in gastroenteritis, 184–186
in non-Caucasians, 33, 133, 203
in premature babies, 11, 184
prenatal development, 11, 33
in protein-energy deficiency, 133
in tropical sprue, 184
Lactose
absorption, 203
malabsorption
in coeliac disease, 150
congenital, 203
in cows' milk intolerance, 153
in gastroenteritis, 184–186
in non-Caucasians, 33
in premature babies, 11, 33, 184
Lactulose, 50
Ladd's bands, 71
Leishmaniasis, 297
Leptospirosis, 300
Lipase
gastric, 19, 205

Lipase (*continued*)
  pancreatic
    colipase and, 31
    congenital deficiency, 205
    function, 30
    normal values, 54, 55
    postnatal development, 13, 34
    prenatal development, 13
Lowe's syndrome, 201
Lupoid hepatitis; *see* Chronic active hepatitis
Lymphangiectasia; *see* Intestinal lymphangiectasia. Protein-losing enteropathies
Lymphosarcoma
  liver, 334
  small intestine, 98
Lysozyme
  function, 22, 167–169
  secreting cells, 22

Malnutrition; *see* Protein-energy deficiency
Malrotation
  associated anomalies, 71
  clinical features and diagnosis, 71–72
  early management following resection, 72
  management and prognosis, 72
  pathogenesis, 4
  protracted diarrhoea and, 188
  symptoms attributed as psychological, 235
Maltase
  function, 29, 202–203
  prenatal development, 11
Maltose
  absorption, 29, 203
  investigation of malabsorption, 50–51
  malabsorption, 184–186
Marasmus; *see* Protein-energy deficiency
Meckel's diverticulum
  cause of intussusception, 92
  general features, 94
  pathogenesis, 4, 93
  peritonitis and, 103
  scanning in diagnosis, 42
Meconium ileus, 73, 337
Meconium peritonitis, 39, 84–85
Meconium plug syndrome, 85
Medium chain triglycerides, use of
  in Crohn's disease, 115
  in cystic fibrosis, 345
  in intestinal lymphangiectasia, 232
  in liver disease, 315
  in protracted diarrhoea, 188
  in Shwachman's syndrome, 347
Megacolon
  anorectal anomalies and, 78–80
  congenital constipation and, 244
  functional, 242–245
  Hirschsprung's disease and, 74–78
  toxic, 110–111
Menetrier's disease
  gastric acid secretion in, 49
  intestinal loss of protein in, 229
Methionine malabsorption, 202
Metronidazole; *see* Flagyl
Microcolon
  in small intestinal atresia, 70
  in small left colon syndrome, 85
Migraine
  recurrent abdominal pain and, 237, 239
  recurrent vomiting and, 236
Milk bolus obstruction, 85
Monosaccharide intolerance
  in congenital glucose-galactose malabsorption, 204
  in kwashiorkor, 137
  in protracted diarrhoea, 186
Motilin, 18

Necrotising enterocolitis, 83, 227
Neonatal hepatitis; *see* Hepatitis syndrome of infancy
Neoplastic disease; *see also* Hepatic tumours
  adenomatous polyps, 99
  aflatoxin and, 135
  Budd-Chiari syndrome and, 320
  carcinoid, 92
  in coeliac disease, 151
  cytomegalovirus hepatitis and, 295
  familial polyposis coli, 98
  hepatitis B virus and, 291
  in hereditary tyrosinaemia, 253
  inferior vena cava obstruction and, 320
  intestinal loss of protein in, 233
  pancreatic cysts and, 350
  pancreatitis and, 349
  Peutz-Jeghers syndrome, 98
  scanning in diagnosis, 41, 42
  small intestinal enteropathy and, 160
  teratoma of stomach, 96
  ulcerative colitis and, 109, 111
  Zollinger-Ellison syndrome, 96–97
Niemann-Pick disease, 331
Norwalk agent, 157, 171, 172

Oesophageal varices; *see* Portal hypertension. Cirrhosis
Oesophagus
  achalasia, 96
  atresia; *see* Tracheo-oesophageal fistula
  diaphragm, 66
  duplications, 80–81
  ectopic mucosa, 66
  fistula; *see* Tracheo-oesophageal fistula
  foreign bodies, 84
  prenatal development, 3–4, 10
  reflux; *see* Gastro-oesophageal reflux
  stricture
    acquired, 95–96
    congenital, 66
  structure, 16
  ulceration, 66, 95
  varices; *see* Cirrhosis. Portal hypertension
  web, 4
Omphalocoele, 82

Pancreas, disorders of,
  annular pancreas, 7, 68, 348

Pancreas, disorders of, (*continued*)
 cystic fibrosis, 336–345
 cysts, 350–351
 ectopic pancreas, 94, 348
 malnutrition, 133–134, 351
 pancreatitis, 348–350
 Shwachman's syndrome, 345–347
 Zollinger-Ellison syndrome, 49, 335
Pancreatic duct obstruction
 in ascariasis, 212, 349
 pancreatic pseudocysts and, 350
Pancreatic insufficiency
 in congenital lipase deficiency, 205
 in cystic fibrosis, 336–345
 in enterokinase deficiency, 201
 in newborn, 13, 34
 in pancreatic duct obstruction, 348
 in pancreatitis, 348–351
 in protein-energy deficiency, 133–134
 in Shwachman's syndrome, 345–347
 in trypsinogen deficiency, 201
Pancreatic pseudocysts, 42, 350–351
Pancreatitis
 acute, 348–349
 acute haemorrhagic, 212, 348, 349
 in ascariasis, 212, 349
 causes, 348
 chronic recurrent, 350
 in cystic fibrosis, 348
 hereditary, 350
 pancreatic pseudocysts and, 350
 portal hypertension and, 318, 319
 scanning in diagnosis, 42
Parasitic hepatitis
 amoebiasis, 219–221, 298–299
 ascariasis, 211–212, 299
 fascioliasis, 223, 299
 hydatid disease, 218–219, 298
 leishmaniasis, 297
 schistosomiasis, 224–225, 299
 toxocariasis, 216–217, 297–298
 toxoplasmosis, 296–297
Parasitic infections; *see also* Hepatic infections, Parasitic hepatitis
 flukes, 223–225
 protozoa, 219–223
 roundworms, 211–217
 tapeworms, 217–219
Pellagra, 131, 132, 201
Pepsin, 10, 19
Pepsinogen, 17, 19
Peptic ulcer
 cause of portal hypertension, 318, 319
 cirrhosis and, 321
 clinical features and diagnosis, 96–97
 Curling's ulcer, 96
 Cushing's ulcer, 96
 in cystic fibrosis, 338
 endoscopy in diagnosis, 48
 gastric acid secretion in, 49
 management, 97
 in Meckel's diverticulum, 94
 portal hypertension and, 321
Peptic ulcer (*continued*)
 in Zollinger-Ellison syndrome, 335
Peptidases
 in coeliac disease, 143
 in cystic fibrosis, 340
 development, 11, 12
 function, 200
 in protein-energy deficiency, 133
Perforation
 amoebiasis and, 220
 appendicitis and, 89–91
 ascariasis and, 212
 bile ducts, 277
 duodenum, 96
 endoscopy and, 48
 gallbladder, 46
 necrotising enterocolitis and, 83
 pancreatic pseudocyst and, 351
 pharynx, 84
 prenatal, 84
 radiological investigation of, 39
 rectum, 40, 47, 84
 small intestinal biopsy and, 44, 148
 stomach, 96
 toxic megacolon and, 110–111, 116
Perianal sepsis, 100
Periodic syndrome, 236, 237, 240
Peritonitis; *see also* Perforation
 abdominal trauma and, 103
 amoebiasis and, 220
 appendicitis and, 89–91
 ascariasis and, 212
 cause of portal hypertension, 319
 hydatid disease and, 298
 liver biopsy and, 46
Peutz-Jeghers syndrome, 98
Phospholipases, 30
Physiological jaundice, 266–268
Plasma cell hepatitis; *see* Chronic active hepatitis
Pneumatosis; *see also* Perforation
 in necrotising enterocolitis, 39, 83
Polycystic disease of liver and kidney, 316–317
Polyps
 adenomatous polyps, 99
 cystic fibrosis and, 337
 familial polyposis coli, 98
 generalised juvenile polyposis, 98
 intussusception and, 92
 juvenile polyps, 99
 Peutz-Jeghers syndrome, 98
 ulcerative colitis and, 107–108
 umbilical, 93
Porphyrias, 263–264
Portal hypertension; *see also* Cirrhosis
 causes, 318
 classification, 317
 in cystic fibrosis, 337
 extrahepatic
  clinical features, 319–320
  portal vein obstruction, 319
  veno-occlusive disease, 321
 intrahepatic, 320
 investigations, 318–319

Portal hypertension (*continued*)
management, 321–322
postsinusoidal
Budd-Chiari syndrome, 320
obstruction inferior vena cava, 320–321
in schistosomiasis, 224
Postnatal development structure and function
absorption of macromolecules, 34–35
bacterial flora, 35
bile salts, 34
enzymes, 33–34
gastric acid, 34
intestinal transit, 35
Postnecrotic cirrhosis; *see* Cirrhosis
Prenatal development of structure and function
early development fertilised ovum, 1–3
functional development
swallowing, 10
stomach, 10
small intestine, 10–11
colon, 12
liver, 12–13
pancreas, 13–14
gross structural development
pharynx and oesophagus, 3–4
stomach, 4
small and large intestine, 4–5
liver and biliary system, 5–6
pancreas, 7–8
histological development
oesophagus, stomach, intestine, 8–9
liver, 9
pancreas, 9
Protein; *see also* Protein-energy deficiency. Protein-losing enteropathies
absorption, 17, 19, 26, 29, 200
macromolecular absorption, 34–35
malabsorption
in blue diaper syndrome, 201
in cystic fibrosis, 338
in cystinuria, 201
in enterokinase deficiency, 201
in Hartnup disease, 201–202
in iminoglycinuria, 201
investigation of, 52
in Lowe's syndrome, 201
in methionine malabsorption, 202
in premature babies, 10
in protein-energy deficiency, 136
in stagnant loop syndrome, 126
in trypsinogen deficiency, 201
in protein-energy deficiency, 136
Protein-energy deficiency, 130–139
Protein-losing enteropathies, 227–234
Protozoa
amoebiasis, 219–221
giardiasis, 221–223
Protracted diarrhoea
differential diagnosis, 187–188
management, 188–191
pathophysiology, 184–187
Pseudo-Hirschsprung's disease, 74
Psychological disturbances
faecal elimination disorders, 240–245
recurrent abdominal pain, 235–237
recurrent vomiting, 237–240
Pyloric atresia, 66
Pyloric stenosis; *see* Hypertrophic pyloric stenosis

Rectal prolapse
in cystic fibrosis, 100, 337, 338
general features, 100
in juvenile polyps, 99
in trichuriasis, 215
Rectocloacal fistula, 78–80
Rectovaginal fistula, 78–80
Rectovestibular fistula, 78–80
Recurrent abdominal pain; *see also* Psychological disturbances
in cystic fibrosis, 338
diagnosis, 238–239
epilepsy and, 238
general features, 237–238
migraine and, 237, 239
pathophysiology, 240
peptic ulcer and, 237, 240
in porphyrias, 264
prognosis, 239
treatment, 239
Recurrent vomiting, 235–237; *see also* Psychological disturbances
epilepsy and, 236
migraine and, 236
Regional enteritis; *see* Crohn's disease
Rendu-Weber-Osler disease; *see* Hereditary telangiectasia
Resection of intestine
absorption of bile salts and lipids, 121–122
absorption of water and electrolytes, 124
absorption of water-soluble vitamins, and iron, 123–124
adaptation of remaining intestine, 72, 120–121
causes, 119
in Crohn's disease, 116
in duodenal atresia and stenosis, 68–69
in enterocolitis, 83
in Hirschsprung's disease, 75–76
hormonal changes, 125
hyperoxaluria and, 126–127
in intussusception, 93
long-term effects, 119–129
in malrotation and volvulus, 71–72
management, 119–129
in meconium ileus, 73
physical and intellectual development in, 125–126
stagnant loop syndrome and, 126
in ulcerative colitis, 105–111
Reye's syndrome, 301
Rhabdomyosarcoma of liver, 332–333
Rickets, 208, 253
Riedel's lobe, 6
Rotavirus, 171, 172
Rotor syndrome, 261

Roundworms
ankylostomiasis, 213–214
ascariasis, 211–212
Capillaria philippinensis, 212
enterobiasis, 215–216
strongyloides, 212–213
toxocariasis, 216–217
trichuriasis, 214–215
Rubella virus; *see also* Hepatitis syndrome of infancy
cause of diarrhoea, 171
extrahepatic biliary atresia and, 279

Salmonella
antibiotics and faecal excretion, 178
effect on adenyl cyclase, 170
gastric acid and, 166
hepatitis and, 299
role in gastroenteritis, 169–171
schistosomiasis and, 224
spread of infection, 173
Schistosomiasis, 224–225
Secretin
bile secretion and, 32
gastrin secretion and, 19
investigation of pancreatic function, 54
pancreatic secretion and, 30
secreting cells, 18, 30
Selective B_{12} malabsorption, 206
Selective inborn errors of absorption
carbohydrates, 202–204
electrolytes, 206–208
fat, 204–205
minerals, 208
proteins and amino acids, 200–202
vitamins, 205–206
Shigella
role in gastroenteritis, 169–171
S. dysenteriae toxin, 170
spread of infection, 173
Shwachman's syndrome
clinical and laboratory features, 346–347
differentiation from cystic fibrosis, 342, 345
histology, 347
pathogenesis, 346
treatment, 347
Soy protein intolerance, 154
Stagnant loop syndrome; *see also* Bile salts. Anaerobic bacteria
cause of protracted diarrhoea, 187
following resections, 126
in protein-energy deficiency, 135–136
relationship to motility of intestine, 167
Starch
absorption, 202–203
composition, 202
Stenosis of anus, 78–80
Stenosis of rectum, 78–80
Strongyloides, 212
Structure and function
gallbladder, 32–33
large intestine, 27–28
liver, 30–32
Structure and function (*continued*)
oesophagus, 16
pancreas, 29–30
salivary glands, 28–29
small intestine, 19–27
stomach, 17–19
Sucrase-isomaltase
congenital deficiency, 203
function, 29, 203
prenatal development, 11
Sucrose
absorption, 29, 203
investigation of malabsorption, 50–51
malabsorption, 184–186, 203
Supraumbilical hernia, 102
Sweat electrolytes
in adrenal insufficiency, 342
in allergic diseases, 342
in cystic fibrosis, 342
in diabetes insipidus, 342
in ectoadrenal dysplasia, 342
in glycogen storage disease, 342
in malnutrition, 342
in salt loading, 342
Sweat test, 342

Taeniasis, 217–218
Tapeworms
Diphyllobothrium latum, 219
hydatid disease, 218–219
hymenolepiasis, 219
taeniasis, 217–218
Teratoma of stomach, 96
Test meal
bile salts and, 54–55
pancreatic function and, 54–55
Testes, undescended, 341
Toxic megacolon, 110–111, 116
Toxocariasis, 216–217, 297–298
Toxoplasmosis, 274, 296–297
Tracheo-oesophageal fistula
with atresia, 3, 64–65
without atresia, 65–66
Transcobalamin I deficiency, 206
Transcobalamin II
congenital deficiency, 206
in protein-energy deficiency, 138
Trehalase deficiency, 204
Trichobezar, 102–103
Trichuriasis, 214–215
Tropical sprue, 158–159, 228
Trypsin
function, 200
normal values, 54, 55
postnatal development, 13, 34
prenatal development, 13
stool trypsin, 343
Trypsinogen
activation, 29, 31, 200
deficiency, 201
prenatal development, 13
Tuberculosis
differentiation from Crohn's disease, 112

Tuberculosis (*continued*)
  hepatitis and, 299
  intestinal loss of protein and, 233
  neonatal hepatitis and, 273
  peritonitis, 103
Tyrosine
  biochemistry, 251–252
  cystic fibrosis and, 252
  hereditary tyrosinaemia, 253–254
  hyperthyroidism and, 252
  neonatal tyrosinaemia, 252–253
  prenatal metabolism, 12
  scurvy and, 252

Ulcerative colitis
  aetiology, 106
  chronic active hepatitis and, 311
  clinical features, 106
  complications, 110–111
  diagnosis, 107
  epidemiology, 105
  extraintestinal manifestations, 107
  hepatitis and, 299
  management, 108–110
  protein loss in, 227
Ulcerative enteritis; *see also* Crohn's disease. Ulcerative colitis
  in amoebiasis, 220
  in enterobiasis, 215–216
  in fascioliasis, 223
  in schistosomiasis, 224
  in strongyloides, 213
  in trichuriasis, 215
Umbilical hernia, 102
Urea cycle disorders, 254–255

Vasoactive intestinal peptide hormone, 19, 27, 336
Veno-occlusive disease, 321
Verner-Morrison syndrome, 49, 335–336
Vibrio cholera
  adenyl cyclase and, 11, 27, 170–171
  gastroenteritis, 169–171
  spread of infection, 173
Vibrio parahaemolyticus, 170
Villikinin, 22
VIP; *see* Vasoactive intestinal peptide hormone
Vitamins
  B_{12}
    absorption, 18, 23, 26, 205
    congenital malabsorption, 205–206
    Diphyllobothrium latum and, 219
    intestinal lymphangiectasia and, 230
    intestinal resection and, 120, 123, 127
    investigation of malabsorption, 53
    protein-energy deficiency and, 138
    pyogenic hepatic abscess and, 299
    Schilling test, 53
Vitamins
  B_{12} (*continued*)
    stagnant loop syndrome and, 53, 126
  folic acid
    coeliac disease and, 148
    congenital malabsorption, 206
    Crohn's disease and, 112–117
    intestinal lymphangiectasia and, 230
    intestinal resection and, 123
    in investigation of malabsorption, 53
    protein-energy deficiency and, 131, 138
  vitamin A
    cystic fibrosis and, 338
    protein-energy deficiency and, 138
    test of fat malabsorption, 52
    treatment of liver disease and, 278
  vitamin D
    resistant rickets, 208
    treatment of liver disease and, 278
    treatment of rickets and, 208
  vitamin E
    abetalipoproteinaemia and, 204
    cystic fibrosis and, 323, 338, 340
    intestinal lymphangiectasia and, 230
  vitamin K
    coeliac disease and, 150
    cystic fibrosis and, 337, 338
    hyperbilirubinaemia and, 267
    liver disease and, 57
    treatment of liver disease and, 254, 278
Vitello-intestinal duct remnants
  fibrous cord, 93
  Meckel's diverticulum, 93–94
  umbilical cyst, 93
  umbilical polyp, 93
  vitello-intestinal fistula, 93
Volvulus
  clinical features and diagnosis, 71–72
  duplications and, 80–81
  management and prognosis, 72
  vitello-intestinal duct remnants and, 93

Weil's disease; *see* Leptospirosis
Wilson's disease, 262
Wolman's disease, 255–256

Xylose
  coeliac disease and, 148
  investigation of malabsorption, 51
  protein-energy deficiency and, 136, 137

Yellow fever, 296
Yersinia enterocolitica, 117, 170

Zinc
  acrodermatitis enteropathica and, 159
  protein-energy deficiency and, 137
Zollinger-Ellison syndrome, 49, 97, 335